AF845553

Contemporary Healthcare Issues in Sub-Saharan Africa

Contemporary Healthcare Issues in Sub-Saharan Africa

Social, Economic, and Cultural Perspectives

Edited by
Edward Nketiah-Amponsah
and Oluwatoyin A. Odeku

LEXINGTON BOOKS
Lanham • Boulder • New York • London

Published by Lexington Books
An imprint of The Rowman & Littlefield Publishing Group, Inc.
4501 Forbes Boulevard, Suite 200, Lanham, Maryland 20706
www.rowman.com

6 Tinworth Street, London SE11 5AL, United Kingdom

Copyright © 2021 by The Rowman & Littlefield Publishing Group, Inc.

All rights reserved. No part of this book may be reproduced in any form or by any electronic or mechanical means, including information storage and retrieval systems, without written permission from the publisher, except by a reviewer who may quote passages in a review.

British Library Cataloguing in Publication Information Available

Library of Congress Cataloging-in-Publication Data

Names: Nketiah-Amponsah, Edward, editor. | Odeku, Oluwatoyin Adepeju, 1966- editor. | Conermann, Stephan, writer of foreword.
Title: Contemporary healthcare issues in Sub-Saharan Africa : social, economic, and cultural perspectives / edited by Edward Nketiah-Amponsah and Oluwatoyin A. Odeku.
Description: Lanham, Maryland : Lexington Books, 2021. | "This compendium is a product of a DAAD Alumni workshop that was held in Accra, in November 2019"—Foreword. | Includes bibliographical references and index.
Identifiers: LCCN 2021005522 (print) | LCCN 2021005523 (ebook) | ISBN 9781793633699 (cloth) | ISBN 9781793633705 (epub)
Subjects: LCSH: Medical care—Africa, Sub-Saharan. | Health services accessibility—Africa, Sub-Saharan. | Medical policy—Africa, Sub-Saharan.
Classification: LCC RA395.A5548 C66 2021 (print) | LCC RA395.A5548 (ebook) | DDC 362.10967—dc23
LC record available at https://lccn.loc.gov/2021005522
LC ebook record available at https://lccn.loc.gov/2021005523

Contents

List of Figures and Tables

FIGURES

TABLES

Foreword

Stephan Conermann

This compendium is a product of a DAAD Alumni workshop that was held in Accra, in November 2019. I was privileged to participate in the opening ceremony as it coincided with the visit of a team from the University of Bonn, of which I was the leader, to the University of Ghana to sign a Memorandum of Understanding (MoU) and further explore collaborations with other Ghanaian Universities. And I was particularly excited about the commitment of both young and experienced scholars from about a dozen African countries who have come together to discuss the continent's topical healthcare issues from a multidisciplinary perspective. Edited by Edward Nketiah-Amponsah and Oluwatoyin A. Odeku, this latest publication is most timely as Africa marches toward realization of the Sustainable Development Goals in the area of healthcare. I would thus very much like to thank the individual contributors and editors for putting this interesting volume together.

The book *Contemporary Healthcare Issues in Sub-Saharan Africa: Social, Economic and Cultural Perspectives* is a collection of well-researched, policy-oriented papers organized into chapters that provide insight into the major health challenges confronting the region and the prospects for improving healthcare delivery. This book is particularly intriguing because the chapters are entirely written and edited by African scholars and experts who have empirical knowledge of the health concerns discussed in the book. The book addresses topical healthcare issues on the continent including drug quality, malaria, health insurance, geriatric care, the environment and health, the relationship between intimate partner violence and maternal-child health, food safety, the prevalence of child tuberculosis, and cardio-vascular disease. This book reveals that inadequate financial resources alone do not explain the state of health and healthcare delivery in the region, but rather cultural and behavioral factors are in play as well. While discussing health challenges and health system deficiencies, the book also offers workable proposals for improving healthcare delivery on the continent. For instance, while COVID-19 has exposed the vulnerability of the health systems the world over, the pandemic has also provided a glimmer of hope for improved healthcare in the very near future, as it has reawakened African governments to the need to improve human health infrastructure. Ghana, Kenya, Ethiopia, Nigeria, and South Africa, among other countries, have already initiated or implemented policies for improving health infrastructure to ensure an adequate response to future pandemics.

This fascinating volume addresses salient new topics as well, such as the prevalence of poor-quality and unregulated drugs and their health implications, the efficacy of plant medicine in the treatment of diabetes, the importance of harmonizing provider payment systems for countries about to introduce a social health insurance scheme, strengthening health systems to accommodate aging populations and the societal health toll of prevalent TB and cardiovascular disease.

Offering profound analysis of contemporary healthcare issues on the continent in writing that ideally blends theory and practice, this book will undoubtedly represent advancement in knowledge in the fields of health and healthcare delivery. I highly recommend this book as a companion work for academics, health policy practitioners, and students across the globe.

Prof. Stephan Conermann, Vice-Rector of International Affairs & Director of the Institute of Oriental and Asian Studies (IOA), University of Bonn, Germany.

Preface and Acknowledgments

The idea of this edited book was conceived when one of the editors won a grant under the "small alumni" grant from the German Academic Exchange Service (DAAD), Bonn, Germany, to organize a workshop titled "Contemporary Healthcare Issues in Sub-Saharan Africa-Social, Economic and Cultural Perspectives, in Accra, Ghana for DAAD Alumni trained in Germany and in-country. The two-day workshop which was held in November 2019 from 22 to 23, necessitated the presentation of insightful research papers by experienced and young scholars on diverse health and healthcare issues on the African continent. The participants, during the closing ceremony and workshop review endorsed the idea of compiling an edited volume to disseminate our findings to the global public. This book is, therefore, a product of the generosity of DAAD funding as well as the ingenuity of the workshop participants. It is also worth-mentioning that some of the chapters were solicited from scholars who did not participate in the workshop, especially against the backdrop that some of the initial contributor's defaulted as they could not meet the deadlines.

The book, which contains twelve chapters, begins with an introduction that motivates the various chapters of the book. A careful scrutiny of the various chapters indicates that sub-Saharan Africa has made some marginal progress in improving the health of the population, yet the region lags behind all the other continents on almost every health indicator. The well-researched chapters provide an introspective view about the state of poor health in the region, which is a product of the existing healthcare system. The book further highlights the need to urgently address the health challenges facing the continent. The various chapters in the book contain policy recommendations, to make the volume policy relevant. There are few outstanding chapters on topical health issues such as the Ebola and the current Coronavirus pandemic (COVID-19), chronic renal failure, and the sociology of aging that did not make it to this volume because of the stringent timelines; hence, a second volume of this book is under consideration.

Our sincerest appreciation goes to the twenty contributors who believed in this project and showed a lot of enthusiasm in meeting the deadlines. The realization of this edited volume is a testament of the authors' genuine desire to contribute to scholarship in Africa and beyond. We are also highly indebted to the reviewers of the various chapters assembled in this book; Dr. Emmanuel Codjoe, Dr. Ama Fenny, Dr. Gloria Afful-Mensah, and Dr. Robert Kaba Alhassan need special mention in this regard. We very much appreciate Prof. Dr. Stephan Conermann for generously accepting to write the foreword to this book as well as Prof. Dr. Mathias Kifmann and Prof. Dr. Ulrika Enemark for their endorsement of the volume. Our acquisition editors, Trevor F. Crowell, Joseph Perry, Judith Lakamper, and Shelby Russell need special mention for the editorial support during the acquisition and production of the book. We are equally indebted to Regina Enyonam Adagbedu an Assistant Registrar of the College of Humanities, University of Ghana, for her kind assistance in the formatting of the various chapters. Moreover, we thank the DAAD very much for funding the alumni workshop which gave impetus to this book.

Lastly, our greatest gratitude goes to the Almighty God, for giving us the strength and mental toughness to complete the book project amidst the COVID-19 pandemic.

Introduction

Contemporary Healthcare Issues in Sub-Saharan Africa: Social, Economic, and Cultural Perspectives

Edward Nketiah-Amponsah
and Oluwatoyin Odeku

INTRODUCTION AND MOTIVATION

Sub-Saharan Africa (SSA) is confronted with a myriad of health challenges that seem to have persisted over the past decades. The region continues to record large cases of preventable diseases and deaths each year. Compared to other regions, SSA is ranked worst for almost every health indicator with health status ranked lower than the global average, making the health of people in SSA a major global concern (WHO, 2019). Maternal and child mortality rates remain high in the region despite the progress in the last two decades. Life expectancy, or better still healthy life expectancy at birth, continues to be the lowest in comparison with other WHO regions. For instance, Africa is the only region with a healthy life expectancy below 60 years (52.3 years), which is in fact, about 10 years lower than the global average of 63 years (World Health Statistics, 2017). Also, over 90 percent of malaria cases reported globally every year occur in Africa with its concomitant productivity implications. Moreover, children below age 5 are the worst affected a phenomenon that has the potential to undermine future human capital (WHO, 2020).

The prevalence of HIV/AIDS, malaria, and tuberculosis has affected the region's economic performance resulting in sluggish economic growth in most countries. In more recent times, the upsurge in chronic diseases (diabetes and hypertension), stoke, cancer, and Cardiovascular Diseases (CVDs) is imposing excess financial burden on households and governments. The concern about the depletion of potential GDP due to ill health is evident in the well-established relationship between health and economic growth

(Bryan, et al., 2010; Lovász and Schipp, 2009; Nketiah-Amponsah et al., 2019; Sarpong et al., 2020). Moreover, the increased disease burden in the region imposes significant strain on the already outstretched health systems.

The health challenges in Africa have been compounded in more recent times by the emergence of more devastating infectious diseases, in particular Ebola and the novel Coronavirus (COVID-19), with their attendant health and economic ramifications. Whilst Ebola affected only few countries in the West and Central African subregions of the continent few years ago, the current COVID-19 pandemic has affected all the fifty-four countries in Africa, the latest being Lesotho. According to the most recent statistics by the Johns Hopkins University and Africa Centre for Disease Control, the affected 54 countries have recorded 81, 608 cases, with South Africa being the most hit. The related mortality rate has also soared to 2,708 while 31,122 recoveries have been recorded (Africa News, 2020). The UNECA (2020) has estimated that a one month full lockdown of the continent will erode its GDP by 2.5 percent which translates to about 65 billion, making it more difficult to effectively fight the current and future pandemics due to resource constraints (UN ECA, 2020).

Although some modest efforts have been made over the period to address the numerous health challenges facing the continent with various degrees of successes, the onset of the Covid-19 pandemic has further exposed the state of unpreparedness and vulnerability of the various health systems. No doubt, the developed and more resourced countries have not been spared the ills of the pandemic given the high rates of infections in countries such as the USA, Italy, Brazil, France, Russia, Spain, and the UK. The African region is projected to suffer greatly if the necessary interventions and protocols are not put in place and enforced in time. This apocalypse partly stems from Africa's lack of essential health resources to combat the pandemic—hospitals, life-saving medical facilities such as ICUs, adequate and qualified medical staff, testing and diagnostic centers and equipment, and isolation centers for treating and managing the virus *inter alia*.

One of the most conspicuous challenges facing the health system in Africa is inadequate funding. To date, only few African countries have met the recommended target of spending 15 percent of government expenditure on health as envisioned by the Abuja Declaration (WHO, 2011). In the area of healthcare spending, half of the countries in the region have per capita health expenditures of less than 140 with only 9 countries registering per capita health expenditure of 500 or better in US$ PPP terms (World Health Statistics, 2017). Consequently, out-of-pocket payment for healthcare is high, while insurance in the sector is a recent phenomenon; thus, undermining the quest for universal health coverage. Even with the few countries operating some form of insurance in their health sectors, there are some challenges regarding targeting and sustainability. Therefore, access to healthcare and utilization of appropriate health services are low, contributing to many needless deaths. Patients in rural areas typically choose to either rely on traditional and alternative medicine, or travel longer distances to access modern healthcare in the major cities and towns leading to congestion particularly in public health facilities where healthcare is relatively affordable. In spite of all these constraints, some progress has been made in a number of health indicators. For example, polio is near eradication; river blindness is no longer a public health concern; and there is massive improvement in the management of guinea worm and leprosy (Africanews, 2020).

Although the continent failed to realize the targets for the Millennium Development Goals (MDGs), its sequel, the Sustainable Development Goals (SDGs), provide another window of opportunity for Africa, especially SSA, to meet the set targets for population health by 2030. The slow pace of Africa's development could be partly blamed on its poor health, mainly orchestrated by a huge disease burden, coupled with inadequate access to healthcare. In line with contemporary global public health discourse, African governments are working toward attaining Universal Health Coverage (UHC), although the pace is slow. The key dimensions of UHC encompass expanding package of services, increasing population coverage, and protecting against financial risk (WHO, 2010). Healthcare financing is vital for health systems to be able to maintain and improve the health of populations. Consequently, there is an upsurge in the commitment of African governments in improving health infrastructure while at the same time creating mechanisms that ensure that individuals are not impoverished or plunged into "financial catastrophe" due to out-of-pocket expenditures on health (financial risk protection). For those households that are already entrapped in poverty, it is important that they are protected so as not to plunge them into extreme poverty. A testament to the commitment of African governments in ensuring UHC can be seen in the proliferation of social health insurance schemes (e.g., Ghana, Rwanda, Kenya Tanzania, Burkina Faso, Senegal, Tanzania, South Africa) on the continent over the past one and half decades with varying degrees of successes. In addition to the lack of health resources, the subregion is further derailed by pervasive sociocultural and behavioral barriers that undermine healthcare delivery. A more recent example of this constraint is the agitation and negative publicity mounted by some individuals and civil society against the piloting and implementation of the new malaria vaccine among children below 6 months old in Ghana (WHO, 2020). In addition, life style diseases such as hypertension and diabetes are steadily becoming public health concerns in the region. These may thwart efforts in achieving the health-related SDG goals.

There is thus an urgent call for revamping the health system in Africa to adequately respond to current and future health needs beyond the COVID-19 pandemic. It is against this backdrop that health experts and academics from various fields across the continent have contributed thought-provoking and policy relevant chapters in this edited book, all aimed at contributing their quota to help improve and strengthen the health system. In this way, the health system will be more responsive to the needs of the population.

WHAT IS IN THIS BOOK?

This collection brings together diverse and yet congruent selected health issues in sub-Saharan Africa. The book envisages that the full impact of health policies is only realized if health is approached from an all-encompassing perspective by synthetizing knowledge from social, economic, and cultural dimensions in the decision-making process. The diverse background of the contributors to the book underpins this objective. It spans authors with clinical background to pharmacists, economists, anthropologists, public health workers, and social scientists.

In the maiden chapter, Asante and Dzudzor provide a reflection on the key dimensions of social, economic, and cultural perspectives of health, drawing several examples from the literature to buttress how these indicators can promote or prohibit population heath. The authors opine among others that issues of affordability and accessibility of healthcare as well as health inequality largely determine quality healthcare delivery in Africa. Moreover, cultural barriers to healthcare delivery are pervasive among a significant proportion of the population in the region, and these usually manifest in misconceptions regarding the causes of illness as being medical or metaphysical. In particular, some infectious diseases like HIV/AIDS, Tuberculosis and Ebola, alongside mental health, are conceived as supernatural in nature and possible afflictions by the gods for wrong doing. Therefore, the choice between allopathic healthcare and alternative medicine is largely influenced by the perceived causes of diseases. The chapter concludes that political will and commitment are essential to bring about the needed change particularly in the absence of strong institutions to drive change.

Chapters 2 and 3 share a common theme in the quality and efficacy of pharmaceutical products and traditional medicine, respectively, in the treatment of diseases. In chapter 2, Odeku and Ola underscore the pervasiveness of substandard, spurious, falsely labeled, falsified and counterfeit medicines, a major public health concern in West Africa. The chapter argues that poor quality and unregulated drugs sold on the market can result in treatment failure, adverse effects, increased morbidity, mortality and development of drug resistance. The prevalence of poor-quality drugs is identified in a number of reasons such as lack of manufacturing process automation and control, and improper understanding of the product and process parameters. The chapter highlights the policies that have been put in place at the international, regional and national levels to fight this canker. For instance, the Nigerian National Agency for Food and Drug Administration and Control (NAFDAC) and Ghana Food and Drug Authority are agencies responsible for setting standards that would guarantee drug quality. The chapter contributes to the drug quality assurance literature by highlighting the causes, effects, and potential remedies to cross-border trade in poor-quality drugs.

Chapter 3 highlights the increasing prevalence of diabetes in SSA and the role of plant medicine in the treatment and management of the disease. In this chapter, Onyekere, Ifeanyi, and Peculiar-Onyekere affirm that the African continent has the highest number of undiagnosed diabetes with an estimated 19.4 million adult population living with the disease. Yet, access to diabetic care is constrained by inadequate access to modern healthcare due to financial, cultural, and social factors *inter alia*. The authors thus highlight the efficacy of herbal medicinal products as an affordable and alternative treatment of diabetes in Africa. Drawing from a pool of literature and clinical trials, the authors catalogue a number of plant medicinal products that have proven efficacious in the treatment of diabetes in the region. The discussion encompasses the protocols that should be observed to identify plants with anti-diabetic elements. It is recommended that pharmacists, social scientist, nutritionists, biologists, botanists, and pharmacologists should be collaborative and work in tandem to discover and promote globally acceptable anti-diabetic medical plants to curb diabetes in Africa and beyond.

Given the devastating impact of malaria on the health system and the economy at large in malaria endemic regions, Fenny and Akuffo provide an interesting retrospective and prospective discourse on malaria control in Ghana. The global- and country-specific policies alongside huge financial investments in the fight against malarial in Ghana notwithstanding, Ghana remains the country with the worlds' firth worst malaria burden, with malaria as the major cause of mortality in Ghana. The discussion in this chapter embraces the history, research agenda, and the progress made pre- and post-implementation of National Malaria Control Programs. The chapter highlights the societal and cultural practices that have the tendency to promote or hinder the fight against the disease in Ghana. The chapter proposes that the fight against the menace calls for an active interaction and engagement among all stakeholders—malaria control experts, disease modelers, and community leaders.

Intimate partner violence (IPV) is considered the most common form of violence experienced by women, accounting for about 2.5 percent of global deaths. In Uganda, up to 54 percent of women experience IPV in their lifetime compared to the global average of 36 percent. In chapter 5, Namuli highlights the causes and effects of spousal violence as well as the nexus between spousal violence and maternal-child health in Uganda. Key among the factors responsible for spousal violence are women with higher education, unemployed male partners, poverty, justification of wife beating by partners and previous exposure to IPV, which has the tendency to engender intergenerational IPV. With regard to the effect on maternal health, low birth weight, unwanted pregnancies, pregnancy complications, mental health, sexually transmitted diseases, depression and suicide were identified as obvious health consequences of IPV. The chapter recommends that findings on spousal violence from Ugandan national surveys like Demographic and Health surveys should be disseminated to the general public to heighten the awareness of the ills of IPV via media sources like radios, televisions (TV), newspapers, and local government notice boards. Corruption especially among authorities where women are supposed to report cases of abuse such as the police service should be eliminated to encourage victims of IPV to report cases of abuse instead of suffering in silence.

In chapter 6, Codjoe discusses the all-important but often neglected issue of geriatric care in Africa. The improvement in life expectancy over the past two decades has resulted in a noticeable increase in the population of the aged on the continent. The continent is thus confronted with the obvious challenge of meeting the current and future health needs of the vast majority of the aging population. There is also the need to provide other psychological and social safety nets to avert the empty nest syndrome associated with old age. In contributing to the scant literature on the phenomenon, the author discusses some of the pertinent issues that ought to be addressed in society's quest to improve the welfare of the aged. Obviously, older people on the continent lack or have inadequate health insurance coverage, and this ultimately limits their access to healthcare. The most critical intervention in caring for the aged lies in improving clinical care. It is recommended that governments invest in and scale-up existing healthcare infrastructure and enhance the standards and quality of geriatric. Besides, other support systems such as housing, transportation, water and sanitation should be improved to meet the basic needs of the growing ageing population on the continent.

One of the contemporary healthcare issues worth discussing in this book is healthcare financing and how provider payment mechanisms influence the quality of healthcare delivery. Ghana is one of the pioneers of social health insurance schemes on the continent, having implemented a National Health Insurance Scheme in 2004. Currently, about 42 percent of the population of Ghana are actively enrolled on the scheme. The cost escalation experienced under the fee-for-service and to some extent the Diagnostic Related Grouping (DRG) few years after the implementation of the scheme prompted the need for provider payment reforms. In chapter 7, Andoh-Adjei provides up-to-date reflections on the relevance, effectiveness, impact, and sustainability of the capitation payment mechanism under Ghana's National Health Insurance Scheme. The discussion covers the politics and politicization of capitation payment policy in Ghana and also proffers suggestions to remedy the ills and misconceptions associated with capitation, which by far remains the best cost-containment provider payment mechanism. The chapter concludes that more education on the positive attributes of capitation payment method and active involvement of healthcare providers in the (re)-design, development and implementation of the policy could render capitation payment a more viable payment method for primary care services in Ghana's health delivery system.

Chapter 8 examines the esoteric relationship between the environment and invention of healthcare strategies among the cattle nomads of Oyo north, Nigeria. The chapter sheds light on how pastoral nomads in Oyo north employ cultural negotiation to exploit the environment for their healthcare needs. In addressing this relationship, Ajala and Akinsete prompted an ethnographic data collection among the cattle nomads in Oyo north, aimed at examining how the processes of negotiation can lead to invention of new healthcare strategies. The study shows that when the need for healthcare beckons, four types of healthcare systems are available to cattle nomads in Oyo north—modern healthcare, faith-based healing, self-medication, and use of quack doctors and drug hawkers. Notably, conceptualization of diseases in terms of their origin or cause essentially determines the choice of healthcare system. For instance, 73 percent of the study's key informants conceive that most of the diseases that afflict the nomads cannot be medically explained. Such diseases are attributable to preternatural forces such as witchcraft and enemies either within or outside the bands. The chapter concludes that the health challenges associated with the semi-arid environment of Oyo north is a threat to pastoralists' survival, and thus pastoralists regularly engage with the environment to invent "new" healthcare strategies.

Safe food systems provide opportunities to improve nutrition, health, and income and drive economic growth in SSA. In chapter 9, Ngigi and Mureithi deliberate on emerging food safety risks in food systems in Africa and in the process highlight solutions to food safety concerns. The chapter identified emerging food safety risks in traditional markets—mycotoxins contamination, residue of agricultural chemicals, wastewater use, and antibiotic residues in animal-source foods. Using a case study on risk of antibiotic residues in dairy supply chain in Kenya, it is revealed that 42 percent of dairy farmers are aware of the health and economic risks of antibiotic residues in milk and that awareness is influenced by years of schooling, perceptions of food safety, and frequency of milk testing at collection points. The authors recommend the need to create awareness to farmer officers and animal health service providers on health risks of antibiotic residues and possible measures to reduce food safety risks. In this regard, strengthening national regulatory frameworks to enhance laws and regulations and encouraging adherence to food-safety standards by all actors in the food chain is nonnegotiable.

The last three chapters of the book are intertwined as they discuss interesting maternal-child health concerns that have far-reaching policy implications. In chapter 10, Afful-Mensah, Nketiah-Amponsah, and Alhassan investigate the impact of indoor air pollution on child health using Demographic and Health Survey (DHS) data from sixteen countries. Using a 2SLS econometric technique to address the problem of endogeneity of the type of cooking fuel used, the study reports that children from households that rely on biomass fuels for cooking are more likely to suffer from acute respiratory infection. The effect is even more pronounced after accounting for country fixed effects. Even among less efficient cooking energy sources, the use of raw biomass as cooking fuels has more negative health effects than charcoal/kerosene/coal. The study contributes to the literature on household energy use and its associated implications on households' welfare as well as the effects of environmental quality on child health.

The African region has the second highest TB cases, accounting for 24 percent of the global burden. TB is a major public health concern in Ghana. Even more so, many cases of the disease in children remain undiagnosed within clinical settings. In chapter 11, Ivy-Mensah examines how TB case detection in children in Ghana can be increased by leveraging the sociocultural settings in Ghana. This is against the backdrop that TB is described as a social disease with a medical component and thus any successful intervention in terms of healthcare access should embrace the social, economic, and environmental dimensions of the disease. The findings from this study show that the TB burden in Ghana is threefold higher in the population above 15 years than previously reported. Also, the prevalence in children is on the ascendancy. The chapter concludes by recommending increased TB case detection in children by targeting screening outside of the healthcare system. This could be achieved by employing innovations such as digital address systems, high mobile phone penetration, and high preschool and basic school attendance to provide the setting for increased screening and detection of cases.

Cardiovascular diseases (CVDs) are the leading cause of global deaths, accounting for 31 percent of all deaths. However, the fight against the disease in SSA is derailed by lack of data and coherent national policies. In the last chapter of the book, Blay reviews the relationship between maternal nutrition and the risk of cardiovascular disease in offspring, focusing on how research findings could be implemented to improve population health. Based on the review, the author concludes that there is ample and reproducible evidence supporting the developmental origins of health and disease, and the effect of maternal nutrition on CVDs in offspring later. The review emphasizes the complementarity between clinical and pharmaceutical therapies, and nutritional interventions in dealing with CVDs in adult life, given the high prevalence of maternal malnutrition in the region. The chapter recommends that CVDs should be considered a top public health priority in SSA because of their impact on economies—loss of life during peak productive years and the financial implications of healthcare and management. The author calls for a coordinated effort among the medical fraternity, researchers and public health officials and experts in the region to come up with interventions that can be implemented to address the rising CVD prevalence. Moreover, SSA governments and health services, as well as nongovernmental organizations, will need to muster the needed political and economic will to propel action.

Finally, this book contains relevant contributions with far-reaching policy implications. What is striking is the depth of analyses that blend theory and practice. Another appeal of the book is the diversity of the contributors-scholars and public health practitioners from different African countries with rich experiences in health research. The book will particularly be useful to undergraduate and graduate students as well as policy makers on the continent. Foreign scholars who wish to undertake comparative health systems could get a better appreciation of the health systems in Africa by reading this book.

REFERENCES

Africanews. 2020. Africa COVID-19 Stats. https://www.africanews.com/2020/05/17/coronavirus-in-africa-breakdown-of-infected-virus-free-countries/. Retrieved on May 17, 2020.

Lovász, Enrico and Schipp, Bernhard. 2009. The impact of HIV/aids on economic growth in sub-Saharan Africa. *South African Journal of Economics*, 77 (2), 245–256.

Nketiah-Amponsah, Edward, Abubakari, Mohammed and Twumasi-Baffour, Priscilla. 2019. Effect of HIV/AIDS on Economic Growth in Sub-Saharan Africa: Recent Evidence. *International Advances in Economic Research,* 25(4): 469–480

Sarpong, Bernard, Nketiah-Amponsah, E. and Owoo, Nkechi Srodah. 2020. Health and Economic Growth Nexus: Evidence From Selected Sub-Saharan. *Global Business Review,* 21(2): 328–347.

UNECA. 2020. COVID-19 Lockdown Exit Strategies for Africa. United Nations Economic Commission for Africa, Addis Ababa.

World Health Organization. 2011. The Abuja Declaration: Ten years On. https://www.who.int/healthsystems/publications/abuja_report_aug_2011.pdf?ua=1, Retrieved May 20, 2020.

World Health Statistics. 2017. Monitoring Health for the SDGs, Sustainable Development Goals, World Health Statistics, Geneva.
World Health Organization. 2020a. The African Regional Health Report. https://www.who.int/bulletin/africanhealth/en/, Retrieved May 15, 2020.
World Health Organization. 2020b. Malaria Vaccine Pilot Launched in Ghana. WHO Regional Office for Africa, Congo.

Chapter 1

A Reflection on Contemporary Economic, Social, and Cultural Healthcare Issues in Sub-Saharan Africa (SSA)

Felix Ankomah Asante and Makafui Isaac Dzudzor

Writing this chapter on contemporary health issues in sub-Saharan Africa in the midst of a global coronavirus (COVID-19) pandemic is enough justification of the relevance of the subject. Health, especially public health strategies and approaches, is once again at the forefront of the fight against the pandemic. Interventions range from self-isolation, quarantine to partial and full lockdown of cities and countries. Public health considerations are overriding economic and other strategic considerations of countries. The WHO has recommended standardized protocols for member countries to follow to curb the spread of COVID-19. However, individual member countries have tailored their responses to the social, cultural, sociopolitical, and economic systems of their respective countries. Thus, it is critical to always situate subjects that permeate all sectors of society like health in their appropriate context.

Health is an important dimension of development (Preston, 1975; Strauss & Thomas, 1998; Bloom, Canning & Jamison, 2004; Bloom, Canning & Sevilla, 2004; Duflo, 2012). It is a basic human right (World Health Organization [WHO], 1948) and is pivotally interrelated with other dimensions of development. Health is important in achieving other dimensions of development such as economic growth, education, improved life expectancy and maternal mortality, and gender equality (Duflo, 2012; WHO, 2012a). Development is important in achieving good health. Good health promotes sustainable development. There is an intricate positive relationship between economic development and health (Preston, 1975; Strauss & Thomas, 1998; Bloom, Canning & Sevilla, 2004; Duflo, 2012). The intricate linkage between health and development places health on the global development agenda. Sustainable Development Goal 3 (SDG-3) highlights the global position of health. SDG-3 seeks to ensure healthy lives and to promote well-being for all at all ages (United Nations [UN], 2015). It brings into sharp focus a wide range of targets which, if met, will improve global health. These targets include reducing maternal mortality ratios and improving child health, ending epidemics like AIDS, tuberculosis, malaria and other communicable diseases, promoting mental health and well-being, strengthening the prevention and treatment of substance abuse, and achieving universal health coverage (UN, 2015; UN, 2016).

HEALTH SYSTEMS IN AFRICA

The status of Africa's health sector is captured succinctly as follows:

> Sub-Saharan Africa (SSA) has been beset with poor health for years with its health status being lower than the aggregate levels for most less developed regions of the world. The region's health sector is confronted with a myriad of problems including shortage of health workers and poor health infrastructure. Also, child and maternal mortality rates are high while life expectancy at birth remains low. The health challenges in SSA are further aggravated by the prevalence of HIV/AIDS, malaria and civil conflicts, culminating in erratic economic performances over the years. Most people in the region have limited access to healthcare with residents in the rural areas, in particular, relying substantially on traditional and alternative medicines. Others travel longer distances to access modern healthcare in the major cities and towns.(Concept note, DAAD Alumni workshop, Accra, Ghana, 2019)

The above description of health care in Africa has unfortunately been the story over the past decades. Amidst the gloom, there are pockets of success stories dotted around the continent—for example, improvement in infrastructure, financing, human resource development, and technology. African countries have improved access to antimalarial drugs, insecticide-treated mosquito nets, and other interventions, leading to a 22 percent reduction in the incidence of malaria between 2010 and 2018 (WHO, 2019a). Notwithstanding these strides, the top ten malaria-burdened countries in Africa recorded an estimated increase of 3.5 million malaria cases between 2016 and 2017 (Economic and Social Council [ECOSOC], 2019). Furthermore, the WHO African Region accounts for at least 90 percent of global malaria cases and deaths between 2016 and 2019 (WHO, 2019a). The story is no different for other communicable diseases like HIV/AIDS and tuberculosis and maternal mortality. According to the Economic and Social Council of the United Nations (ECOSOC), the channeling of more funds toward evidence-based interventions in the fight against HIV is yielding dividends. Consequently, infections per 1,000 uninfected people between 15 and 49 years in sub-Saharan Africa declined from 3.39 in 2010 to 2.14 in 2017 (ECOSOC, 2019). A lot of strides have been made over the past three decades to improve healthcare. But looking at the frontiers of healthcare and health systems, the continent still has a lot of work to do.

But it is critical to note that health on the continent is not homogenous. There is an uneven distribution of health across the continent and even within countries, among different socioeconomic groups, and demographics. There is also a difference between rural and urban areas (WHO, 2012b).

GLOBAL HEALTH THREATS

The World Health Organization (WHO) has highlighted some global threats to health as has other stakeholders in the sector. The convergence of stakeholders on these threats is reflected in global interventions like the SDGs, especially SDG-3. The ten biggest threats to global health in 2019 identified by the WHO include air pollution and climate change, noncommunicable diseases, global influenza pandemic, fragile and vulnerable settings, antimicrobial resistance, Ebola and other high-threat pathogens, weak primary healthcare, vaccine hesitancy, dengue fever, and HIV (WHO, 2019b). Furtherance to these threats, at the turn of the decade, the health challenges expected to engage governments and policy makers include elevating health in the climate debate, delivering health in conflict and crises, making healthcare fairer, expanding access to medicines, stopping infectious diseases, preparing for epidemics, protecting people from dangerous products, investing in health professionals, keeping adolescents safe, earning public trust, harnessing new technologies, protecting the medicines that protect us, and keeping health care clean (WHO, 2020).

HEALTH ISSUES IN AFRICA

A number of health issues confront sub-Saharan African countries. There is a broad spectrum of issues that are critical to the provision of effective health care on the continent. They can be described as soft issues (such as changing behaviors, social and cultural beliefs) and hard issues (such as health infrastructure, medicines, and equipment). So, the subject of health in Africa is multidimensional and multifaceted with many intricate nuances.

In 2014, health ministers on the continent, under the auspices of the African Union (AU) and WHO, committed to the adoption of identified health issues crucial to the development of health care and systems in Africa. The ministers committed to implementing universal health coverage, an African medicine agency, strategies and policies to address the risk factors of noncommunicable diseases, ending preventable maternal and child deaths, establishing an African center for disease control and prevention, and establishing an accountability mechanism to assess the effectiveness, efficiency, impact, and sustainability of commitments made (African Union Commission & World Health Organization [AUC&WHO], 2015).

Rapid growth in noncommunicable diseases (NCD), weak primary healthcare and high prevalence of infectious diseases (e.g., Ebola, dengue fever and, more recently, corona virus, COVID-19) pose new challenges to stakeholders in the health sector on the continent. NCDs are a growing public health concern. NCDs such as neoplasms (e.g., cervical, breast, and liver cancers), cardiovascular diseases (e.g., heart attack and strokes), diabetes and kidney diseases, chronic respiratory diseases, and neurological, mental and substance use disorders are increasing on the continent. Demographic transition which culminates in the increase in life expectancy and the growing rate of unhealthy lifestyle by people underpin the rise in NCDs on the continent (Gouda et al., 2019; Fenollar & Mediannikov, 2018; Huber, Finelli & Stevens, 2018; AUC & WHO, 2015). Climate change and its attendant problems are altering the ecosystem and biodiversity and, thus, has increased the outbreak of certain diseases (Smith et al., 2014). Given the seemly weak health systems and the level of development across the continent, coupled with poverty levels and harsh climatic and environmental conditions, the incidence rate, severity, effect, and impact of these threats are direr and more manifest in Africa than in other parts of the world.

Against this background, government and stakeholder actions and responses are determined by a cocktail of considerations. Some of the issues will require distinct solutions while others require a cocktail of economic, social, and cultural solutions. This chapter provides economic, social, and cultural perspectives on contemporary health issues in sub-Saharan Africa. It is based on reflections, observations from stakeholders in the health sector, and scholarly materials from research.

Economic Perspective

Undoubtedly, a significant portion of the threats and challenges to the health system in sub-Saharan Africa is economic and financial in nature. Governments' restricted fiscal space is fundamental to most economic arguments on the health system on the continent. According to the United

Nations Economic Commission for Africa (UNECA) in collaboration with GBCHealth and the Aliko Dangote Foundation (ADF), about $114 billion is required annually to finance health care in Africa. However, only $46 billion is spent annually, resulting in a financing gap of about $66 billion. More than half of this amount is required by Egypt ($12 billion) and Nigeria ($21 billion). To provide more context, Africa provided less than 2 percent of global expenditure on health in 2015. In 2015, global expenditure on health was approximately $9.7 trillion (United Nations Economic Commission for Africa, GBCHealth, & Aliko Dangote Foundation [UNECA, GBCHealth & ADF], 2019). The continent accounts for 16 percent of the global population and 26 percent of the global disease burden. Countries on the continent spent between 5 and 6 percent of GDP between 2000 and 2015 on health (equivalent to $150 to $292 per capita in PPP$). Twenty countries are either severely or very health-stressed and need to be prioritized for immediate attention (UNECA, GBCHealth & ADF, 2019).

High-income countries continue to spend higher on health than low- and middle-income countries (table 1.1). Low, lower, and upper middle-income countries spent $41, $130 and $471 per capita respectively on health compared to $2,937 by high-income countries (WHO, 2019c).

Aside the limited fiscal space, the limited funds are not judiciously applied. There are concerns about the incoherent and disjointed nature public funds are allocated and applied by governments on the continent (WHO, 2016). Most African countries have not been able to appropriately target funds to make sure they get to those who need them the most and the projects they

Table 1.1 2017 Key Health Expenditure Indicators by Income Group

	Low (n=30)	*Lower middle (n=45)*	*Upper middle (n=54)*	*High (n=58)*	*Global (n=187)*
Health spending (% of GDP)	6.3%	5.3%	6.6%	7.8%	6.6%
Health spending per capita (US$)	41	130	471	2,937	1,085
Government spending per capita (US$)	10	60	277	2,021	723
Donor spending (% of health spending)	29%	12%	4.1%	-	-
Out-of-pocket (% of health spending)	41%	39%	32%	22%	32%
Out-of-pocket spending per capita (US$)	18	46	132	565	228

Note: 2017 World Bank income groups. In this table, unweighted averages are reported.
Source: Adapted from WHO (2019c)—Global spending on health: a world in transition.

Table 1.2 Healthcare Spending in Africa, 2000–2015

	Current Health Expenditure (CHE)*		Domestic government health spending as % of CHE	Out-of-pocket spending as % of CHE	External assistance for health as % of CHE	Prepaid private spending as % of CHE
Year	Per capita PPP	As % of GDP				
2000	150.4	5	36.7	45.4	11.7	6.2
2005	186.5	5.5	35.4	41.6	15.9	7.1
2010	244.7	5.8	33.2	39.9	20.7	6.2
2015	292.3	6.2	34.7	36.1	22.3	6.9

Note: * Total health spending comprises capital and current health expenditure.
Data from WHO Global Health Expenditure Database.
Source: Adapted from UNECA, GBCHealth and ADF, 2019.

are needed for. Also, the proper execution of budgeted projects to ensure value for money and optimally using public funds for the intended purpose are issues that have not been adequately addressed by most countries on the continent (WHO, 2016; Ebegbulem, 2012; Ndikumana & Boyce, 2011).

The culmination of these economic issues contributes to the poor health infrastructure on the continent. From primary through tertiary and quaternary health infrastructure, facilities are lacking in most countries. Where they exist, they are concentrated in urban and peri-urban areas to the detriment of the rural poor. The few facilities that are available are overburdened and are at the verge of collapse (Doctor, Nkhana-Salimu & Abdulsalam-Anibilowo, 2018; WHO, 2012b).

Notwithstanding the limited fiscal space and disjointed allocation and disbursement of funds, healthcare expenditure on the continent has increased. Data from the WHO Global Health Expenditure database shows that between 2000 and 2015 (table 1.2), current health expenditure (CHE) as a percentage of GDP increased from 5 percent to 6.2 percent. However, this expenditure is dominated by Out-of-Pocket Expenditure (OPE). Over the same period, OPE was between 45.4 percent and 36.1 percent of CHE. Domestic government expenditure decreased by 2 percent from 36.7 percent to 34.7 percent of CHE. External contributions to CHE increased from 11.7 percent to 22.3 percent (UNECA, GBCHealth and ADF, 2019).

Health shocks at the household level does not only cost the household in terms of healthcare spending but can also result in loss of productive time leading to income losses (Alam & Mahal, 2014; Atake, 2018). Households in these circumstances adopt different coping strategies to mitigate the impact of these shocks. Due to low economic development and poverty, households' health decisions are compromised. Households on the continent are characterized by high curative health expenditure and minimal investment in preventive healthcare (Lépine, 2015). Households spend their money on other competing interests than invest in preventive healthcare.

Linked to the lack of investment in preventive health care by households is the lack of effective public health insurance schemes on the continent. As indicated in table 1.1, table 1.2 and figure 1.1, most households on the continent spend directly from their pockets when they fall ill. Healthcare financing through out-of-pocket spending is not a sustainable approach to financing health care. Studies have shown that public health insurance affords the poor in society the opportunity to get appropriate health care (WHO, 2019c; McIntyre, Obse, Barasa, & Ataguba, 2018; Bonfrer, Breebaart & Van de Poel, 2016). Effective public health insurance promotes equitable distribution of healthcare services such that the vulnerable in society can access healthcare services that they could not afford if they had to pay from their pockets (McIntyre et al., 2018; Bonfrer et al., 2016; Aikins, Kushitor, Koram, Gyamfi & Ogedegbe, 2014).

Cost of treatment is high relative to household income. This puts enormous strain on household income for other activities. Households are relatively price-inelastic relative to medical treatment (curative) (Lépine, 2015; Srivastava & McGuire, 2015; Sauerborn, Nougtara & Latimer, 1994). When a household member falls sick, the family has no choice than to pay the full cost of treatment while, on the other hand, they are price-elastic when it comes to preventive healthcare (Cohen & Dupas, 2010; Kremer & Miguel, 2007). The family has to decide whether to buy a treated mosquito net for a pregnant mother or to spend the money on buying inputs for their farming activities.

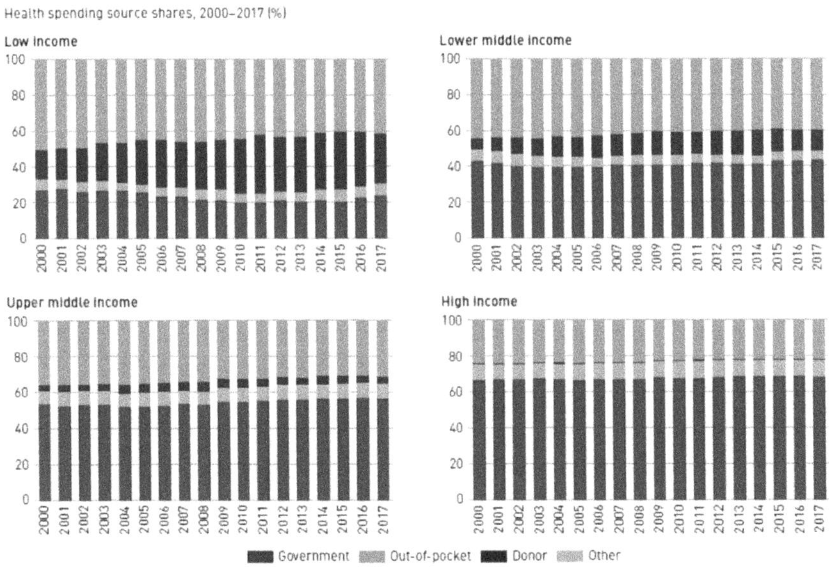

Figure 1.1 Health Spending Source Shares, 2000–2017. Adapted from WHO, 2019c—Global Spending on Health: A World in Transition.

The insufficient production of essential drugs on the continent is a growing concern because of their critical role in the health system and delivery of healthcare services. Pharmaceutical imports are estimated at US$14 billion and this constitutes about 70 percent of the pharmaceutical market (UNECA, GBCHealth & ADF, 2019). The market is projected to be worth between $40 billion and $60 billion by 2020 (Mckinsey&Company, 2015). Pharmaceutical companies on the continent are relatively smaller in size and lack the capacity and human resource to produce required drugs. Issues of patent rights and licenses also limit their expanding drives. In the absence of patent right and licenses constraints, fiscal constraints set in. Due to financial constraints, pharmaceutical companies are unable to do the right investments in technology and research to upgrade their operations to produce some essential generic medicines (Mckinsey&Company, 2015; United Nations Industrial Development Organization [UNIDO], 2019). Creating the conditions for local manufacturing companies to strive in this space will not only reduce the import bill but also have the potential to create 16 million jobs. By 2030, the continent's health market will be worth $259 billion (UNECA, GBCHealth & ADF, 2019). Most households pay out of pocket for medicines. Thus, it is crucial that essential drugs are priced appropriately. They also ought to be available, affordable, quality and safe for consumers.

A challenge to the pharmaceutical sector is fake drugs flooding the market (WHO, 2017; Nayyar, Breman, Newton & Herrington, 2012). The Africa Medicines Agency (AMA) is to provide a regulatory framework through which access to quality medicines and medical products can be guaranteed. The agency is also meant to harmonize the various regulations and legislations at the country and subregional levels. The recognition of traditional medicine as an integral part of the production and provision of drugs is a step in the right direction (AUC&WHO, 2015). Use of traditional and herbal medicine is a common feature among households on the continent (James, Wardle, Steel & Adams, 2018; Kahumba et al., 2015). Thus, its integration into national health policies is important. For example, Ghana has the Center of Plant Medicine Research (CPMR). This center promotes the research and development of herbal products that meet scientific standards.

The double burden of both malnutrition and disease is a growing concern on the continent (Gouda et. al., 2019; Development Initiative, 2018; Dalal et. al., 2011) due to factors like demographic change (youthful, longer life expectancy), urbanization, consumption of more processed foods, sedentary lifestyles, and epidemiological changes (Gouda et al., 2019). The percentage of infectious diseases is still high. However, the rate of growth in noncommunicable diseases (NCD) is rapid. The changes have cost implications for the financing of healthcare and the maintenance of a healthy and productive population.

Health systems need to improve to provide a good healthcare system that is responsive to the expectation of people and meet equitable financial contribution standards. Some "old" issues continue to linger on the continent: persistence of inadequate number of health professionals, malaria, tuberculosis (TB), HIV/AIDS, maternal and infant mortality, and malnutrition.

Social Perspective

From a social perspective, a health system should facilitate the safety of society. With the current system, a number of health issues come up in the health architecture in sub-Saharan Africa that impedes the smooth running of society. The functionality of the healthcare system is fraught with a number of inefficiencies that compromise its ability to deliver its core mandate (i.e., providing good healthcare that meets the needs and aspirations of the society in a timely manner). In an inefficient health system, economic development is low because the society is not optimally healthy to increase productivity.

Social inequality is a barrier to quality health care (Heaton, Crookston, Pierce & Amoateng, 2016; Marmot, 2005). It stifles human development (UNDP, 2019). Different demographic groups receive different treatments when they access healthcare services (Asamoah, Moussa, Stafström & Musinguzi, 2011; Magadi, Agwanda & Obare, 2007). The quality and access to healthcare is influenced by gender, societal status, geography, age, education, and so on (Marmot, 2005). Urban dwellers tend to have more health services compared to those in rural areas (WHO, 2012a). It is a mixed bag for the continent on the performance in reducing inequality. There is growing income inequality within and across some countries while the reverse also holds for some countries. For example, between 1993 and 2011, countries like Ghana, Kenya, and South Africa recorded increasing levels of inequality compared to countries like Burkina Faso, Senegal, and Ethiopia that recorded decreases in inequality (UNDP, 2019; Cornia, 2017). Access to resources is skewed in favor of the rich. But at the same time, there has been a drop in child marriage (ECOSOC, 2019) which will help the girls stay in school longer. Educating women and their full participation in the job market promote socioeconomic empowerment which has the potential to translate into improved productivity in the economy (Duflo, 2012). Sub-Saharan Africa has seen a drop in the loss of human development due to inequality. It dropped from 35.1 percent in 2010 to 30.5 percent in 2018. However, the continent is the biggest loser in human development due to inequality (UNDP, 2019). Thus, the performance of countries to curb inequality has been mixed.

There is still a sizable segment of the population that carries the notion and misconception that certain sicknesses are beyond medical reasons. For example, infectious diseases like HIV/AIDS, tuberculosis, Ebola, and mental health are believed by some to be supernatural in nature and a possible punishment for wrongdoing. Therefore, certain sicknesses become the construction of society. A person with that sickness is expected by society to behave in a prescribed way. These misconceptions lead to stigmatization which compounds the fight against some of these sicknesses by healthcare professionals. The healthcare system's recognition of these issues in society and their provision of appropriate social support systems for victims are a necessity in addition to medical treatment of the sicknesses.

Violence against women and girls is a major public health issue. Psychological, economic, physical, and sexual violence are the worst forms of violence perpetrated against women and girls (Cools & Kotsadam, 2017; Garcia-Moreno et al., 2015; Chrisler & Ferguson). Women and girls are abused psychologically, harassed sexually, and discriminated against at their work places and in educational institutions and their misery is compounded by intimate partner violence in the home. In Ghana, about $19 million is spent by households on violence-related expenditures annually (ISSER, Ipsos MORI, International Center for Research on Women-ICRW, NUI Galway, 2019). Society is not supportive of the victims when they confront their abusers (Cools & Kotsadam, 2017). Also, harmful traditional practices such as female genital mutilation (FGM) are still alarmingly high on the continent. Some countries have passed legislations to criminalize such acts but they are practiced on the quiet. About two million girls annually between the ages of 4 and 12 years suffer from the ordeal of FGM (WHO, 2012a).

African women do not enjoy the best of healthcare services. Women on the continent bear a high load of the global burden of disease and death. For example, African women accounted for about 66 percent of global maternal deaths in 2017. Over the same period, the maternal mortality ratio (MMR) on the continent was 542 per 100,000 livebirths (1 in 37 lifetime risk maternal death), while their counterparts in Europe and North America had 10 per 100,000 livebirths (1 in 6,500 lifetime risk maternal death) and 18 per 100,000 livebirths (1 in 3,100 lifetime risk maternal deaths) respectively (WHO, 2019d). Malaria continues to be endemic in Africa and pregnant women and children are the most vulnerable. In 2018, 11 million pregnant mothers were exposed to malaria infections in sub-Saharan Africa. West and Central Africa had the highest levels of exposure. Equally, global infant mortality from malaria was highest on the continent (WHO, 2019a). The continent has to rally around the framework of SDG-5-gender equality and empower all women and girls to promote inclusiveness.

The quality of healthcare accessed by women is constrained by some social constructs. Gender-sensitive subjects like reproductive health are sometimes handled by male health professionals because of the shortage of qualified female health professionals. Some pregnant women are hesitant to seek appropriate antenatal and postnatal health care because they do not want to be examined by male physicians (WHO, 2012a). The health of a woman goes a long way to affect the health of her children. A malnourished pregnant woman will likely give birth to a malnourished child who will be underweight (low birthweight) and lacking essential nutrients at birth. It is well documented that malnutrition can lead to irreversible cognitive deficiency in children (De Onis & Branca, 2016; Abuya, Ciera & Kimani-Murage, 2012; Berkman, Lescano, Gilman, Lopez & Black, 2002; Brown & Pollitt, 1996). The ramification is that the next generation of the human resource base on the continent is compromised right from the onset.

Private involvement in the provision of healthcare in some places has excluded the poor and vulnerable from accessing the quality healthcare services provided by the private sector. With minimal safety nets, out-of-pocket health expenditures are taking a toll on the vulnerable. Refugees and migrants are also a vulnerable part of society. Even in the absence of conflict, people will move within countries and across borders for economic reasons. According to the UNHCR global report for 2018, sub-Saharan Africa accounts for about 6.3 million refugees and 17.7 million internally displaced people (IDP). Conflict and climatic conditions like drought are the underlying reasons for the movement of these individuals (UNHCR, 2019). The human rights of these vulnerable individuals need to be protected at all times and these include access to appropriate healthcare. Also, their susceptibility to all manner of diseases underscores the need for a robust and inclusive healthcare system.

Cultural Perspective

Health from a cultural perspective in sub-Saharan Africa is a nuanced subject to discuss. Culture plays a major role in how people in sub-Saharan Africa view and relate to health. It shapes people's perception and perspectives on health in terms of what constitute health, and how their health needs and aspirations are met. The cultural system entails a diversity of values, customs, norms, and beliefs which influence the most basic decisions at the household level such as "who eats more meat?," and in national conversations such as "sexual and reproductive health legislations." Thus, the sustainable delivery of quality health to people on the continent ought to be situated in the appropriate cultural context.

Women and children are a vulnerable group. Yet, they are the most underserved group when it comes to the distribution of resources and access to goods and services including health (Odusola, Cornia, Bhorat & Conceição, 2017; WHO, 2012a). Although women are the main caregivers at home and in the formal healthcare system, they do not receive the best of care themselves when they need it (Sharma, Chakrabarti & Grover, 2016; WHO, 2012a). Economically, women are negatively discriminated against through various norms (Odusola et al., 2017). The impact of out-of-pocket expenditure on them is more debilitating.

Reproductive health empowerment for women and girls may go against some power relations in society (Ouedraogo & Ouedraogo, as cited in United Nations Development Program [UNDP], 2019) and thus can face resistance but its benefits at both the micro and macro levels are enormous. Reproductive health education of particularly adolescents empowers them to take control of their reproductive life (Yakubu & Salisu, 2018; Phillips & Mbizvo, 2016). In sub-Saharan Africa, women mostly need the approval of men to take reproductive health decisions such as the number of children they want to have and the time to start childbirth (Atake & Ali, 2019; Phillips & Mbizvo, 2016). Empowering women and girls' reproductive knowledge facilitate reduction in sexually transmitted diseases (STDs) (including HIV/AIDS) and in teenage pregnancy (Asaolu et al., 2018; Phillips & Mbizvo, 2016; Pratley, 2016; Jewkes, Morrell & Christofides, 2009).

Sub-Saharan African countries are integrating "traditional medicine/healthcare" alongside the orthodox medicine/healthcare in their mainstream health delivery (AUC & WHO, 2015). The commitment of countries to enact these polices is commendable but not all countries have appropriate policies and regulatory institutions to effectively monitor and regulate the sector (Ndomondo-Sigonda, Miot, Naidoo, Dodoo & Kaale, 2017; WHO, 2010). Quality and safe medicines, and the likelihood of conflicting diagnoses and prescription between traditional and orthodox healthcare professionals are matters that need urgent attention.

The widespread misconception about certain groups of diseases, especially the infectious ones, have contributed to the spread of these diseases and the ineffectiveness of measures put in place by governments to curtail their spread. For example, HIV is considered by some communities as punishment from the "gods" or as a result of witchcraft (Gershman, 2016; Sovran, 2013; Gausset, 2001; Hrdy, 1987). Others are judged to be promiscuous and their punishment is the infection with the HIV virus. The shame and stigmatization associated with these diseases discourage individuals and families from voluntary testing. Unfortunately, this is a recurring story in many places on the continent. Similar stories of shame, stigmatization of patients, fear of banishment and accusation of witchcraft were reported in the recent Ebola outbreak in sub-Saharan Africa, especially in West Africa (Overholt, et al., 2018; Van Bortel et al., 2016; Karamouzian & Hategekimana, 2015; Davtyan, Brown & Folayan, 2014).

When there is a conflict between cultural beliefs and conventional scientific processes, it can breed mistrust. The growing mistrust between health professional and communities is and will continue to be a challenge going forward (Elston et al., 2016; Karamouzian & Hategekimana, 2015; Thiam et al., 2015). There are communities that are firmly rooted in their cultural and spiritual beliefs and thus do not wholly subscribe to scientific explanations given by health professionals for some of the outbreaks, especially infectious epidemics and the solutions to curb them.

Some cultural norms and belief systems on the continent are also a major blockade to the provision of adequate health care. There are communities that believe the cause of certain illnesses like mental disorders are punishment from the "gods" or from the ancestors (Daniel, Njau, Mtuya, Okelo & Mushi, 2018). The practice of sorcery and witchcraft, or other religious beliefs supersedes seeking medical care. The consequence of this cultural undertone is stigmatization and victim shaming. These practices discourage victims from seeking proper medical care. The element of stigmatization still exists in some societies about people living with HIV/AIDS. The recent outbreak of the Ebola virus also witnessed stigmatization and victim shaming. This contributed to families' reluctance to send members to healthcare facilities (Thiam et al., 2015; Overholt et al., 2018; Davtyan, Brown & Folayan, 2014). The recent pandemic outbreak of COVID-19 is also witnessing stigmatization of cured patients.

The skepticism and mistrust between locals and health professionals are also leading to vaccine hesitancy among communities. Communities refused to receive the Ebola vaccine because they had reservations about the intent of the drugs (Karamouzian & Hategekimana, 2015). In northern parts of Nigeria, communities refused to receive the polio vaccines because of similar misinformed positions of community members (Micheal et al., 2014; Ghinai, Willott, Dadari & Larson, 2013; Jegede, 2007).

Mental health has assumed a global status. Going forward, much attention and resources should be committed to mental health in sub-Saharan Africa. Culturally, mental disorders and challenges are frowned upon and not accepted in some societies (Daniel et al., 2018; Stefanovics et al., 2016). This has permeated into the broader decision making of policy makers that adequate financial resources are not committed to the fight. The economic perspective is closely linked to the cultural belief system of the society. Mental health is a significant arm of general health. The subject of mental health is faced with social and cultural challenges which affect how governments and communities relate to the subject on the continent. Mental health goes beyond mental disorders. However, communities associate mental health with witchcraft, stigmatization, and shame (Daniel et al., 2018; WHO, 2013; Read, Adijbokah & Nyame, 2009). Some of these underlying issues translate into the unpopularity of the subject and thus affect the urgency they deserve. It is critical not to lose sight of mental health issues in sub-Saharan Africa.

Survivors of some traumatic illnesses like Ebola, and child soldiers who survive wars are scarred from their experience. Sometimes the guilt that they survived and their family members died, or as in the case of child soldiers the killing they witnessed compromises their mental health. Violence, especially psychological and sexual violence, also exposes especially women to mental health challenges (Pannetier, Lert, Roustide & Du Loû, 2017; Cortina, Sodha, Fazel & Ramchandani, 2012; Vinson & Chang, 2012; Njenga, Nguithi & Kang'ethe, 2006).

According to the WHO, mental health is "a state of well-being in which every individual realizes his or her own potential, can cope with the normal stresses of life, can work productively and fruitfully, and is able to make a contribution to his or her community" (WHO, 2018). In summary, the well-being and development of society equally hinge on the mental health status of its members. Unfortunately, the risk factors of mental health are rife in Africa. Aside the genetic factors responsible for mental health, risk factors such as conflict and wars, violence and trauma, socioeconomic pressures, unemployment, poverty, and hunger are common occurrences on the continent (WHO, 2018; WHO, 2013). The WHO comprehensive mental health action plan for 2013–2020 has steered some needed attention and action in this area. Individual African countries are developing their mental health laws and are integrating mental health into the mainstream health policy of the state.

CONCLUSION

Contemporary health issues have evolved over the years but some issues have persisted. New issues like the growing rate of noncommunicable diseases, production of essential medicines and mental health and older ones like infectious diseases, effects of malnutrition and maternal mortality continue to engage stakeholders in the sector. Regional leaders are converging toward harmonizing policies and interventions to tackle the emerging issues at the regional level rather than at the various national levels. Addressing health issues in the proper context and perspectives to bring out policies and interventions that meet the needs and aspirations of the citizenry is important.

Universal health coverage is still elusive. A lot still needs to be done to achieve universal healthcare for all. Given the high proportion of the marginalized and vulnerable on the continent, the attainment of universal health coverage will enhance equity in healthcare delivery. Healthcare and its implications permeate all facets of society. Therefore, its effective implementation requires multisectoral and multidisciplinary approaches and engagements.

Continuous training of the requisite human resource (knowledge and skills) and building infrastructure, especially primary health infrastructure and public health education, cannot be overemphasized. All segments of the health sector are understaffed. Thus, aggressive training of health staff across all disciplines and proper remuneration to retain them on the continent should be a priority.

The investment gap in the health sector provides a good opportunity for the private sector to be brought on board. Public–private partnerships for health should be promoted to bridge the funding gap. A lot can be done through collaboration between the public and private sector—from financing to introduction of new technologies. Countries can equally pool resources together to undertake projects that are capital intensive and optimize the economies of scale.

Leveraging innovation and technology can help achieve the needed impact. In this regard, investment in technology is key to the provision of adequate and essential and generic medicines to meet the demand of the continent. Technological innovation would also help provide fair and equitable distribution of healthcare infrastructure and services, research into neglected tropical and infectious diseases to provide prompt responses during outbreaks, and respond effectively to climate change effects.

Women reproductive health education needs more attention. Multisectoral approach to develop policies and interventions designed to improve women's health status is required. More resources should be committed to an education that involves the training of more female health workers in areas like gynecology so that cultural norms to prevent women from seeking these specialized services can be overcome.

Finally, the impact of all the gaps in the health system and the threats to the system are exacerbated by climate change effects. Thus, a concerted effort on the part of all is needed to bridge the gaps and improve the health systems on the continent. All these interventions and solutions will not be realized without political will and commitment. Political will and commitment are needed to bring about the needed change particularly in the absence of strong institutions to drive change.

REFERENCES

Abuya, Benta A., James Ciera, and Elizabeth Kimani-Murage. 2012. "Effect of mother's education on child's nutritional status in the slums of Nairobi." *BMC Paediatrics* 12(1): 80. https://doi:10.1186/1471-2431-12-80.

Africa Union Commission, and World Health Organization. 2015. "First meeting of African Ministers of Health jointly convened by the AUC and WHO Luanda, Angola, 14–15 April, 2014, No. 2."

Aikins, Ama de-Graft, Mawuli Kushitor, Kwadwo Koram, Stella Gyamfi, and Gbenga Ogedegbe. 2014. "Chronic non-communicable diseases and the challenge of universal health coverage: insights from community-based cardiovascular disease research in urban poor communities in Accra, Ghana." *BMC Public Health* 14:S2:S3.

Alam, Khurshid, and Ajay Mahal. 2011. "Economic impacts of health shocks on households in low and middle income countries: a review of the literature." *Globalization and Health* 10(1): 1–18.

Asamoah, Benedict O., Kontie M. Moussa, Martin Stafström, and Geofrey Musinguzi. 2011. "Distribution of causes of maternal mortality among different socio-demographic groups in Ghana; a descriptive study." *BMC Public Health* 11(1): 159.

Asaolu, Ibitola O., Halimatou Alaofè, Jayleen KL Gunn, Akosua K. Adu, Amanda J. Monroy, John E. Ehiri, Mary H. Hayden, and Kacey C. Ernst. 2018. "Measuring women's Empowerment in sub-Saharan Africa: exploratory and confirmatory factor analyses of the demographic and health surveys." *Frontiers in Psychology* 9: 994.

Atake, Esso-Hanam. 2018. "Health shocks in Sub-Saharan Africa: are the poor and uninsured households more vulnerable?." *Health Economics* Review 8(1): 26.

Atake, Esso-Hanam, and Pitaloumani Gnakou Ali. 2019. "Women's empowerment and fertility preferences in high fertility countries in Sub-Saharan Africa." *BMC Women's Health* 19(1): 1–54.

Berkman, Douglas S., Andres G. Lescano, Robert H. Gilman, Sonia L. Lopez, and Maureen M. Black. 2002. "Effects of stunting, diarrhoeal disease, and parasitic infection during infancy on cognition in late childhood: a follow-up study." *The Lancet* 359(9306): 564–571.

Bloom, David E., David Canning, and Dean T. Jamison. 2004. "Health, wealth, and welfare." *Finance and Development* 41: 10–15.

Bloom, David E., David Canning, and Jaypee Sevilla. 2004. "The effect of health on economic growth: a production function approach." *World Development* 32(1): 1–13.

Bonfrer, Igna, Lyn Breebaart, and Ellen Van de Poel. 2016. "The effects of Ghana's national health insurance scheme on maternal and infant health care utilization." *PLoS One* 11(11): e0165623.

Brown, J. Larry, and Ernesto Pollitt. "Malnutrition, poverty and intellectual development. 1996." *Scientific American* 274(2): 38–43.

Chrisler, Joan C., and Sheila Ferguson. 2006. "Violence against women as a public health issue." *Annals of the New York Academy of Sciences* 1087(1): 235–249.

Cohen, Jessica, and Pascaline Dupas. 2010. "Free distribution or cost-sharing? Evidence from a randomized malaria prevention experiment." *Quarterly Journal of Economics* 125(1): 1.

Cools, Sara, and Andreas Kotsadam. 2017. "Resources and intimate partner violence in Sub-Saharan Africa." *World Development* 95: 211–230.

Cornia, Giovanni Andrea & Odusola, Ayodele & Bhorat, and Haroon & Conceição, Pedro. 2017. "Income inequality trends in sub-saharan africa divergence, determinants and consequences: introduction, motivation and overview." *UNDP Africa Reports* 267639, United Nations Development Programme (UNDP).

Cortina, Melissa A., Anisha Sodha, Mina Fazel, and Paul Ramchandani G. 2012. "Prevalence of child mental health problems in sub-Saharan Africa: a systematic review." *Archives of Pediatrics & Adolescent Medicine* 166(3): 276–281.

Dalal, Shona, Juan Jose Beunza, Jimmy Volmink, Clement Adebamowo, Francis Bajunirwe, Marina Njelekela, Dariush Mozaffarian, et al. 2011. "Non-communicable diseases in sub-Saharan Africa: what we know now." *International Journal of Epidemiology* 40(4): 885–901.

Daniel, Monica, Bernard Njau, Chauka Mtuya, Elialilia Okelo, and Declare Mushi. 2018. "Perceptions of mental disorders and help-seeking behaviour for mental health care within the Maasai community of northern Tanzania: an exploratory qualitative study." *EA Health Research Journal* 2(2): 103–111.

Davtyan, Mariam, Brandon Brown, and Morenike Oluwatoyin Folayan. 2014. "Addressing Ebola-related stigma: lessons learned from HIV/AIDS." *Global Health Action* 7(1): 26058.

De Onis, Mercedes, and Francesco Branca. 2016. "Childhood stunting: a global perspective." *Maternal & Child Nutrition* 12: 12–26.

Deutscher Akademischer Austauschdienst (DAAD). 2019. "Concept note: contemporary healthcare issues in Sub-Saharan Africa: social, economic and cultural perspectives". DAAD Alumni Workshop in Accra, Ghana.

Doctor, Henry V., Sangwani Nkhana-Salimu, and Maryam Abdulsalam-Anibilowo. 2018. "Health facility delivery in sub-Saharan Africa: successes, challenges, and implications for the 2030 development agenda." *BMC Public Health* 18(1): 765.

Duflo, Esther. 2012. "Women empowerment and economic development." *Journal of Economic literature* 50(4): 1051–1079.

Ebegbulem, Joseph C. 2012. "Corruption and leadership crisis in Africa: Nigeria in focus." *International Journal of Business and Social Science* 3(11): 221–227.

Economic and Social Council-United Nations. 2019. Special Edition: Progress towards the Sustainable Development Goals Report of the Secretary-General. *Advanced unedited version. New York (US): United Nations.*

Elston, J. W. T., A. J. Moosa, F. Moses, G. Walker, N. Dotta, Ronald J. Waldman, and J. Wright. 2016. "Impact of the Ebola outbreak on health systems and population health in Sierra Leone." *Journal of Public Health* 38(4): 673–678.

Fenollar, Florence, and Oleg Mediannikov. 2018. "Emerging infectious diseases in Africa in the 21st century." *New Microbes and New Infections* 26: S10–S18.

García-Moreno, Claudia, Kelsey Hegarty, Ana Flavia Lucas d'Oliveira, Jane Koziol-McLain, Manuela Colombini and Gene Feder. 2015. "The health-systems response to violence against women." *The Lancet* 385(9977): 1567–1579.

Gausset, Quentin. 2001. "AIDS and cultural practices in Africa: the case of the Tonga (Zambia)." *Social Science & Medicine* 52(4): 509–518.

Gershman, Boris. 2016. "Witchcraft beliefs and the erosion of social capital: Evidence from Sub-Saharan Africa and beyond." *Journal of Development Economics* 120: 182–208.

Ghinai, Isaac, Chris Willott, Ibrahim Dadari, and Heidi J. Larson. 2013. "Listening to the rumours: What the northern Nigeria polio vaccine boycott can tell us ten years on." *Global Public Health* 8(10): 1138–1150.

Gouda, Hebe N., Fiona Charlson, Katherine Sorsdahl, Sanam Ahmadzada, Alize J. Ferrari, Holly Erskine, Janni Leung et al. 2019. "Burden of non-communicable diseases in sub-Saharan Africa, 1990–2017: results from the Global Burden of Disease Study 2017." *The Lancet Global Health* 7(10): e1375–e1387.

Heaton, Tim B., Benjamin Crookston, Hayley Pierce, and Acheampong Yaw Amoateng. 2016. "Social inequality and children's health in Africa: a cross sectional study." *International Journal for Equity in Health* 15(1): 92.

Hrdy, Daniel B. 1987. "Cultural practices contributing to the transmission of human immunodeficiency virus in Africa." *Reviews of Infectious Diseases* 9(6): 1109–1119.

Huber, Caroline, Lyn Finelli, and Warren Stevens. 2018. "The economic and social burden of the 2014 Ebola outbreak in West Africa." *The Journal of Infectious Diseases* 218(5): S698–S704.

Institute of Statistical, Social and Economic Research, Ipsos MORI, International Centre for Research on Women-ICRW, NUI Galway. 2019. *Economic and Social Costs of Violence Against Women in Ghana: Summary Report*. Galway: NUI Galway

Iwelunmor, Juliet, Sarah Blackstone, Dorice Veira, Ucheoma Nwaozuru, Collins Airhihenbuwa, Davison Munodawafa, Ezekiel Kalipeni, Antar Jutal, Donna Shelley, and Gbenga Ogedegbe. 2015. "Toward the sustainability of health interventions implemented in sub-Saharan Africa: a systematic review and conceptual framework." *Implementation Science* 11(1): 43.

James, Peter Bai, Jon Wardle, Amie Steel, and Jon Adams. 2018. "Traditional, complementary and alternative medicine use in Sub-Saharan Africa: a systematic review." *BMJ Global Health* 3: 5.

Jegede, Ayodele Samuel. 2007. "What led to the Nigerian boycott of the polio vaccination campaign?" *PLoS Med* 4(3): e73.

Jewkes, Rachel, Robert Morrell, and Nicola Christofides. 2009. "Empowering teenagers to prevent pregnancy: lessons from South Africa." *Culture, Health & Sexuality* 11(7): 675–688.

Kahumba, Joseph, Tsiry Rasamiravaka, Philippe Okusa Ndjolo, Salvius Amuri Bakari, Leonidas Bizumukama, Martin Kiendrebeogo, Mondher El Jaziri, E. M. Williamson, and Pierre Duez. 2015. "Traditional African medicine: from ancestral knowledge to a modern integrated future." *Science* 350(6259): S61–S63.

Karamouzian, Mohammad, and Celestin Hategekimana. 2015. "Ebola treatment and prevention are not the only battles: understanding Ebola-related fear and stigma." *International Journal of Health Policy and Management* 4(1): 55.

Kremer, Michael, and Edward Miguel. 2007. "The illusion of sustainability." *The Quarterly Journal of Economics* 122(3): 1007–1065.

Lépine, Aurélia. "Is Health a Necessity in sub-Saharan Africa? An Investigation of Income-Elasticity of Health Expenditures in Rural Senegal. 2015. " *Journal of International Development"* 27(7): 1153–1177.

Magadi, Monica Akinyi, Alfred O. Agwanda, and Francis O. Obare. 2007. "A comparative analysis of the use of maternal health services between teenagers and older mothers in sub-Saharan Africa: evidence from Demographic and Health Surveys (DHS)." *Social Science & Medicine* 64(6): 1311–1325.

Marmot, Michael. 2005. "Social determinants of health inequalities." *The Lancet* 365(9464): 1099–1104.

McKinsey and Company. 2015. Insights into pharmaceuticals and medical products in Africa: a continent of opportunity for pharma and patients, April. McKinsey & Company.
McIntyre, Diane, Amarech G. Obse, Edwine W. Barasa, and John E. Ataguba. 2018. "Challenges in financing universal health coverage in sub-Saharan Africa." In *Oxford Research Encyclopedia of Economics and Finance*. DOI:10.1093/acrefore/9780190625979.013.28.
Meki Kombe, Charity Lengwe, and Chaya Herman. 2017. "Can education innovations be sustained after the end of donor funding? The case of a reading intervention programme in Zambia." *Educational Review* 69(5): 533–553.
Michael, Charles A., Ikechukwu U. Ogbuanu, Aaron D. Storms, Chima J. Ohuabunwo, et al. "An assessment of the reasons for oral poliovirus vaccine refusals in northern Nigeria. 2014. "*The Journal of Infectious Diseases*" 210 (1): S125–S130.
Nayyar, Gaurvika ML, Joel G. Breman, Paul N. Newton, and James Herrington. 2012. "Poor-quality antimalarial drugs in southeast Asia and sub-Saharan Africa." *The Lancet Infectious Diseases* 12(6): 488–496.
Ndikumana, Léonce, and James K. Boyce. 2011. "Capital flight from sub-Saharan Africa: linkages with external borrowing and policy options." *International Review of Applied Economics* 25(22): 149–170.
Ndomondo-Sigonda, Margareth, Jacqueline Miot, Shan Naidoo, Alexander Dodoo, and Eliangiringa Kaale. 2017. "Medicines regulation in Africa: current state and opportunities." *Pharmaceutical Medicine* 31(6): 383–397.
Njenga, Frank G., Anna N. Nguithi, and Rachel N. Kang'ethe. 2006. "War and mental disorders in Africa." *World Psychiatry* 5(1): 38.
Odusola, A. F., Cornia, G. A., Bhorat, H., and Conceição, P. (Eds.). 2017. *Income inequality trends in sub-Saharan Africa: divergence, determinants and consequences*. United Nations Development Programme, Regional Bureau for Africa.
Overholt, Luc, David Alain Wohl, William A. Fischer, Daniel Westreich, Sam Tozay, Edwina Reeves, Korto Pewu, et al. 2018. "Stigma and Ebola survivorship in Liberia: results from a longitudinal cohort study." *PLoS One* 13: 11.
Pannetier, Julie, France Lert, Marie Jauffret Roustide, and Annabel Desgrées du Loû. 2017. "Mental health of sub-Saharan African migrants: the gendered role of migration paths and transnational ties." *SSM-Population Health* 3: 549–557.
Phillips, Sharon J., and Michael T. Mbizvo. 2016. "Empowering adolescent girls in Sub-Saharan Africa to prevent unintended pregnancy and HIV: A critical research gap." *International Journal of Gynecology & Obstetrics* 132(1)1: 1–3.
Pratley, Pierre. 2016. "Associations between quantitative measures of women's empowerment and access to care and health status for mothers and their children: a systematic review of evidence from the developing world." *Social Science & Medicine* 169: 119–131.
Preston, Samuel H. 1975. "The changing relation between mortality and level of economic development." *Population Studies* 29(2): 231–248.
Read, Ursula M., Edward Adiibokah, and Solomon Nyame. 2009. "Local suffering and the global discourse of mental health and human rights: An ethnographic study of responses to mental illness in rural Ghana." *Globalization and Health* 5(1): 13.

Sauerborn, Rainer, Adrien Nougtara, and Eric Latimer. 1994. "The elasticity of demand for health care in Burkina Faso: differences across age and income groups." *Health Policy and Planning* 9(2): 185–192.

Sharma, Nidhi, Subho Chakrabarti, and Sandeep Grover. 2016. "Gender differences in caregiving among family-caregivers of people with mental illnesses." *World Journal of Psychiatry* 61: 7.

Smith, Kirk, Alistair Woodward, Diarmid Campbell-Lendrum, D. Chadee, Yasushi Honda, Qiyong Liu, Jane Olwoch et al. "Human health: impacts, adaptation, and co-benefits." In *Climate Change 2014: impacts, adaptation, and vulnerability. Part A: global and sectoral aspects. Contribution of Working Group II to the fifth assessment report of the Intergovernmental Panel on Climate Change*, pp. 709–754. Cambridge University Press, 2014.

Sovran, Steven. "Understanding culture and HIV/AIDS in sub-Saharan Africa. 2013." *Sahara-J: Journal of Social Aspects of HIV/AIDS* 10(1): 32–41.

Srivastava, Divya, and Alistair McGuire. 2015. "Patient access to health care and medicines across low-income countries." *Social Science & Medicine* 133: 21–27.

Stefanovics, Elina A., Hongbo He, Maria Cavalcanti, Helio Neto, Angelo Ofori-Atta, Meaghan Leddy, Adesuwa Ighodaro, and Robert Rosenheck. 2016. "Witchcraft and biopsychosocial causes of mental illness: attitudes and beliefs about mental illness among health professionals in five countries." *The Journal of Nervous and Mental Disease* 204(3): 169–174.

Strauss, John, and Duncan Thomas. 1998. "Health, nutrition, and economic development." *Journal of Economic Literature* 36(2): 766–817.

Thiam, Sylla, Alexandre Delamou, Soriba Camara, Jane Carter, Eugene Kaman Lama, Bara Ndiaye, Josephat Nyagero, John Nduba, and Mor Ngom. 2015. "Challenges in controlling the Ebola outbreak in two prefectures in Guinea: why did communities continue to resist?" *The Pan African Medical Journal* 22(1): 22.

United Nations Industrial Development Organisation. 2019. Pharmaceutical industry in sub-Saharan Africa. A guide for promoting pharmaceutical production in Africa. United Nations Industrial Development Organisation.

United Nations. 2016. *The Sustainable development goals report 2016*. United Nations.

United Nations. 2015. Transforming Our World: The 2030 Agenda for Sustainable Development, A/RES/70/1.

United Nations Development Programme. 2019. *Human Development Report 2019: Beyond Income, Beyond Averages, Beyond Today: Inequalities in Human Development in the 21st Century*. United Nations Development Programme, 2019.

United Nations Economic Commission for Africa, GBCHealth, and Aliko Dangote Foundation. 2019. *Healthcare and economic growth in Africa*. Addis Ababa, Ethiopia.

United Nations High Commissioner for Refugees. 2020. The Global Report 2018.

Van Bortel, Tine, Anoma Basnayake, Fatou Wurie, Musu Jambai, Alimamy Sultan Koroma, Andrew T. Muana, Katrina Hann, Julian Eaton, Steven Martin, and Laura B. Nellums. 2016. "Psychosocial effects of an Ebola outbreak at individual, community and international levels." *Bulletin of the World Health Organization* 94(3): 210.

Vinson, Gregory A., and Zoua Chang. 2012. "PTSD symptom structure among West African War trauma survivors living in African refugee camps: A factor-analytic investigation." *Journal of Traumatic Stress* 25(2): 226–231.

World Health Organisation. 2020. Urgent health challenges for the next decade. Accessed January 13, 2020.

World Health Organisation. 2019a. World malaria report 2019. Geneva: World Health Organization; 2019. Licence: CC BY-NC-SA 3.0 IGO.

World Health Organisation. 2019b. Threats to global health 2019. Accessed January 13, 2020.

World Health Organisation. 2019c. *Global spending on health: a world in transition* (No. WHO/HIS/HGF/HFWorkingPaper/19.4). World Health Organization.

World Health Organisation. 2019d. Trends in maternal mortality 2000 to 2017: estimates by WHO, UNICEF.

World Health Organisation. 2018. Mental health: strengthening our response. Fact sheet. *World Health Organization.* Accessed January 13, 2020.

World Health Organisation. 2017. WHO global surveillance and monitoring system for substandard and falsified medical products.

World Health Organisation. 2016. *Public financing for health in Africa: from Abuja to the SDGs* (No. WHO/HIS/HGF/Tech. Report/16.2). World Health Organization.

World Health Organisation. 2013. Mental health action plan 2013-2020.

World Health Organisation. 2012a. *Addressing the challenge of women's health in Africa: report of the Commission on Women's Health in the African Region.* World Health Organization.

World Health Organisation. 2012b. Health systems in Africa-Community perception and perspectives. The report of a multi-country study. June 2012.

World Health Organisation. 2010. Assessment of medicines regulatory systems in sub-Saharan African countries. An overview of findings from 26 assessment reports. *Geneva: WHO.*

World Health Organisation. 1948. Constitution of the World Health Organization.

Yakubu, Ibrahim, and Waliu Jawula Salisu. 2018. "Determinants of adolescent pregnancy in sub-Saharan Africa: a systematic review." *Reproductive Health* 15(1): 15.

Chapter 2

Medicine Quality in West Africa

Impact of Trans-Border Trade

Oluwatoyin Adepeju Odeku and Christie Bose Ola

Drugs play a crucial role and impact the quality of life by reducing morbidity and mortality. Therefore, a reliable good-quality drug supply is essential for health and well-being. Falsified and substandard drugs have resulted in treatment failure, poisoning, and, sometimes, death. For this reason, safety, quality, and efficacy of drugs are the three most important criteria used by governments to regulate pharmaceuticals (MCA, 1997; WHO, 2017a).

The pharmaceutical sector in any economy plays a prominent role in the general health of the populace since they are saddled with the responsibility of producing quality drugs needed for the treatment of diseases and maintenance of health. The pharmaceutical industry develops, produces, and markets drugs and medical devices licensed for use. The global pharmaceuticals market was worth \$1.2 trillion in 2018, up by \$100 billion from 2017 (\$934.8 billion in 2017) and it is estimated that by 2023, the global pharmaceutical industry will be worth \$1.57 trillion (Proshare Intelligent Investing, 2019).

This growth is fueled by the growing and aging population in key markets. It has been predicted that the world's population is likely to rise to 9.3 billion by 2050 and around 21 percent of this population is expected to be aged 60 and above (UN, 2019). In addition to the improvements in purchasing power and access to quality healthcare and pharmaceuticals by poor and middle-class families worldwide and the rising focus of pharmaceuticals companies to tap the rare and specialty diseases market, the growth in the pharmaceutical market will be further propelled by consumers' willingness to use alternative therapies or distrust of taking drugs and government policies affecting reimbursement (and insurance company) regulations, which can be significant (Navadhi Market Research, 2019). In addition, the availability of an appropriate treatment, for instance, during an epidemic, will further propel drug discovery and development, which will further propel the market.

MEDICINE QUALITY

Medicine quality is important since poor-quality medicines jeopardizes national, regional, and global attempts to improve access to effective health-care since they can lead to avoidable morbidity, and contribute to drug resistance. The number of substandard and counterfeit medications that have made their way into trusted pharmacies and subsequently to patients' medicine cabinets has been on the increase and has become a concern not only to patients, but also to pharmacists and pharmaceutical companies.

There are two main categories of poor-quality medicines:

i. *Substandard drugs*: Substandard drugs have been defined as "pharmaceutical products that do not comply with quality standards and specifications at release and throughout the product shelf-life required by the territory of use" (WHO, 2009). These standards and specifications are normally reviewed, assessed, and approved by the relevant regulatory agency before the medicine is authorized for marketing. Substandard medicines could be as a result of poor manufacturing practices, inadequate quality-control processes, incorrect storage or inappropriate packaging, or a combination of these factors. This can affect both branded and generic medicines. Whether or not a drug product is substandard because of criminal intent or because of failures in manufacturing, storage is immaterial to the patient because the impact on their health will be the same, regardless of cause (UNODC, 2010).
ii. *Counterfeit/Falsified/Fake drugs*: Counterfeit/falsified/fake/spurious "drugs are medicines that are deliberately and fraudulently mislabeled with respect to identity and/or source" (WHO, 2003). Both branded and generic products may be counterfeited. "Counterfeit medicines may include products with the correct ingredients or with the wrong ingredients, without active ingredients, with insufficient or too much active ingredients, or with fake packaging. However, because of the potential misunderstanding of the term 'counterfeit'—which, in the context of intellectual property, refers specifically to trademark infringement—the phrase 'falsified medicines' is used by some authorities, particularly in Europe."

The WHO has estimated that 10 percent of global pharmaceutical commerce or $21 billion worth involves counterfeit drugs, and about 1 percent of counterfeit medications are sold in the United States (WHO, 2017b). Most U.S. counterfeit medications are purchased online; however, others have gained access to legitimate supply chains. Drugs that are mostly counterfeited are high-demand and expensive medications such as erectile dysfunction drugs, weight loss aids, chemotherapeutic drugs, antibiotics, antivirals, analgesics, vaccines, hormones, steroids, antihistamines, and antianxiety drugs (Ziance, 2008; FDA, 2011; Chambliss, 2012). The European Union Intellectual Property Office (EUIPO) recently released a report that shows that the EU pharma industry loses €16.5bn in sales to counterfeit drugs, with about 80,459 employment loss (EUIPO, 2019).

Developing countries are confronted with a growing menace from poor-quality medicines, which are made worse by the failing economic conditions, and poor implementation of existing pharmaceutical and customs regulations (Cockburn et al., 2005; Caudron, 2008). The sales of medicines of uncertain quality and origin are on the rise, especially, with the expansion of illegal markets in urban areas, where medicines are sold and treated as mere commodities often stored in very harsh weather conditions (sunlight and high humidity). Most victims of this illicit trade are the world's poorest populations that cannot afford to purchase quality drugs through the right or private sector distribution channels. Globalization of the pharmaceutical industry has contributed to the rapid spread of poor-quality medicines worldwide.

Poor-quality medicines can lead to:

i. *Increased morbidity and mortality*: Poor-quality medicines increase risks of morbidity by prolonging illnesses and increase treatment failure, poisoning, and adverse drug reactions, which can eventually result in mortality. The impact of poor quality medicines becomes fatal if it contains toxic incorrect active ingredients as tragically illustrated by the death of about 500 children after ingestion of paracetamol containing a renal toxin. Paracetamol adulterated with diethylene glycol, a renal toxin and a cheaper substitute for propylene glycol or glycerol, caused the death of a number of children in various developing countries (Hanif et al., 1995; Newton, 2006). The British think-tank, International Policy Network, estimates that globally, 700,000 deaths a year are caused by fake malaria and tuberculosis drugs, giving rise to drug-resistant strains of diseases. In Africa, over 100,000 deaths a year are linked to the counterfeit drug trade (WHO, 2017a). A study carried out in sub-Saharan Africa in 2015 shows that more than 122,000 children under the age of five died each year due to substandard anti-malarial drugs (Renschler et al., 2015).

ii. *Adverse effects*: Some substandard drugs contain more active ingredients than stated and, for drugs with narrow therapeutic range, this may increase the incidence of adverse effects (Wondemagegnehu, 1999). Studies have shown that pharmaceutical products containing unexpected ingredients such as co-trimoxazole containing diazepam, reused ceftazidime vials containing streptomycin, counterfeit artesunate tablets containing artemisinin, chloramphenicol, paracetamol, and metamizole, may lead to adverse effects in patients (Wondemagegnehu, 1999). Patients allergic to these concealed pharmaceuticals may experience adverse events, which may be confusing to the prescriber and difficult to treat.

iii. *Development of drug resistance and loss of drug efficacy*: The administration of subtherapeutic doses of active drugs—particularly antibiotics, antimalarial, and antiretroviral drugs—have resulted in the emergence of drug resistance. Counterfeit antimalarial drugs containing subtherapeutic amounts of active ingredients have been reported to increase the risk of emergence and spread of drug-resistant pathogens (Stepniewska and White, 2008). Models used for the emergence and spread of resistance to antimalarial drugs make it very difficult to tease apart the effects of the misuse of antimalarial drugs by health workers, patient adherence, and poor-quality drugs.

iv. *Economic wastage*: Poor-quality medicines cause economic wastage, which increases the costs of treatment for patients and the health system (Wilson and Fenoff, 2011; WHO, 2017a). Some of these costs, such as resources wasted on ineffective therapies and the treatment of additional complications, are borne primarily by consumers and health facilities (WHO, 2017a). Other indirect costs such as decreased economic productivity resulting from prolonged illness, reduced sales and tax revenues, and costs of anti-counterfeiting initiatives, are borne by governments, companies, the pharmaceutical industry, donors, and the society. In addition, substandard and falsified medicines purchased through the use of personal savings, sale of assets, or borrowing can lead to wastage of scarce resources and poverty (WHO, 2017a).

v. *Loss of confidence in health systems and health workers*: Substandard and falsified medicines pose a threat to global treatment effectiveness, and can lead to loss of trust in the health system and its legitimate healthcare professionals. This diminished trust in licensed healthcare professionals, overtime, may further encourage self-medication and informal care-seeking (Østergaard, 2015). Poor health outcomes can also erode trust in the manufacturers of genuine pharmaceutical products; genuine medicines are sometimes difficult to distinguish from substandard and falsified medicines without the use of verification technologies.

SUBSTANDARD/COUNTERFEIT MEDICINES IN AFRICA

Globally, the trade in counterfeit pharmaceuticals is worth about $200bn (£150bn) annually (Cartwright and Baric, 2018). It is difficult to estimate the extent of the counterfeit drug business in Africa due to the lack of systematic and consistent testing, detection, capture, and reporting. In addition, many African countries have long-standing political instability that has led to poor drug procurement practices by the healthcare administrations. Furthermore, there is low literacy and public awareness of the existence of fake drugs. Drugs are often hawked on the streets and displayed as wares without considering the optimum conditions necessary for storage to maintain stability. There are also open drug markets in major cities in Africa and many poor people who cannot afford costly authentic medications procure their medications from these apparently cheaper sources.

The WHO stated that 42 percent of all fake medicines reported between 2013 and 2017 were from Africa (WHO, 2017a). Analysis of a database collating customized summaries of 251 published anti-malarial quality reports shows that, out of 9,348 antimalarials sampled, 30.1 percent (2,813) failed chemical/packaging quality (Tabernero et al., 2014). The report aggregated from surveys of antimalarial quality done between 2001 and 2010 from twenty-one countries in sub-Saharan Africa shows that 35 percent of samples (796 of 2,297) failed chemical analysis (Nayyar et al., 2012). Although many antimalarials purchased in sub-Saharan Africa are of poor quality, the quality varies greatly by location with seventeen of the forty-four malaria-endemic sub-Saharan African countries having no report on antimalarial quality (Tabernero et al., 2014). In 2012, Angola reported about 1.4 million packets of counterfeit of the antimalarial drug, Coartem®, made by Swiss pharmaceutical giant Novartis, found hidden in a shipment of cargo container containing loudspeakers from China (Almuzaini et al., 2013; Tabernero et al., 2014). Had they been genuine, the fake drugs were enough to treat more than half of Angola's annual malaria cases. This is part of the proliferation of bogus malaria drugs in Africa that threatens to undermine years of progress in tackling the disease. Many of the substandard and fake pharmaceuticals make their way to Africa from countries such as China and India (Faucon et al., 2013). A report in 2009 reveals that over 45 million antimalarial drugs valued at over $438 million were shipped from India and China to West Africa alone (Bennett, 2010). Nearly half (48.7 percent) of the documented cases of drug counterfeiting were reported in developing countries of the Western Pacific (China, the Philippines, and Vietnam); this is followed by developing countries in Africa with 18.7 percent and the industrialized countries with 13.6 percent reported cases (WHO, 2017a).

PHARMACEUTICAL PRODUCTION IN AFRICA

Africa has a rapidly growing pharmaceutical market with a value of $20.8 billion in 2013 and $28.56 billion in 2017. The value is predicted to rise to $56–$70 billion by 2030 (WHO 2012). African countries import around 70–90 percent of the pharmaceutical products consumed. The continent overall has roughly 375 drug manufacturers, most in North Africa, to serve a population of around 1.3 billion people (Michael et al., 2019).

By comparison, China and India, each with roughly 1.4 billion in population, have about 5,000 and 10,500 drug manufacturers, respectively (Cartwright and Baric, 2018). The sub-Saharan African market's value is still relatively small, at roughly $14 billion compared with roughly $120 billion overall in China and $19 billion in India. Only thirty-four of fifty-five African countries have some level of pharmaceutical production capability. Those in sub-Saharan Africa are located in nine of forty-six countries, and they are mostly small, with operations that do not meet international standards. Only Kenya, Nigeria, and South Africa have a relatively sizable industry, with dozens of companies producing for their local markets and, in some cases, for export to neighboring countries.

Almost all local drug producers in sub-Saharan Africa are drug-product manufacturers (i.e., they purchase active pharmaceutical ingredients [APIs] from other manufacturers and formulate them into finished products such as tablets, syrups, creams, and capsules). Up to 100 manufacturers in sub-Saharan Africa are limited to packaging: purchasing tablets and other finished drug products in bulk and repackaging them into consumer packs. Only three companies, two in South Africa, and one in Ghana, produce APIs, and none has significant R&D activity. Poor infrastructure, coupled with a lack of expertise, forces African countries to import up to 70 percent of their pharmaceutical products. Nearly half of the continent's population still lacks access to good quality essential medicines, and burgeoning trade deficits make importing medicine extremely unsustainable (Harris et al., 2009).

In 2017, South Africa, Egypt, and Nigeria, topped importers of Chinese pharmaceutical products with imported medicines worth $300 million each, while Senegal imported $181 million worth of pharmaceutical products (Michael et al., 2019).

With a growing population and continuing health challenges posed by malaria, HIV, and tuberculosis, the pharmaceutical industry is a growth industry that has continued to attract investments. There is extensive trade in pharmaceuticals between countries in West Africa. Nigeria has the most important drug market in the West African region with countries like Togo, Benin, Chad, Niger, and Cameroon buying their drugs from them. Given this flow of trade, the status of drug supply in Nigeria, in terms of quality and security, is to some degree mirrored in many of the other West African countries.

TRANS-BORDER TRADE

Borders serve a wide variety of functions in the areas of security, economics, politics, and social interactions. Despite contemporary challenges to sovereignty, borders still delineate areas of legal competence and it encompasses the territoriality necessary to the concept of the "state" (Jean-Paul Rodrigue 2020). They provide a key element in the structure of the global system, mapping the number and arrangement of the territorial units upon which all humans live. Borders both facilitate and constrain human interaction in conflict and trade, in war and in peace (Newman, 2003). They prevent the entry of undesired elements (people, goods, arms, drugs). The determination of what can be transferred through borders is dependent on the given society or country's views on the functions of borders (Jean-Paul Rodrigue 2020).

Globalization implies increasing flow of people and goods across international borders. Thus, passenger and freight transportation operations must cope with borders as impediments to mobility. A state's attitude to its boundaries is influenced by many factors such as security, cross-border population movements, trade, and illegal activities across the borders.

In traditional African communities, people see themselves as one and they commute from one community to another to visit relatives, engage in business transactions, social trips and for safety during political unrest in their home towns. In modern African societies, the political border imposed by the colonial imperialists has created impediments toward free movement of people across the international boundaries and consequently discouraged their relationship with the neighboring countries. This problem has not been properly addressed by some of the researchers on transborder movement which gives room to smuggling, human trafficking, and stealing, violence, organized crime, terrorism, and drug abuse and other social vices among the communities' borders (UNODC, 2020).

Cross-border criminal activities are often linked to persons or organizations located well beyond the African continent.

Over the past few years, West Africa has become an increasingly important venue for international drug trafficking and organized crime with tons of drugs transiting through the region to Europe (UNODC, 2020).

In the same vein, counterfeit and substandard drugs have been transported across the West African smuggling routes linking inland markets to seaports in Benin, Ghana, and Togo (WHO, 2003). Drugs and other commodities are shipped through seaports of countries with limited restrictions and then distributed through the land borders. The WHO has reported that counterfeit medicines potentially make up more than 50 percent of the global drug market, with a significant proportion of these fake products being encountered in developing countries (WHO, 2013). This is largely due to the lack of effective regulation and weak enforcement capacity existing in these countries, with an increase in this trade resulting from the growing size and sophistication of drug counterfeiters.

West Africa, made up of fifteen countries, namely: Benin, Burkina Faso, Cape Verde, Cote D'Ivoire, Gambia, Ghana, Guinea, Guinea-Bissau, Liberia, Mali, Niger, Nigeria, Senegal, Sierra Leone, and Togo, belongs to a regional economic community called ECOWAS (The Economic Community of West African States). The ECOWAS countries have a rapidly growing population but very limited economic resources. They are also faced with similar diseases and critical issues affecting drug production and distribution. Transborder trade of poor-quality medicines is flourishing across the West African countries because the health authorities are ill-equipped to adequately address the situation. Key factors that have been identified as contributing to the transborder trade of substandard medicines include corruption and lack of political will (WHO, 2008), absent or weak national drug regulating authority (WHO, 2008), inadequate legislations or loopholes in existing legislations (Mackey and Liang, 2011), poor cooperation among different stakeholders in the countries (WHO, 2008; 2013), lucrative drug business due to continued high demand for medicines and low production costs (WHO, 2013), lack of awareness about ill-effects of counterfeit medicines among the general community/healthcare professionals/pharmacists (Abdoulaye et al., 2006; Chauvé, 2008), poor socioeconomic status (Mackey and Liang, 2011), health illiteracy (Abdoulaye et al., 2006; Mackey and Liang, 2011), globalization and free trade policies (WHO, 2008), and availability of medicines outside conventional and government-regulated networks, viz., internet pharmacies (WHO, 2008).

The sale of fraudulent medicines from East Asia and the Pacific to Southeast Asia and Africa alone amounts to about $5 billion per year and a sizable amount of money is being fed into the illicit economy (UNODC, 2013). In a survey conducted by Gallup in 2011 to gauge the experience of about 1,000 people in sub-Saharan Africa with poor-quality medicines, about one in five adults across all surveyed countries or members of their household have been "victims" of fraudulent medicines with the percentages varying from as high as 43 percent in Sierra Leone to as low as 3 percent in South Africa (Gallup, 2011). There have also been several reports of drug seizures in recent years, which give an indication of the size of the problem in West Africa. A BBC report indicates that 19 tons of counterfeit medicines were seized in Ivory Coast, Guinea-Bissau, Liberia, and Sierra Leone in 2018; 12 tons of counterfeit pharmaceuticals smuggled from Ghana were intercepted in Ivory Coast in 2019; more than 420 tons of illicit pharmaceutical products were seized in Interpol-led operations in seven West African countries in 2017; nearly 19.88 tons of fake medicines were seized in Mali between

2015 and 2018 (Mwai, 2020). Some of these drugs are transported through the porous land borders and since the regulation is weak, the quality of these medicines cannot be ascertained. These drugs are sold by unlicensed and unregulated vendors, selling medications off the streets and such medications are easily accessible to the poor. Lack of necessary legislation, regulatory enforcement, and appropriate drug laws are some of the issues identified to be crippling the fight against drug counterfeiting. In addition, corruption, bribery, and conflict of interest have ensured that government officials fail to enforce laws and subsequently refrain from arresting individuals engaging in drug counterfeiting. The desperate demand for drugs in many African countries, coupled with global drug shortages to meet such demands, has made such enterprise to flourish in Africa.

IMPROVING MEDICINE QUALITY

The proliferation of substandard/spurious/falsified/fake/counterfeit medicines in Africa is a public health crisis that can no longer be ignored. The WHO has focused on the public health implications of these medicines, and has been providing support for the establishment of the framework to facilitate information exchange and to foster international collaboration to combat poor-quality medicines (WHO, 2017b). In addition, member states have embarked on the development of direction tools and capacity building to establish global monitoring systems, and assessment of risk in the allocation of resources in their national context (Rajapandian et al., 2013; Tremblay, 2013). National pharmaceutical programs promoting universal access to essential generic medicines at reasonable cost have been identified as one of the methods to curb the problem. A system based on strict, rational pharmaceutical purchasing, and distribution policies with quality assurance at every level of the supply chain is needed to guarantee that patients receive safe, effective, and high-quality healthcare products (Rajapandian et al., 2013). The quality of medicine can be improved by:

Improved Quality Production

Good manufacturing practice (GMP) is the part of quality assurance that ensures medicines are consistently produced and controlled to the quality standards appropriate to their intended use and as required by the marketing authorization (Lezotre, 2014). GMP is aimed primarily at diminishing the risks involved in any pharmaceutical production that cannot be eliminated through testing of the final product. Thus, GMP covers all aspects of production: from the starting materials, premises, and equipment, to the training and personal hygiene of staff. It is therefore important for pharmaceutical industries to observe GMP in order to ensure that substandard products are not produced by the manufacturers. To ensure improved quality medicine, periodical inspections of the production facilities is necessary, especially in contract manufacture of medicines involving companies based in other countries. This requires the active involvement of the medicine regulatory agencies in the various countries to conduct proper inspection and approval of the medicines for importation.

Other factors that have been associated with the production and sale of poor-quality antimalarials include inaccessibility and high price of quality antimalarials, limited regulatory oversight, lack of penalties, self-prescribing practices, poor knowledge about product authenticity, and a large unregulated private sector for purchasing pharmaceuticals (Newton et al., 2010; WHO, 2013; Renschler et al., 2015). The WHO estimated that 30 percent of countries lack any capacity to oversee medicine manufacture, importation, or distribution (WHO, 2013). To date, South Africa, Kenya, and Tanzania are the only malaria-endemic African countries with WHO-prequalified laboratories for drug quality testing (Tabernero et al., 2014). Nigerian manufacturers invested over N400 billion in the last twenty years in upgrading facilities to acquire the WHO prequalification needed for international competition. Only one (Swiss Pharma Nigeria Limited, Swipha) of the four pharmaceutical companies in Nigeria listed for WHO prequalification was prequalified making it the first pharmaceutical manufacturer in sub-Saharan West Africa to have demonstrated an acceptable level of compliance with WHO GMP; one went bankrupt in the process and the other companies are still working to meet up with the standard (WHO, 2014). Thus, many drug manufacturers still do not have WHO prequalification that would enable them compete in international tenders financed, inter alia, by the Global Fund (UNIDO, 2011). Hence, most of the drugs donated to Africa by international agencies are still manufactured from the Asian countries and imported to Africa.

Supply Chain

The complexity of the supply chain for pharmaceuticals has been identified as contributing to the market for counterfeit medicines (Rajapandian et al., 2013). There should be a supply chain in place in every country that would ensure the safe supply of medicines. This supply chain begins with the raw materials and ends with the finished products delivered to the patients, ensuring that there has been no tampering, diversion, falsification, substitution, or adulteration (Tremblay, 2013). Pharmacists, because of their position in the supply chain and their expertise in drugs and drug products, play an important role in securing the supply chain.

In most developing countries, counterfeit medicines can be found in street markets and legitimate pharmacies belonging to the formal supply chain (Sewing, 2007). The network of criminals involved in counterfeit medicines distribution have the intimidating and corruptive power to introduce counterfeit products into the market while they can also undertake street selling to lure potential victims with low-priced drugs. As a result, patients in these countries can hardly trust the product they are buying and simply have no choice but to purchase them, unless they have enough money to buy from the official pharmacies, where they have the hope that the supply procedures and regulations have been respected by all actors and, the medicine obtained is actually genuine. In the case of street/local markets in poorer countries, the diffusion of counterfeit medicines can also be linked to their appealing price that attracts patients with lower financial possibilities (Sewing, 2007). Thus, to ensure medicine quality, it is important that the supply chain is regulated to ensure that quality medicines that have been stored under proper conditions get to the hands of consumers.

Medicine Regulatory Authorities

The WHO estimated that 30 percent of countries have no drug regulation (WHO, 2012). Each country should have a medicine regulatory agency such as the Nigerian National Agency for Food and Drug Administration and Control (NAFDAC) and Ghana Food and Drug Authority, saddled with the responsibility of setting standards that would ensure medicine quality. Medicine Regulatory Authorities (MRAs) should be strengthened to carry out their functions. It is crucial to have a sustained political will and financial support for the coordinated action from the police, customs officials, and MRAs. A recent forensic investigation into the trade of fake Artesunate demonstrated that the police, the pharmaceutical industry, scientists, governments, and the WHO can work together to combat these problems.

At a regional level, harmonization of medicine registration and regulatory activities should be done to determine the quality of medicines imported to ECOWAS member states (UNIDO, 2011). The harmonization of medicine registration (e.g., by the African Medicines Regulatory Harmonization Initiative) would address the issue of poor-quality and counterfeit medicines as the standards can be harmonized across the region. In addition, the global interconnectedness must be mirrored by regulatory structures that allow national authorities to exchange information and skills quickly and efficiently.

Equipping officials with tools to identify counterfeit medicines is another way to curb the trafficking of medicines across international borders. Custom and MRA officers at the borders should be trained to identify counterfeit drugs and be able to confiscate counterfeit drugs before they reach consumers. Anticounterfeit measures using the Short Messaging Service verification system was effective in developing countries including Ghana. Nigeria and Kenya announced in early 2012 that more than one million people had used this system to verify the authenticity of their medicines (Agbaraji et al., 2012).

International organizations such as UNODC regional cooperation networks should work with INTERPOL and other relevant organizations to provide the ideal platform to trace counterfeit drugs and make seizures through the supply chain and to track down and investigate criminal networks involved in this illicit trade. The International Medical Products Anti-counterfeiting Taskforce (IMPACT), which brings together some 193 countries and transnational organizations such as INTERPOL, set up in 2006 has been a successful model for cross-country collaborative effort (UNICRI, 2012). There is the need to enhance border management capacities across the region at strategic locations and to provide improved national and cross-border coordination between law enforcement agencies. This would enable efficient tracking of medicines imported to different countries. The capacities to collect, analyze, and disseminate information, and detect fraudulent and fraudulently obtained travel documents/import license should be strengthened. There is also the need to foster international collaboration to conduct cross-border investigations and better exchange of information between consular offices abroad (UNODC, 2020).

Transnational cooperation and global surveillance of the supply chains of medicinal products should be linked with global legislation/litigation in order to enhance Africa's capacity to track counterfeit/substandard medicines (Dégardin et al., 2014).

CONCLUSION

Available evidence suggests that poor-quality essential medicines have grievous effects on public health in developing countries. The actions necessary to combat poor-quality medicines may be more straightforward if criminal deception is not involved. There is the need for increased provision of free or inexpensive medicines for key diseases to undercut counterfeiters and reduce criminal financial incentives. Regulations are also needed at international, regional, and national levels to strengthen the fight against the menace. Countries need to set up medicine regulatory agencies with the responsibility of setting standards and monitoring the quality of medicines produced, imported, and sold. This is to ensure that quality medicines get to the citizens. Cross-border trade (parallel trade, reimportation, or importation) within the West African subregions should be regulated to ensure that substandard medicines are not circulated across the region. It is clear that transnational cooperation and improved global surveillance of the supply chains of medicinal products are crucial in the trade in quality drugs.

REFERENCES

Abdoulaye I., Chastanier H., Azondekon A., Dansou A., Bruneton C. 2006. Evaluation of public awareness campaigns on counterfeit medicines in Cotonou, Benin. *Med Trop* (Mars);66:615–8.

Agbaraji E. C., Ochulor D. O., Ezeh G. N. 2012. Food and drug counterfeiting in the developing nations: The implications and way-out. *Academic Research International*;3:24–31.

Almuzaini T., Choonara I., Sammons H. 2013. Substandard and counterfeit medicines: a systematic review of the literature. *BMJ* Open;3(8):e002923.

Bennett S. 2010. *Scratch and win war on Africa's counterfeit malaria medicines gets under way*. Bloomberg Press. 2010.

Business Day Weekender 2019. Nigerian Pharmaceutical Industry: Big steps, setbacks, prospects. https://businessday.ng/real-sector/article/nigerian-pharmaceutical-industry-big-steps-setbacks-prospects/. Accessed 3 March 2020.

Cartwright R., Baric A. 2018. The rise of counterfeit pharmaceuticals in Africa Robin. Available from: https://enact-africa.s3.amazonaws.com/site/uploads/2018-11-12-counterfeit-medicines-policy-brief.pdf, 2018. Accessed 3 March 2020.

Caudron J. M. 2008. Substandard medicines in resource-poor settings: a problem that can no longer be ignored. *Trop. Med. Int. Health*. 2008;13:1062–1072.

Chambliss W., Carroll W., Yelvigi M., et al. 2012. Role of the pharmacist in preventing distribution of counterfeit medications. *J Am Pharm Assoc.*;52(2):195–199.

Chauvé M. 2008. The fight against counterfeit medicines in Africa: Experience and role of pharmacists. *C R Biol.*;331:982–5.

Cockburn P., Newton P. N., Agyarko E. K., Akunyili D., White N. J. 2005. The global threat of counterfeit drugs: why industry and governments must communicate the dangers. *PLoS Med.*;**2**:e100.

Dégardin K, Roggo Y., Margot P. 2014. Understanding and fighting the medicine counterfeit market. *J Pharm Biomed Anal.*;87:167–75.

EUIPO. 2019. European Union Intellectual Property Office, https://www.outsourcing-pharma.com/Article/2019/06/18/Economic-cost-of-counterfeit-drugs?utm_source=copyright&utm_medium=OnSite&utm_campaign=copyright 2019. Accessed 3 March 2020

Faucon B, Murphy C, Whalen J. 2013. Africa's Malaria Battle: Fake Drug Pipeline Undercuts Progress. https://bambooinnovator.com/2013/05/29/africas-malaria-battle-fake-drug-pipeline-undercuts-progress

FDA. 2011. Food and Drug Administration. Reporting serious problems to FDA. www.fda.gov/Safety/MedWatch/HowToReport/default.htm, 6 January 2011. Accessed 29 March 2020.

Gallup. 2011. Fake Medicine Common in Many Sub-Saharan African Countries. Available from: https://news.gallup.com/poll/149942/Fake-Medicine-Common-Sub-Saharan-African-Countries.aspx 5 October 2011. Accessed 3 March 2020

Glass B. D. 2014. Counterfeit drugs and medical devices in developing countries. *Res Reports Trop Med.*;5:11–22.

Hanif M., Mobarak M. R., Ronan A., Rahman D., Donovan J. J. J., Bennish M. L. 1995. Fatal renal failure caused by diethylene glycol in paracetamol elixir: the Bangladesh epidemic. *BMJ*;311:88–91.

Harris J., Stevens P., Morris J. 2009. Keeping it real. Combatting the spread of fake drugs in poor countries. *International Policy Network*, 2009.

Jean-Paul Rodrigue 2020. The Geography of Transport Systems, fifth edition, New York: Routledge, 456 pages. ISBN 978-0-367-36463-2 https://transportgeography.org/?page_id=3978. Accessed 3 March 2020.

Michael C., Tania H., Adam S., Irene Y.S., 2019. Should sub-Saharan Africa make its own drugs? A comprehensive analysis of the business, economic, and public-health impact finds the potential for local production of pharmaceuticals to be a mixed bag. https://www.mckinsey.com/industries/public-sector/our-insights/should-sub-saharan-africa-make-its-own-drugs# Accessed 3 March 2020.

Proshare Intelligent Investing 2019. Assessing Efficiency in the Pharmaceutical Sector of Nigeria. https://www.proshareng.com/news/Health/Assessing-Efficiency-in-the-Pharmaceutical-Sector-of-Nigeria/44194) Accessed 3 March 2020.

Lezotre P. L. 2014. State of Play and Review of Major Cooperation Initiatives. In: International Cooperation, Convergence and Harmonization of Pharmaceutical Regulations. *Global Perspective.*;7–170. https://doi.org/10.1016/C2013-0-12774-2

Mackey T. K., Liang B. A. 2011. The global counterfeit drug trade: Patient safety and public health risks. *J Pharm Sci.*;100:4571–9.

MCA. 1997. *Towards safe medicines. A guide to the control of safety, quality and efficacy of human medicines in the United Kingdom.* Revised edition 1997. London: Medicines Control Agency (MCA),1–93.

Mwai P. 2020. Fake drugs: How bad is Africa's counterfeit medicine problem? BBC 2020. Available from: https://www.bbc.com/news/world-africa-51122898. Accessed 20 January 2020

Navadhi Market Research. 2019. https://www.reportlinker.com/p05761205/U-S-Pharmaceuticals-Industry-Analysis-and-Trends.html?utm_source=GNW. Accessed 3 March 2020

Nayyar G. M., Breman J. G., Newton P. N., Herrington J. 2012. Poor-quality antimalarial drugs in southeast Asia and sub-Saharan Africa. *Lancet Infect Dis.*;12(6):488–96.

Newman D. 2003. On borders and power: A theoretical framework. *Journal of Borderlands Studies*;18(1):13–25.

Newton P. N. 2006. Counterfeit anti-infective medicines. *Lancet Inf. Dis.*;6:602–613.

Newton P. N., Green M. D., Fernández F. M. 2010. Impact of poor-quality medicines in the developing world. *Trends Pharmacol. Sci.*;31:99–101.

Østergaard L. R. 2015. Trust matters: a narrative literature review of the role of trust in health care systems in sub-Saharan Africa. *Glob Public Health.*;10(9):1046–1059.

Rajapandian G., Narayanan N., Maheswaran A., Chanchal P. 2013. Dangerous world of counterfeit drugs–Pharmacist's role and its prevention. *Int J Pharm Sci Rev Res.*;4:1709–1713.

Renschler J. P., Walters K. M., Newton P. N., Laxminarayan R. 2015. Estimated under-five deaths associated with poor-quality antimalarials in sub-Saharan Africa. *Am J Trop Med Hyg.*;92(6 Suppl):119–126.

Sewing P. 2007. Counterfeit Drugs in Africa. Causes, Magnitudes and Impacts, UNODC, November, p. 1.

Stepniewska K., White N. J. 2008. The pharmacokinetic determinants of the window of selection for antimalarial drug resistance. *Antimicrob Agents Chemother.*;52:1589–1596.

Tabernero P., Fernández F. M., Green M., Guerin P. J., Newton P. N. 2014. Mind the gaps-the epidemiology of poor-quality anti-malarials in the malarious world-analysis of the Worldwide Antimalarial Resistance Network database. *Malar J.*;13:139.

Tremblay M. 2013. Medicines counterfeiting is a complex problem: A review of key challenges across the supply chain. *Curr Drug Saf.*;8:43–55.

UN. 2019. United Nations, Department of Economic and Social Affairs, Population Division (2019). World Population Prospects 2019: Highlights (ST/ESA/SER.A/423). https://www.ined.fr/en/everything_about_population/demographic-facts-sheets/focus-on/world-population-prospects-2019/. Accessed 3 March 2020.

UNICRI. 2013. United Nations Interregional Crime and Justice Research Institute, 2012. counterfeit medicines and organised crime. http://www.unicri.it/topics/counterfeiting/medicines/report/Ctf_medicines_and_oc_advance_unedited2013.pdf Accessed 3 March 2020.

UNIDO. 2011. Pharmaceutical Sector Profile: Nigeria. https://www.unido.org/sites/default/files/2011-04/Nigeria_Pharma%20Sector%20Profile_032011_Ebook_0.pdf Accessed 3 March 2020.

United Nations Office on Drugs and Crime 2020. West and Central Africa. Border Control. https://www.unodc.org/westandcentralafrica/en/newrosenwebsite/TOC/border-control.html. Accessed 3 March 2020.

UNODC. 2020. Border Control-United Nations Office on Drugs and Crime. https://www.unodc.org/westandcentralafrica/en/newrosenwebsite/TOC/border-control.html, Accessed 3 March 2020.

UNODC. 2013. United Nations Office on Drugs and Crime, "Transnational Organized Crime in East Asia and the Pacific: A Threat Assessment", p. 129, 2013. Available from http://www.unodc.org/documents/southeastasiaandpacific//Publications/2013/TOCTA_EAP_web.pdf. Accessed 3 March 2020.

UNODC. 2010. United Nations Office on Drugs and Crime. World Drug Report 2010, 2010. Available athttp://www.unodc.org/documents/wdr/WDR_2010/World_Drug_Report_2010_lo-res.pdf. Accessed 18 December 2019.

Wilson J., Fenoff R. 2011. *The Health and Economic Effects of Counterfeit Pharmaceuticals in Africa*. East Lansing: Michigan State University; 2011.

Wondemagegnehu, E. 1999. Counterfeit and substandard drugs in Myanmar and Viet Nam. WHO Report. WHO/EDM/QSM/99.3. Geneva: WHO. 1999.

World Health Organization. 2020. First Nigerian manufacturer considered compliant with WHO GMP. https://extranet.who.int/prequal/news/first-nigerian-manufac turer-considered-compliant-who-gmp; 2014. Accessed 3 March 2020.

World Health Organization. 2019. Counterfeit medicines: frequently asked questions, 2009. Available athttp://www.who.int/medicines/services/counterfeit/faqs/QAC ounterfeit-October2009.pdf Accessed 18 December 2019.

World Health Organization. 2019. Substandard and counterfeit medicines. Fact sheet No. 275, 2003. Available at http://www.who.int/mediacentre/factsheets/2003/fs2 75/en/ Accessed 18 December 2019.

World Health Organization. 2017. A Study on the Public Health and Socioeconomic Impact of Substandard and Falsified Medical Products. Geneva, Switzerland: World Health Organization; 2017.

World Health Organization. 2017. WHO Global Surveillance and Monitoring System for Substandard and Falsified Medical Products. Geneva, Switzerland: World Health Organization; 2017.

World Health Organization. 2013. General information on counterfeit medicines. 2013. Available from: http://www.who.int/medicines/services/counterfeit/overv iew/en . Accessed 3 March 2020.

World Health Organization. 2013. What Encourages Counterfeiting of Medicines? 2013. https://www.wiltonpark.org.uk/wp-content/uploads/WP1185-WHO-What-encourages-counterfeiting-of-medicines.pdf Available at. Accessed October 3, 2013.

World Health Organization. 2012. International Regulatory Harmonization. International conference of drug regulatory attitudes. *WHO Drug Inform.*; 26:339–352 www.nigeriamanufacturingexpo.com › Pages › site160_33589_en_ file1 Accessed 3 March 2020.

World Health Organization. 2008. Counterfeit drugs kill. 2008. Available from: http: //www.who.int/impact/FinalBrochureWHA2008a.pdf . Accessed 3 March 2020.

World Health Organization. 1999. *Effective drug regulation: what can countries do?* Geneva: WHO, 1999; 1–53.

Ziance R. J. 2008. Roles for pharmacy in combatting counterfeit drugs. *J. Am. Pharm. Assoc;*48:e71–e88.

Chapter 3

Tackling Diabetes in Sub-Saharan Africa

The Medicinal Plant Approach

Peculiar Feenna Onyekere, Felix Ifeanyi Nwafor, and Chioma Obianuju Peculiar-Onyekere

Diabetes is among the world's most chronic diseases and sub-Saharan Africa is one of the worst affected regions globally. According to the International Diabetes Federation, over 463 million adults are currently living with diabetes and this may rise to 700 million by 2045 (IDF, 2019).

Diabetes mellitus is a chronic metabolic syndrome associated with insulin resistance, insufficiency of insulin secretion, or both (WHO, 2010). It is an endocrine disorder that impairs glucose homeostasis, leading to diabetic complications, including retinopathy, neuropathy, and nephropathy. In 2016, the multifactorial disease was ranked seventh among death-causing diseases and third when its complications are considered globally (Merlin et al., 2005; Sharma et al., 2010). It is diagnosed when fasting plasma glucose level is ≥7.0 mmol/L (126 mg/dL) or glycated hemoglobin (A_{IC}) at ≥6.5 percent or a random plasma glucose ≥11.1 mmol/L. It is mainly classified as type 1 and type 2. Type 1 occurs due to autoimmune destruction of β-cells of the pancreas, which invariably leads to absolute insulin deficiency. In type 2, the beta-cells of the pancreas can produce insulin but the insulin produced is ineffective due to resistance (Aroda et al., 2002). The percentage of people with type 2 diabetes is on the rise in most countries of the world with over 75 percent of diabetic adults living in low- and middle-income countries—one of the reasons sub-Saharan Africa is bedeviled by the menace.

Despite the existence of an array of pharmacological agents for the management of the disorder, it is usually difficult to achieve optimal glycemic control. Moreover, the available drugs are associated with a number of adverse effects. Researchers are increasingly seeking for novel therapeutic agents from medicinal plants that are safer, more efficacious, and more affordable (Onyekere et al., 2020).

There are different approaches in the management of diabetes including pharmacological, non-pharmacological, and the green approach (medicinal plant approach). The pharmacological approach involves the use of insulin and other oral hypoglycemic agents, while the non-pharmacological approach which is both prophylactic and synergistic in action, involves diet, physical exercise, and reduction of the risk factors such as smoking and alcohol. Type 1 diabetes is conventionally managed with insulin while type 2 is managed with oral hypoglycemic agents such as sulfonylureas, biguanides, gliptins, among others (Osadebe et al., 2014; Onyekere et al., 2020).

Natural products have remained sources of therapeutic agents with numerous beneficial uses (Arkshada et al., 2019). Those obtained from plants and animals are called crude drugs and are produced in the living cells of plants or animals. It is important to note that majority of the naturally derived drugs are from plant sources, while others are from animal or mineral sources (Ibezim et al., 2018).

Medicinal plants are proven sources of pharmaceuticals for the treatment of various ailments. The World Health Organization reported that over a thousand plant species worldwide have demonstrated potential anti-diabetic activity and a significant number of them have shown measurable efficacy on laboratory evaluation (Rajasekhar et al., 2010). Sub-Saharan Africa is endowed with natural products especially medicinal plants. While some have been scientifically evaluated for their anti-diabetic activity, many are yet to be discovered, explored, and validated. For instance, some plants in Nigeria have been studied for their hypoglycemic and anti-diabetic activity including *Acanthus montanus* (Odoh and Ezugwu, 2005); *Anthocleista vogelii* (Osadebe et al., 2014; Onyekere et al., 2017); *Combretum dolichopetalum* (Uzor et al., 2015), *Psydrax horizontalis* (Onyekere et al., 2020) among others.

Phytomedicines and plant-based drugs have wider acceptability, availability, tolerability, and affordability over their synthetic or semisynthetic counterparts. There is a great need to explore and harness the potentials of the rich African forest of herbs, trees, and common medicinal plants in tackling diabetes.

CLASSIFICATION OF DIABETES MELLITUS

Diabetes can be classified into three: type 1 diabetes (formerly called Insulin-Dependent Diabetes Mellitus), type 2 diabetes (formerly called Non-Insulin-Dependent Diabetes Mellitus), and gestational diabetes.

Type 1 diabetes mellitus occurs due to cellular mediated autoimmune destruction of pancreatic β-cells, which invariably lead to absolute insulin deficiency. Severe clinical manifestations appear almost immediately and they include: polyphagia (excessive hunger), polyuria (excessive urination), polydipsia (excessive thirst), and weight loss. Since the beta cells are responsible for insulin secretion, as its mass decreases, the insulin secretion reduces until it reaches a level where the insulin available can no longer maintain the normal blood glucose levels (American Diabetes Association, 2014).

Type 2 diabetes mellitus is the most common form of diabetes mellitus accounting for 85 to 95 percent of cases in developed nations and an even higher percentage in developing nations. The beta-cells of the pancreas are capable of producing insulin but become so resistant that the insulin produced is ineffective (Aroda et al., 2017). It may range from predominantly insulin resistance with relative insulin deficiency to a predominantly secret defect with or without insulin resistance. The majority of patients with this form of diabetes are obese, and obesity causes or aggravates insulin resistance (Han et al., 2013; Samuel and Shulman 2016).

Gestational Diabetes Mellitus (GDM) is defined as any degree of glucose intolerance with onset or first recognition during pregnancy (Metzger and Coustan, 1998). The prevalence may range from 1 to 14 percent of all pregnancies, depending on the population studied and the diagnostic tests employed (American Diabetes Association, 2014). It is important to note that GDM develops during the second or third trimester of pregnancy in about 3–10 percent of pregnancies. Hence, care must be taken to avoid risk of obesity, overweight, and sedentary lifestyle during the second and third trimester of pregnancy. Older women of 45 years and above are more susceptible to GDM; hence, age is also a risk factor.

SIGNS/SYMPTOMS AND COMPLICATIONS OF DIABETES MELLITUS

The classical signs and symptoms of diabetes are also associated with hyperglycemia and they are known as "hyperglycemic triad"—polyuria (frequent urination), polydipsia (increased thirst), and polyphagia (increased hunger). Others include xerostomia (dry mouth), fatigue, weight loss, skin and genital itching, stomatitis, visual disturbances, peripheral neuropathy, poor wound healing, recurrent vaginal infection, and erectile dysfunction in men. Complications could be acute or chronic in nature. The major acute complications include hypoglycemia, diabetic ketoacidosis, and hyperglycemic hyperosmolar non-ketotic coma. Unlike the acute complications, chronic complications affect major vital organs and systems of the body. They range from diseases of major blood vessels (such as coronary artery disease, cerebrovascular, and peripheral artery diseases) to diseases of tiny blood vessels (such as retinopathy).

GLOBAL PREVALENCE OF DIABETES

The global prevalence rate of diabetes in 2019 is estimated at 9.3 percent (463 million people) and is expected to rise to 10.2 percent (578 million) by 2030 and 10.9 percent (700 million) by 2045. According to the International Diabetes Federation Diabetes Atlas, 9th edition, one in two people (50.1 percent) living with diabetes are not aware of their status. The prevalence is higher in urban areas (10.8 percent) than rural (7.2 percent) and in high-income (10.4 percent) than low-income countries (4.0 percent) (IDF, 2019). Moreover, the prevalence of diabetes is higher in men than in women, but there are more women living with diabetes than men. The most important demographic change to diabetes prevalence across the world appears to be the increase in the proportion of people >65 years of age. It is predicted that by 2030 diabetes mellitus may afflict up to 79.4 million individuals in India, 42.3 million in China, and 30.3 million in the United States (Wild et al., 2 004; Whiting et al., 2011). Moreover in figure 3.1, IDF also predicts that in South East Asia about 50 million individuals would be affected while 70 million people might be affected in North America and the Caribbean by 2045. The

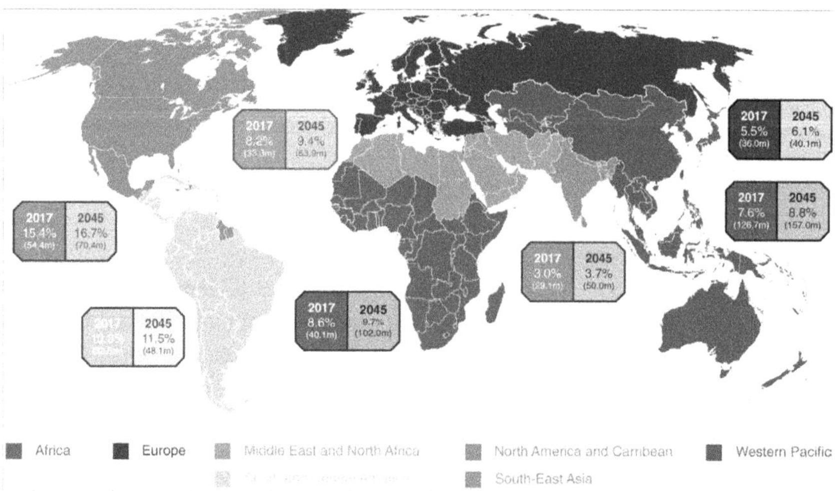

Figure 3.1 Prevalence of Diabetes Across the Globe. Adapted from International Diabetes Federation Atlas Map, 9th edition (2017–2045).

Western Pacific would likely be the most affected. This is due to the increasing risk in obesity, rapid development, and unhealthy lifestyle associated with that region (Juliana et al., 2014).

PREVALENCE OF DIABETES IN SUB-SAHARAN AFRICA

The African continent currently has the highest proportion of people with undiagnosed diabetes on the global scale. According to the *IDF Diabetes (Atlas 9th Edition)*, an estimated 19.4 million adults aged 20–79 years are living with diabetes in the IDF Africa Region in 2019, representing a regional prevalence of 3.9 percent. By 2045, IDF projects that 102.0 million Africans are expected to have diabetes if no radical management approach is adopted as seen in Figure 3.1. A major factor that contributes to a rise in the prevalence of diabetes in sub-Saharan Africa is urbanization (Godfrey and Julien, 2005). The rural-to-urban migration coupled with sedentary lifestyle in the urban regions cannot be overemphasized. Other factors include: increasing obesity—influenced by economic, sociocultural, and nutritional transitions—and increasing age (Werfalli et al., 2015). Besides, the sub-Saharan Africa has greater genetic variation compared to other regions of the world.

APPROACHES TO TACKLING DIABETES

There are various management approaches that can be adopted in the management of diabetes including pharmacological, non-pharmacological, and medicinal plant approaches. However, for good management and treatment to be possible, it is essential that clear diagnosis be carried out using the diagnostic tools as stated earlier. According to WHO (2010), the target objectives of management include but are not limited to the following: to relieve symptoms; to correct associated health problems and to reduce morbidity, mortality, and economic costs of diabetes; to prevent as much as possible acute and long-term complications; to monitor the development of such complications and to provide timely intervention as well as to improve the quality of life and productivity of the individual with diabetes. For the purpose of this chapter, we shall focus more on the medicinal plant (green) approach.

Medicinal Plant Approach

According to WHO, "a medicinal plant is any plant in which one or more of its organs contains substances or compounds that can be used for therapeutic purposes or which are precursors for the synthesis of useful drugs" (Sofowora, 2008). There is an increasing focus on the importance of medicinal plants and traditional medicine in tackling healthcare problems in Africa and the world at large. The WHO has stated that 80 percent of the world's population depends on medicinal plant for their healthcare delivery. This has led to an increased search for novel bioactive compounds from medicinal plants (Ekor, 2013). There is increasing need to scientifically explore the potentials of phytomedicines, phytotherapeutics, ecology, environmental medicine, and clinical pharmacognosy.

Trado-Medical Practice for Management of Diabetes

In Africa, herbal medicines are usually dispensed by a traditional healer who makes use of natural products in treating diseases. The potential anti-diabetic plant(s) is (are) prepared in different forms including concoction, maceration, or decoction using appropriate solvent. Water is the most common solvent that is used for such procedures. This is done to enable extraction of the active principles in the plants. Since the traditional healers do not depend on conventional laboratory techniques, they utilize different trado-medical methods to diagnose diabetes in their patients. They achieve this via identification of diabetic symptoms like frequent urination, swollen legs, hands and stomach, sexual dysfunction, obesity, fatigue, and profuse sweating during the consultation process. In some cases, they direct the patients to urinate on locally prepared concoctions and return after a couple of days with the results of a diagnosis (Mohammed et al., 2014).

Diabetes is among the diseases which are treated with traditional medicines using medicinal plants. The efficacy of some of these medicinal plants are greater than that of orthodox medicines which are associated with adverse reactions. Various ethno-botanical surveys from different regions across sub-Saharan Africa have been carried out to validate this fact. This includes Western Africa (Adebayo, 2009; N'guessa et al., 2009), Eastern Africa (Rutebember et al., 2013. Keter and Mutiso 2012; Moshi and Mbwambo, 2002) Southern Africa (Afolayan and Sunmonu, 2010; Mahop, 2007) and Central Africa (Din et al., 2011).

PRELIMINARY QUALITY CONTROL PROCEDURES FOR SELECTING POTENTIAL MEDICINAL PLANT

There are certain steps that are critical in the use of a plant or plants with potential anti-diabetic activity:

Proper Plant Selection and Identification

Plant selection and identification is one of the critical and foundational elements in medicinal plant research. It is important to note that a plant can bear several different local names or different plants can have the same name. This is common in African traditional medicine and can obviously lead to error in plant collection. Hence, it is expedient that the researcher is well acquainted with the proposed plant. To ensure right plant selection, two things are important—the International Botanical name of the plant and its common or local name in a particular geographical location. The International Botanical Name is the globally accepted nomenclature of plants that gives information on the generic and the specific name including the efficacy of the plant. For instance, the anti-diabetic plant *Allium cepa* L. is commonly known as Onion. It belongs to the Family of Liliaceae. The generic name is *Allium*, while the specific name is *cepa*. This mode of nomenclature makes it easily identifiable and globally acceptable. Currently, most African countries have adopted the use of official monographs known as Pharmacopeia. These are official books that provide information about specific medicinal plants, their photographs, traditional recipes, taxonomic classification, and other standards that are vital in the identification of the supposed plant (Sofowora, 2008).

Proper Plant Collection and Authentication

This is another important step in the use of plants for medicinal purposes. Plants can be harvested from either wild or cultivated sources. The ethnopharmacological information or traditional use of the plant preinforms the collector about the geographical location for the collection of the plant. This is because the geographical location of a medicinal plant can affect the presence (qualitative analysis) and amount (quantitative analysis) of its phytochemicals. According to Sofowora, a plant growing wild in a particular country may not produce the same phytoconstituents and biological action as another plant growing wild in another location (Sofowora, 2008). Ethnopharmacological information can be obtained from villagers, trado-medical herbal sellers or scientific publications. Moreover, students can be used to collate data on medicinal plants with known anti-diabetic activity.

The time of collection can also affect the level of secondary metabolites present in a plant. Leaves are best collected during vegetation stage of the plant while roots are best collected during dry season. Fruits are best collected when there is a binge of yellow in the plant fruit and not when they are fully ripe except when it is used for edible or special purposes. The date and time of collection is needed for reproducibility and ascertaining the best concentration of phytochemicals contained in the plant. It is important to note that during plant collection, unwanted matter and unnecessary bulky materials must be excluded to avoid adulteration. The authentication of the plant is usually done by a herbarium curator or plant taxonomist. A fresh specimen of the plant sample is prepared and fixed in the herbarium for further reference purposes.

Proper Plant Drying and Preservation

The most common and cheapest form of drying is shade/air-drying especially for leaves and flowers because of volatile components that may be present. However, roots and stem bark are dried under the sun. Oven drying at controlled temperature can be used in cases of extreme weather condition. Appropriate plant drying techniques should be employed as this can determine the half-life of the crude drug sample. Improper drying can lead to microbial contamination due to presence of moisture. Microbial load will invariably reduce plant efficacy, purity, and safety. After the plant sample has been well dried, clean and air-dried containers should be used in preserving the sample for further use. Plant samples must be stored under specific conditions and used within known stability period. It is important to note, however, that containers or bottles that are capable of leaching chemicals should be avoided for preservation purposes. Glass containers are usually preferred.

Plant Extraction

Plants are extracted depending on the nature of the plant material and the bioactive principle of interest. The mode of extractions mostly utilized for various parts by organic solvent extractions includes maceration/cold extraction, Soxhlet, distillation, percolation, and sequential extraction (Mohammed et al., 2014). Maceration method and Soxhlet extraction are common methods that are employed for most anti-diabetic plants leaves.

Preliminary Phytochemical Screening

Plants contain various compounds known as phytochemicals which are classified as secondary metabolites. Phytochemicals are chemical compounds of diverse nature that assigns pharmacological activity to plants. They can be found in plant parts such as roots, stem bark, leaves, flowers, seeds, and pulp. Generally, they act as defense mechanism for plants, but in animal or human systems, they treat diseases. These phytochemicals include alkaloids, tannins, saponins, anthraquinones, cardenolides, terpenoids, and steroids, among others. Flavonoids, tannins, and terpenoids have been reported to be responsible for the anti-diabetic activity of some medicinal plants (Onyekere et al., 2020).

Simple standard procedures and chemical tests have been designed for phytochemical screening of medicinal plants (Harborne, 1973). It is important to note that false positive results in this test are possible; hence, confirmatory tests should always be carried out (Trease and Evans, 1996; Sofowora 2008).

MEDICINAL PLANTS WITH KNOWN ANTI-DIABETIC ACTIVITY FROM SUB-SAHARAN AFRICA

Plant-based medicines are easily available, efficacious, less expensive, and serve to develop leads. Interestingly, some known anti-diabetic drugs are obtained from natural sources—metformin from *Galega officinalis* (a traditional herb), insulin and exenatide (from animal), acarbose (from microorganism). The untoward effects of and various limitations associated with synthetic drugs necessitate the search for safer and more efficacious drugs of natural sources particularly from plants (Osadebe et al., 2014).

The following medicinal plants have been scientifically investigated for their anti-diabetic and their putative hypoglycemic activities as depicted in table 3.1 (Mohammed et al., 2014).

Anti-Diabetic Phytocompounds from Sub-Sahara African Medicinal Plants and Their Mode of Action

Over the years, the medicinal plant approach to management and treatment of diabetes in sub-Sahara Africa has improved from traditional medicinal practices to pharmacological investigations and characterization of the bioactive compounds. Medicinal plants such as *Allium sativum*, *Momordica charanthia*, *Catharanthus roseus*, and *Curcuma longa* are among the most researched and explored for anti-diabetic molecules. These molecules are ubiquitously distributed in these plants in different forms and are classified according to their structural makeup and biosynthetic pathway. They include alkaloids, amino acids, amines, glycosides, flavonoids, saponins, carboxylic acids, and so on. As their structural makeups differ, so are their pharmacological modes of action. As glycolysis is the fundamental of carbohydrate metabolism, an attempt at controlling this process is relevant to regulation of the blood sugar level (Singh et al., 2003).

Another approach to diabetic treatment is inhibition of α-glucosidase—which catalysis the cleavage of glucose from disaccharides and oligosaccharides in the small intestine, thereby delaying the time of absorption of glucose. Some phytochemicals exhibit anti-diabetic activity by the holistic approach of regenerating pancreatic β cells and maintaining optimum secretion of insulin (Bharti et al., 2018). Insulin secreted by the pancreatic β cells

Table 3.1 List of Selected Scientifically Investigated Anti-diabetic Medicinal Plants in Some Parts of sub-Saharan Africa

Scientific Name	*Common Name*	*Family*	*Part(s) Used*	*Active Extract/Fraction*	*Type of DM/ Model Used*	*Country*
Abelmoschus esculentus L.	Okro	Malvaceae	Fruit	Aqueous extract	Type 1/Animal	Nigeria
Acaia albida Del	Ana tree	Mimosaceae	Root	Methanol extract	Type 1/ Animal	Nigeria
Acalypha wilkesiana Müll. Arg.	Copperleaf	Euphorbiaceae	Leaf	Aqueous extract	Type 1/ Animal	Nigeria
Acanthus montanus (Nees) T.	Mountain thistle	Acanthaceae	Root	Ethylacetate fraction	Type 1/Animal	Nigeria
Adansonia digitata L.	Baobab	Bombacaceae	Stem bark	Aqueous extract	Type 1/ Animal	Nigeria
Afzelia Africana Smith.	Counter wood	Fabaceae	Root	Aqueous extract	Type 1/ Animal	Nigeria
Ageratum conyzoides L.	Billygoat weed	Asteraceae	Seed	Ethanol extract	Type 1/ Animal	Nigeria
Alchornea cordifolia Müll. Arg.	Christmas bush	Euphorbiaceae	Leaf	Butanol fraction	Type 1/ Animal	Nigeria
Allium cepa L.	Onion	Liliaceae	Bulb	Aqueous extract	Type 1/ Animal	Nigeria
Allium sativum L.	Garlic	Liliaceae	Bulb	Aqueous extract	Type 1/ Animal	Nigeria
Aloe barbadensis	Aloe vera	Liliaceae	Leaf	Ethanol extract	Type 1/Animal	Sudan
Aloe perryi Baker.	-	Liliaceae	Leaf	Ethanol extract	Type 1/ Animal	Nigeria
Anacardium occidentale L.	Cashew	Anacardiaceae	Leaf	Aqueous extract	Type 1 and 2/ Animal	Nigeria
Anisopus mannii N. E. Br.	Dogbane	Asclepiadaceae	Stem	Aqueous extract	Type 1/ Animal	Nigeria
Annona muricata	Soursop	Annonaceae	Leaf/fruit	Methanol /aqueous extract		Nigeria
Anthocleista djalonensis A. Chev.	Cabbage tree	Loganiaceae	Leaf/Stem/ Root	Methanol extract and its fractions	Type 1/ Animal	Nigeria
Anthocleista vogelii	Cabbage tree	Gentianaceae	Stem bark	methanol ,n-hexane extract	Type1/Animal	Nigeria
Axonopus compressus P. Beauv.	Blanket grass	Fabaceae	Leaf	Methanol extract	Type 1/ Animal	Nigeria

Azadirachta indica A. Juss.	Neem	Meliaceae	Leaf	Ethanol extract	Type 1/ Animal	Nigeria/ Ghana
Bauhinia rufescens Lam.	Silver Butterfly tree	Caesalpiniaceae	Leaf	Methanol extract	Type 1/ Animal	Nigeria
Bridelia ferruginea Benth.	Locus bean tree	Euphorbiaceae	Root bark	Methanol extract	Type 1/ Animal	Nigeria
Buchholzia coriacea Engl.	Wonderful kola	Capparidaceae	Fruit/root/ seed	methanol seed extract and butanol fraction	Type 1/Animal	Nigeria
Carica papaya L.	Pawpaw	Caricaceae	Seed/root	Aqueous extract	Type 1/ Animal	Nigeria
Carum carvi L.	Caraway	Apiaceae	Fruit	Aqueous extract	Type 1/ Animal	Nigeria
Cassia italic Mill.	Italian senna	Caesalpiniaceae	Leaf	Aqueous/ethanol extract	Type 1/ Animal	Nigeria
Catharantus roseus L.	Madagascar periwinkle	Apocynaceae	Leaf	Ethanol extract	Type 1/ Animal	Nigeria
Ceiba pentandra L. Gaertn.	Silk-cotton tree	Bombacaceae	Stem bark	Aqueous extract	Type 1/ Animal	Nigeria
Chrysophyllum albidum G.Don	White star apple	Sapotaceae	Leaf/stem/ root/fruit	Ethanol extract		Nigeria
Chrysophyllum cainito L.	Star apple	Anacardiaceae	Leaf	Aqueous extract in drinking water	Type 1/ Animal	Côte d'Ivoire
Cinnamonium zeylanicum Garcin ex Blume	Cinnamon	Lauraceae	Bark	Aqueous extract		Nigeria
Cinchona calisaya Wedd	Peruvian bark	Rubiaceae	Stem bark	Aqueous extract	Type 1/ Animal	Nigeria
Cissampelos mucronata A. Rich.	Heart-leaved vine	Menispermaceae	Leaf	Ethanol extract	Type 1/ Animal	Nigeria
Cissampelos owariensis P. Beauv	Velvet leaf	Menispermaceae	Leaf	Ethanol extract	Type 1/ Animal	Nigeria
Citrus aurantium L.	Bitter orange	Rutaceae	Fruit	Aqueous extract	Type 1/ Animal	Nigeria
Citrus paradise Macfad.	Grapefruit	Rutaceae	Seed	Aqueous extract	Type 1/ Animal	Nigeria
Clausena lansium Lour. Skeels.	Wampee	Rutaceae	Stem bark	Methanol and dichloromethane extract	Type 1/ Animal	Nigeria
Cnestis ferruginea D. C.	Horn of plenty	Connaracea	Leaf	Methanol and ethyl acetate extract	Type 1/ Animal	Nigeria

(Continued)

Table 3.1 List of Selected Scientifically Investigated Anti-diabetic Medicinal Plants in Some Parts of sub-Saharan Africa *(Continued)*

Scientific Name	*Common Name*	*Family*	*Part(s) Used*	*Active Extract/Fraction*	*Type of DM/ Model Used*	*Country*
Combretum micranthum G. Don.	Kikeliba (Benin)	Combretaceae	Leaf	Methanol and ethyl acetate extract	Type 1/ Animal	Nigeria
Combretum dolichopetalum Engl. & Diels	Sun bird's wine	Combretaceae	Leaf	Methanol extract	Type 1/Animal	Nigeria
Commelina africana L.	Common yellow commelina	Commelinaceae	Leaf	Aqueous extract	Type 1/ Animal	Nigeria
Curcumin longa L.	Curcuma	Zingiberaceae	Root	Methanol extract	Type 1/ Animal	Nigeria
Curcumis sativus L.	Cucumber	Cucurbitaceae	Fruit	Methanol /butanol extract		Nigeria
Cymbopogon citratus	Lemon grass	Poaceae	Leaf	Aqueous extract		Nigeria
Da niella oliveri Bull. Misc.	Daniellia	Caesalpiniaceae	Root	Aqueous extract	Type 1/ Animal	Nigeria
Detarium microcarpum Guill. & Perr.	Sweet detar	Caesalpiniaceae		Aqueous extract	Type 1/ Animal	Nigeria
Ficus asperifolia L.	Sand paper tree	Moraceae	Stem	Aqueous extract	Type 1/ Animal	Nigeria
Ficus exasperate Vahl.	White fig tree	Moraceae	Leaf	Aqueous extract	Type 1/ Animal	Nigeria
Ganoderma lucidum Curtis. P. Karst.	Hemlock varnish shelf	Ganodermataceae	Fruit	Ethyl acetate and butanol fractions	Type 1/ Animal	Nigeria
Garcinia kola L.	Bitter kola	Clusiaceae	Nut	Aqueous extract		Nigeria
Gongronema latifolium Benth.	Amaranth globe	Asclepiadaceae	Leaf	Aqueous extract	Type 1/ Animal	Nigeria
Hibiscus sabdariffa L.	Red sorrel	Malvaceae	Calyces	Aqueous and ethanol extract	Type 1/ Animal	Nigeria

Holarrhena floribunda G. Don.	False rubber tree	Apocynaceae	Leaf	Ethanol extract and its solvent fractions	Type 1/ Animal	Côte d'Ivoire
Homalium letestui Pellegr.	Otuo (Nigeria); Mvezork (Gabon), Tembo (Cameroon)	Flacourtiaceae	Root	Ethanol extract	Type 1/ Animal	Nigeria
Hunteria umbellate K. Schum. Hallier f.	Flantueh	Apocynaceae	Stem	Ethanol extract	Type 1/ Animal	Nigeria
Hymenocardia acida Tul	Red-heart	Phyllanthaceae	Leaf	Methanol extract	Type 1/ Animal	Nigeria
Hyptis suaveolens Poit.	Mint weed	Lamiaceae	Leaf	Methanol extract	Type 1/ Animal	Nigeria
Indigofera pulchra L.	Indigofera	Papilionaceae	Leaf	Butanol fraction	Type 1/ Animal	Nigeria
Irvinga gabonensis Aubry-Lecomte ex O'Rorke. Baill	Wild mango	Asteraceae	Stem bark	Aqueous extract	Type 1/ Animal	Nigeria
Khaya senegalensisis Desr. A. Juss.	African mahogany	Meliaceae	Stem	Aqueous extract/oil	Type 1/ Animal	Nigeria
Leptedenia hastate Pers.	-	Leguminosae	Leaf	Ethanol extract	Type 1/ Animal	Nigeria
Loranthus micranthus L.	Mistletoe	Loranthaceae	Leaf	Methanol extract and its fractions	Type 1/ Animal	Nigeria
Mangifera indica L.	Mango	Anacardiaceae	Leaf	Methanol extract	Type 1/ Animal	Nigeria
Mammea africana Sabine.	African apple	Guttiferae	Stem bark	Ethanol extract	Type 1/ Animal	Nigeria
Melanthera scandens Schum. & Thonn.	Black anther	Asteraceae	Leaf	Ethanol extract and its fractions	Type 1/ Animal	Nigeria
Mimosa invisa Mart.	Sleeping plant	Fabaceae	Leaf	Aqueous extract	Type 1/ Animal	Nigeria
Momordica charantia L.	Bitter melon	Cucurbitaceae	Leaf	Methanol extract	Type 1/ Animal	Nigeria
Morinda lucida Benth.	Brimstone tree	Rubiaceae	Stem bark	Aqueous extract	Type 1/ Animal	Nigeria
Moringa oleifera Lam.	Horseradish	Moringaceae	Leaf	Aqueous Extract	Type 1/ Animal	Nigeria
Musa paradisiaca	Plantain	Musaceae	Fruit (unripe)	Methanol extract		Nigeria

(*Continued*)

Table 3.1 List of Selected Scientifically Investigated Anti-diabetic Medicinal Plants in Some Parts of sub-Saharan Africa *(Continued)*

Scientific Name	*Common Name*	*Family*	*Part(s) Used*	*Active Extract/Fraction*	*Type of DM/ Model Used*	*Country*
Musa sapientum L var. *paradisiacal.* Sucker.	Banana	Musaceae		Methanol extract	Type 1/ Animal	Nigeria
Musanga cecropioides R.Br. & Tedlie.	Umbrella tree	Cecropiaceae	Stem bark	Aqueous and ethanol extract	Type 1/ Animal	Nigeria
Nauclea latifolia S.M.	Bishop's head	Rubiaceae	Root/Stem/ Leaf	ethanol and hexane extracts	Type 1/ Animal	Benin/ Nigeria
Newbouldia laevis P. Beauv.	African border tree	Bignoniaceae	Leaf	Ethanol extract	Type 1/ Animal	Nigeria
Ocimum gratissimum L.	African/Clove basil	Lamiaceae	Leaf	Methanol extract	Type 1/ Animal	Nigeria
Ocimum suave Wild.	Hoary basil	Lamiaceae	Leaf	Aqueous extract	Type 1/ Animal	Nigeria
Oxytenanthera abyssinica A. Rich Munro.	Bindura bamboo	Gramineae	Leaf	Ethanol extract	Type 1/ Animal	Benin
Parinari excels (Guinea Plum)	Mubura (Tanzania, Uganda), Inyi (Nigeria)	Chrysobalanaceae	Bark	Aqueous extract	Type 1/ Animal	Senegal
Parkia biglobosa Jacq.	African locust bean	Fabaceae	Seed	Aqueous extract	Type 1/ Animal	Nigeria
Persea Americana Mill.	Avocado	Lauraceae	Seed	Ethanol extract	Type 1/ Animal	Nigeria
Phyllanthus amarus L.	Stone breaker	Euphorbiaceae	Whole plant	Aqueous/hydro-alcoholic extract	Type 1/ Animal	Nigeria/ Togo
Picralima nitida Stapf.	Picralima	Apocyanaceae	Pulp/seed	ethanol and aqueous extract	Type 1/ Animal	Nigeria/ Benin
Psydrax horizontalis Shum. &Thonn	Blister/bump tree	Rubiaceae	Leaf	methanol extract	Type 1/Animal	Nigeria
Rauvolfia vomitoria Afzel.	Swizzle stick	Apocynaceae	Fruit	aqueous extract	Type 1/ Animal	Nigeria

Senna occidentalis L.	Stink weed	Caesalpinaceae	Leaf	methanol extract	Type 1/ Animal	Nigeria
Sphenocentrum jollyanum Pierre.	Sorghum bicolor	Menispermaceae	Leaf	aqueous extract	Type 1/ Animal	Nigeria
Strophanthus hispidus	Kombe seed	Apocyanaceae	Root	Chloroform extract	Type 1/Animal	Nigeria
Tapinanthus globiferas	African mistletoe	Loranthaceae	Leaf	Ethanol extract		Nigeria
Terminalia catappa L.	Bengal almond	Combretaceae	Seed	aqeous extra ct	Type 1/ Animal	Côte d'Ivoire
Vernonia amygdalina Del.	Bitter leaf	Compositae	Leaf	hexane and ethylacetate extract	Type 1/ Animal	Nigeria
Vernonia colorata Schreb	Star-flowered bitter-tea	Compositae	Leaf	aqueous extract	Type 1/ Animal	Senegal
Vitex doniana Wild.	African black plum sweet	Verbenaceae	Stem bark	Aqueous extract	Type 1/ Animal	Nigeria
Viscum album L.	Mistletoe	Loranthaceae	Whole plant	methanol extract	Type 1/ Animal	Nigeria
Zingiber officinale L. Roscoe.	Ginger	Zingiberaceae	Rhizome	ethanol	Type 1/ Animal	Nigeria
East African Region						
Aspilia pluriseta Schweinf.	Dwarf aspilia	Asteraceae	Root	aqueous extract		Kenya
Bidens pilosa L.	Spanish needle	Asteraceae	Leaf	aqueous extract		Kenya
Caylusea absyinica Fresen. Fisch. & Mey.	-	Asteraceae	Leaf	methanol extract		Ethiopia
Catha edulis Vahl.	Bushman's tea	Celastraceae	Root	aqueous extract		Kenya
Erythrina abyssinica Lam	Red-hot-poker	Fabaceae	Stem bark	aqueous extract		Kenya
Ficus sycomorus L.	Fig-mulberry	Moraceae	Stem bark	aqueous extract		Kenya
Moringa stenopetala Baker	Cabbage tree	Moringaceae	Leaf	butanol fraction		Ethiopia
Pappea capensis Eckl. & Zeyh.	Jacket plum	Sapindaceae	Leaf/stem bark	aqueous and ethylacetate extract		Kenya
Pentas schimperina A.Rich	-	Rubiaceae	Leaf	aqeous extract		Ethiopia

(*Continued*)

Table 3.1 List of Selected Scientifically Investigated Anti-diabetic Medicinal Plants in Some Parts of sub-Saharan Africa *(Continued)*

Scientific Name	*Common Name*	*Family*	*Part(s) Used*	*Active Extract/Fraction*	*Type of DM/ Model Used*	*Country*
Strychnos henninsii Gilg. Central African Region	Red bitter berry	Loganiceae	Leaf	aqueous extract		Kenya
Anacrdium occidentale L.	Cashew	Anacardiaceae	Leaf	Methanol and its solvent fraction		Cameroon
Bersama engleriana Gurke	Winged bersama	Melianthaceae	Leaf	aqueous extract	Type 2	Cameroon
Canarium schweinfurthii Engl.	Bush candle tree	Burseraceae	Stem bark	methanol and dichloromethane extract		Cameroon
Ceiba pentandra L.	Silk cotton	Bombacaceae	Stem bark	methylene chloride/ methanol extracts	Type 2	Cameroon
Citrullus lanatus	Watermelon	Cucurbitaceae	Seed	ethanol extract		Cameroon
Cucurbita moschata Duchesne ex Poir.	Butternut squash	Leguminosae	Pods	Aqueous extract		Cameroon
Dichrostachys glomerata Chiov.	Chinese lantern	Cucurbitaceae	Seed	ethanol extract		Cameroon
Dracena arborea Wild.	Dragon tree	Dracaenaceae	Root	ethanol extract		Cameroon
Kalanchoe crenata Andr. Haw	Never ride	Crassulaceae	Whole plant	ethanol extract		Cameroon
Lagenaria siceraria L.	Bottle gourd	Cucurbitaceae	Seed	methanol extract		Cameroon
Sclerocarya birrea A. Rich. Hochst.	Jelly plum	Anacardiaceae	Stem bark	meathnol and dichloromethane extract		Cameroon
Telfairia occidentalis Hook. f.	Fluted pumpkin	Cucurbitaceae	Seed	methanol and dichloromethane		Cameroon
Terminalia superba Engl. & Diels	Ofram tree	Combretaceae	Stem bark	methanol and dichloromethane extract		Cameroon

Source: Adapted from Mohammed et al. (2014): African Medicinal Plants with Antidiabetic Potentials: A Review.

increase glycogen, protein and triacylglycerols syntheses. Therefore, repair of pancreatic β cells by these phytocompounds is a systemic way of enhancing the expression of the insulin gene, promoting insulin secretion and inhibiting their degeneration. Some other compounds like vincristine, vindoline, and catharanthine simply reduce blood sugar levels by free radical scavenging actions (Bharti et al., 2018). Several other examples of anti-diabetic phytochemicals and their modes of action are highlighted below:

Alkaloids

Alkaloids are a class of naturally occurring organic nitrogen-containing bases. They occur primarily in plants and are especially common in certain families of flowering plants such as Solanaceae, Apocynaceae, Loganiaceae, and Ranunculaceae. *Catharanthus roseus* (Apocynaceae) is a rich source of cathranthine, vincristine, vinblastine, vindoline, and vindolinene which are good anti-diabetic compounds (figure 3.1). They act by scavenging free radicals and stimulating immune response (Kar et al., 2003; Bharti et al., 2018). Ginkgolides from *Ginkgo biloba* initiates and promotes secretion of insulin as an attempt to reduce blood sugar levels (Pinto et al., 2009). *Allium sativum* (garlic) is known for its antidiabetic activity. It is a good source of allylpropyl disulfide which is involved in glycogen synthesis and insulin secretion (Kumari and Augusti, 2007). Marmesin and marmelosin from the plant *Aegle marmelos* promote regeneration of the pancreatic β cells and also help in insulin secretion. The anti-diabetic activities of betaine and β-ecdysone (present in *Achyranthus aspera*) lie in their ability to regulate digestion and absorption of carbohydrates (Bharti et al., 2018).

Amino Acids, Amines, and Carboxylic Acid Derivatives

Another group of nitrogen-containing secondary metabolites are the nonproteinous amino acids and amines. They are ubiquitous in diverse plants and are attributed to various biological functions. Their importance in phytomedicine cannot be overemphasized. Allicin, alliin, and apigenin (figure 3.2) from *Allium sativum* (garlic) are good anti-diabetic phytocompounds that regulate cholesterol and glycogen synthesis (Gholap and Kar, 2004) while [-] Hydroxycitric acid present in *Garcinia cambogia* helps in insulin secretion (Bharti et al., 2018). Ferulic acid from *Curcuma longa* exhibits free radical scavenging activities and plays roles in insulin secretion. Reports show that 4-hydroxyisoleucine and n-hydroxyisoleucine isolated from *Trigonella foenum*, nitrosamines (from *Areca catechu*), leucine and isoleucine (from *Aloe vera*) control blood sugar levels by regulating glucose transport and carbohydrate metabolism (Bharti et al., 2018). S-methyl cysteine sulfoxide and S-allyl cysteine sulfoxide are anti-diabetic constituents from *Allium cepa*.

They were found to play some roles in cholesterol synthesis and glycolysis. A study on *Phyllanthus amarus* showed that brevifolin carboxylic acid and ethyl brevifolin carboxylate isolated from the leaves regulate carbohydrate digestion and absorption (Ali et al., 2006).

Anthranoids

Several anthranoids isolated from medicinal plants are popularly used as laxative but a good number of them have been proven to exhibit anti-diabetic activities by promoting insulin secretion and synthesis, and regeneration of pancreatic β cells. Examples include aloin, barbaloin, isobabaloine, emodin, cinnamic acid, and crysophanic acid isolated from *Aloe vera* and *Cassia tora* (Nam and Choi, 2008). Other anti-diabetic anthranoids from *C. tora* include torachrysone, rhein, alatermin and toralactone, and vicine (figure 3.2) from *Momordica charantia. Ocimum canum* and *Syzygium aromaticum* are both rich in anthranoids such as eugenol, camphor, geraniol, limonene, p-cymene, and thujone which also help in insulin secretion and regeneration of pancreatic β cells (Hannan et al., 2006).

Carbohydrates

Carbohydrates are biological molecules that contain carbon, hydrogen, and oxygen in their makeup. They are arguably the most distributed biomolecules in nature. Even though consumption of too much carbohydrate may lead to diabetes, a little carbohydrates may help reduce blood sugars. Together with dietary fiber, they may limit cholesterol absorption by binding bile acids. Glucomannan and caryophylline isolated from *Aloe vera* and *Ocimum sanctum* respectively exhibit anti-diabetic actions by boosting insulin secretion and reducing carbohydrate digestion and absorption (van de Venter et al., 2008). Some protein-bound polysaccharides in these plants also have similar mechanisms of action. Pectin, guar gum, and mucilaginous fiber from *Citrus sinensis*, *Coccinia indica*, and *Trignonella foenum* were attributed glucose transport and carbohydrate metabolism, and as stabilizing agents (Kar et al., 2003). Cellulose and mannose (figure 3.2) extracted from *Aloe vera* control blood sugar intake by regulating carbohydrate digestion and absorption (van de Venter et al., 2008; Bharti et al., 2018).

Glycosides

Glycosides are phytoconstituents that contain a glycone (sugar) moiety and an aglycone (non-sugar) moiety. They are found in plants where they play roles in defense against and treatment of diseases, perform many biological activities as well. Momordin, momordicine, momorcharaside A and B, momorcharin A and B, and charantin from *Momordica charantia* were reported to exhibit anti-diabetic actions by promoting insulin secretion and glycogen synthesis (Chao and Huang, 2003). Tinosporine, cordifolide, tinosporide, cordifole, and columbin (figure 3.2) from *Tinospora* spp. are glycosides with anti-diabetic activity (Kar et al., 2003). They reduce cholesterol synthesis and glycolysis. Mormordin-a, luffin-a (from *Luffa cylindrical*), citrullol, colocynthin, elaterin, colosynthetin (from *Citrullus colocynthis*), leucocyanidin and pelarogonidin (from *Ficus benghalensis*) showed antioxidant and anti-diabetic activities by promoting insulin secretion and glycogen synthesis (Lemus et al., 1999). Taraxacin isolated from *Taraxacum officinale* was also reported to promote insulin secretion (Broadhurst et al., 2000).

Flavonoids

Flavonoids are a class of polyphenolic compounds with fifteen carbon skeletons, consisting of a heterocylic ring and two phenyl rings. Flavonoids have a lot of functions in plants such as organ colouration/pigmentation, but medicinally, they are attributed to many biological activities—anticancer, antioxidant, anti-inflammatory, anti-diabetic and so on. Flavonoids such as α-cephalin, myricetin-3-glucoside and ambrettolide isolated from *Abelmoschus moschatus*, and quercetin, quecetrin and rutin from *Ginkgo biloba* exhibited anti-diabetic actions by promoting insulin secretion (Ngueyem et al., 2009; Bharti et al., 2018). Soy isoflavones from the soybean plant (*Glycine max*) showed anti-diabetic activities by regulating lipid and glucose metabolism and peroxisome proliferator-activated receptor (PPAR) activation. The edible mushroom, *Agaricus campestris*, contains anti-diabetic flavonoids (α-terpineol and hexanol) that promote insulin secretion (Gray and Flatt, 1998). Flavonoids like [+] catechin, [-] epicatechin, chlorogenic acid (figure 3.2) are responsible for insulinomematic anti-diabetic activities of *Pterocarpus marsupium*, *Phyllanthus embelica*, and *Acacia Arabica* (Kar et al., 2003). Other anti-diabetic flavonoids found in sub-Saharan African plants are kaempferol, isorhamnetin (*Ginkgo biloba*), and shamimin (*Biophytum sensitivum*) (Bharti et al., 2018).

Peptidoglycans

Peptidoglycans also called murien, make up the cell walls of most bacteria. They are polymers that comprise sugars and amino acids. Peptidoglycans associated with plants were attributed anti-diabetic activities for their roles in glucose transport and carbohydrate digestion and absorption. Some of the examples documented in the literature are fenugreekine (from *T. foenum-graecum*), gluten, taraxacerin (from *Taraxacum officinale*), and glucosamines (from *Aloe vera*) (Bharti et al., 2018).

Polyphenols

Polyphenols in *Curcuma longa*—curcumin, tumerone, germacrone, and zingiberene exhibit anti-diabetic activities by insulin secretion and carbohydrate digestion and absorption (Kar et al., 2003; Zang et al., 2013). Ellagic acids and its derivatives found in *Phyllanthus niruiri* and *Acacia arabica* also play similar roles (Ueda et al., 2004). Tannins and gallotannic acid in *Syzygium aromaticum* help in regeneration of pancreatic β cells and insulin secretion. Other polyphenols from sub-Saharan African plants with anti-diabetic actions include wedelolatone, dimethyl wedelolactone (from *Eclipta alba*), carvacrol, linalool (from *Ocimum sanctum*) and mangiferin, a catechol from *Salacia* spp. and *Mangifera indica* (Yoshikawa et al., 2001).

Saponins

Saponins are non-nitrogenous secondary metabolites with vast diversity in plants. They have the ability to form stable foam when agitated in aqueous solutions. Their wide range of biological activities include anti-inflammatory, anti-viral, antimutagenic, hemolytic, and anti-diabetic properties. Anti-diabetic saponins are recognized by their ability to quicken regeneration of pancreatic β cells and promote insulin secretion. A few examples from sub-Saharan African plants are andrographolide (from *Andrographis paniculata*) (Yu et al., 2003), lactucain C (from *Lactuca indica*), trigonellin (from *T. foenum-graecum*), diterpene and triterpenes (from *Salacia* spp. and *Croton cajucara*). Diosgenin is also found in *T. foenum-graecum* and exhibits anti-diabetic actions by facilitating glucose transport and regulating carbohydrate metabolism (Bharti et al., 2018).

PHARMACOLOGICAL SCREENING STUDIES

Acute toxicity and lethality test

The acute-toxicity and lethality (LD_{50}) of the crude extract is determined using the method described by Lorke (1983) via the oral route.

Phase one: The mice are divided into three groups of three animals each and treated orally with the crude methanol extract at doses of 10, 100 and 1000 $mgkg^{-1}$ body weight. They are observed for 24 hours for signs of toxicity.

Phase two: The doses used in this phase are determined by the number of deaths per dose recorded in phase one. If no death occurred in all the doses of phase one, three different doses—1600, 2900, and 5000 $mgkg^{-1}$ are administered orally to other groups of animals at one dose per animal. The treated animals are observed for number of deaths in 24 hours. The LD_{50} is determined by calculating the geometric mean of the least and most toxic doses, that is, the median lethal dose (LD_{50}).

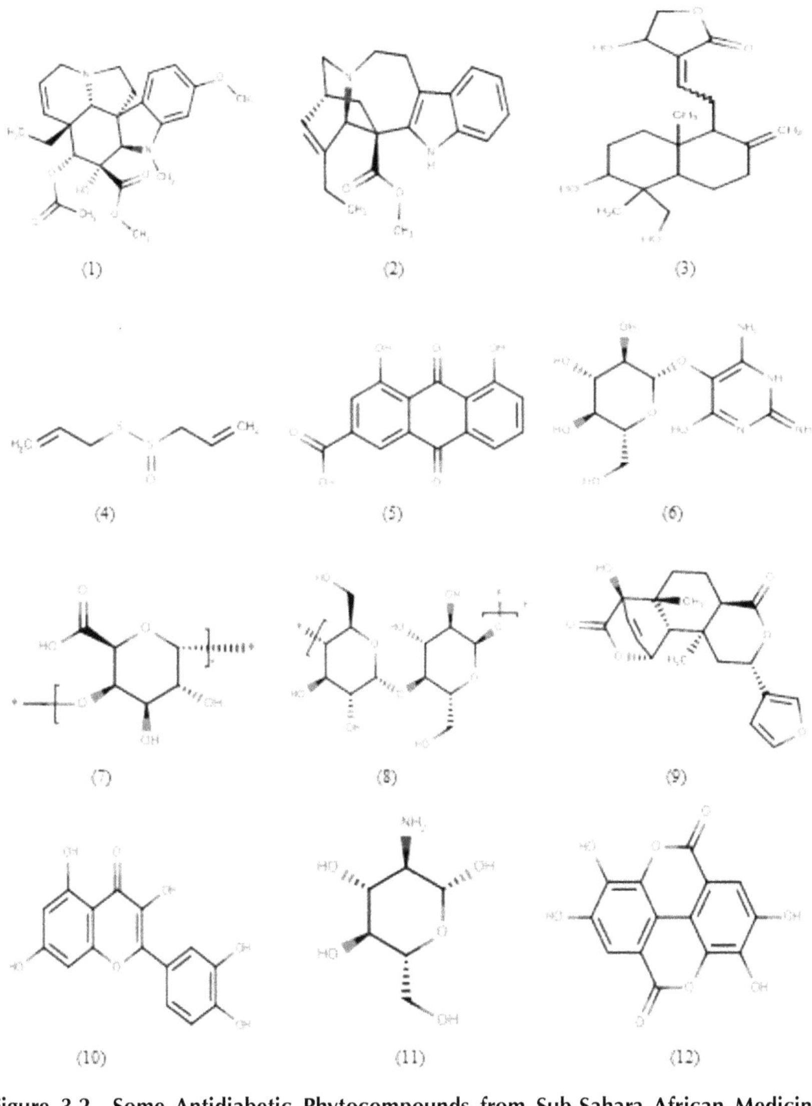

Figure 3.2 Some Antidiabetic Phytocompounds from Sub-Sahara African Medicinal Plants. Authors' own conceptualization.

In vivo models

Most experiments in diabetes employ rodents; however, some studies make use of larger animals (Bell and Hye, 1993). Rodents that have been used include rats, mice, and rabbits (Srinivasan and Ramarao, 2007). Currently, the murine model is one of the most popular models due to the availability of over 200 well-characterized inbreed strains. Other animal types used in diabetes experiment include obese mouse: Diabetic mouse (Psammomys obesus), Spiny mouse (Acomys cahirinus), BB rats, KK mouse, Yellow mouse, Yellow KK mouse, New Zealand obese mouse, Tuco-tuco (clenomys talarum)—they are burrowing rodents from Argentina, Chinese hamster (Cricetulus griseus), NOD mouse, Japanese wistar rat (Goto rat), and so on (Srinivasan and Ramarao, 2007; WHO Report, 1985; Rees and Alcolado, 2005).

Evaluation of the hypoglycemic or anti-diabetic effect of a test sample can be done in vivo using the following models (Bell and Aye, 1993): Normoglycemic rats, diabetic animals, or Oral Glucose Tolerance Test (OGTT).

Hypoglycemic Activity in Normoglycemic Rats

Normoglycemic rats are randomly grouped and labeled accordingly. They are fasted overnight for 12 hours and then their fasting blood glucose levels are checked with a sensitive glucometer. Various treatments are administered orally according to the body weight. The control group is usually administered with a standard anti-diabetic drug while others receive different doses of the plant extract. A negative control group is also essential.

DIABETIC ANIMALS

Chemical induction of Diabetes Mellitus

The chemicals that are commonly used in experimental induction of diabetes are Alloxan monohydrate, Streptozotocin (STZ), and Pyrinuron (Pyriminil). Alloxan and STZ are the most frequently used due to their proven usefulness in providing detailed information of the disease. They exert diabetogenic actions when administered parenterally, intravenously, intraperitoneally, or subcutaneously. They act by partial destruction of the β-cells of islet of langerhans leading to hyperglycemia (Lenzen, 2008). This results in decreased insulin level and hyperglycemia leading to type 1 diabetes. However, it is important to know that animal models differ significantly from one another and none can exactly reproduce the essentials of human diabetes (Rerup, 2005).

Surgical Induction of Diabetes Mellitus

Another technique used to induce diabetes is the complete removal of the pancreas known as pancreatectomy. Few researchers have employed this model in the last few years to explore effects of natural products on animal species such as rats, pigs, dogs and primates.

Diet-Induced Diabetes

This model is clinically similar to type 2 diabetes mellitus in humans. It involves inducing type 2 diabetes in some strains of mice, although there is usually risk of associated obesity (De' Souza et al., 2005). It is important to note that genetic predisposition to diet-induced diabetes is a criterion for the animals that are used in this model. According to De' Souza et al. (2005), the fat rich diet is composed of protein (24 g percent), carbohydrate (41 g percent) and fat (24 gpercent). Adult Swiss mice are fed with fat-rich diet for at least eight weeks, after they become diabetic, hyperinsulinemic, insulin resistant, and even obese.

In vitro models

These methods may serve as complementary tools to explore findings obtained in *in vivo* models.

Studies Using Isolated Pancreatic Islet Cell Lines

Insulin secretion occurs when pancreatic beta cells utilize glucose to generate ATP from ADP. The resulting increase in cytoplasmic ATP/ADP ratio closes ATP-sensitive potassium channels, causing depolarization of the plasma membrane which activates voltage-dependent Ca^{2+} channels. This results in elevation of the intracellular Ca^{2+} concentration which triggers insulin secretion. In type 2 diabetes, pancreatic beta cells exhibit atypical ion channel activity and an abnormal pattern of insulin secretion. The most widely used insulin secreting cell lines are RIN, HIT, beta-TC, min6, and ins-1 cells. These cell lines release mainly insulin and small amount of glucagon and somatostatins.

Studies on Glucose Uptake

Elevated intracellular lipid concentrations of the adipose tissue promote lipotoxicity; hence, the critical link between obesity and type 2 diabetes. Insulin resistance either at the adipocyte or skeletal muscle level can lead to hyperglycemia. However, adipocyte from different sites of the body may have various pathological effects. Pathways related to insulin resistance may be studied in cell lines of adipocytes such as murine 3T3-L1 and rat L6 muscle engineered to over-express GLUT4 and may be employed as tools to evaluate the effects of test substance on glucose uptake (Schnedl et al., 1994). A standard procedure for the determination of glucose uptake by rat hemidiaphragm has been reported (Chattopadhyay and Bandyopadhyay, 2005; Jadhav and Puchchakayala, 2012).

Glucose diffusion test

This procedure involves the use of intestinal segment as the semipermeable membrane for measurement of glucose transport inhibitory activity with and without the test agent (Jadhav and Puchchakayala, 2011).

Alpha amylase and alpha glucosidase inhibition

Alpha amylase and apha glucosidase enzymes are involved in metabolism of complex carbohydrates. The ability of the test sample or plant extract to inhibit the activities of these enzymes is an indication of their anti-diabetic activity. For instance, the anti-diabetic drug, acarbose, inhibits alpha glucosidase enzyme. Procedures for the evaluation of the activities of these enzymes have been reported (Narkhede et al., 2011).

CONCLUSION

Sub-Saharan Africa is endowed with a great number of medicinal plants with potential anti-diabetic compounds. The gains of using medicinal plant far outweigh those of the synthetic drugs in the management of diabetes. Some of these plants have been scientifically investigated while others are yet to be explored. Pharmacists, researchers, nutritionists, biologists, botanists, and pharmacologists have key roles to play in the collaborative effort in curbing diabetes in Africa and beyond. The closer we get to nature, the better the health of the African man. Africans should learn to appreciate and promote one of the best natural endowments they have—our medicinal plants.

REFERENCES

Adams Peter. 2013. "The impact of brief high-intensity exercise on blood glucose levels". *Diabetes, Metabolic Syndrome and Obesity: Targets and Therapy,* 6: 113–122.

Adebayo Gbolade. 2009. "Inventory of antidiabetic plants in selected districts of Lagos State, Nigeria." *Journal of Ethnopharmacology,* 121: 135–139.

Afolayan Anthony and Sunmonu Toafik. 2010. "In vivo Studies on Antidiabetic Plants Used in South African Herbal Medicine". *Journal of Clinical Biochemistry and Nutrition,* 47: 98–106.

Akshada Amit Koparde, Rajendra Chandrashekar Doijad and Chandrakant Shripal Magdum. 2019. "Natural Products in Drug Discovery". In: Shagufta Perveen and Areej Al-Taweel: *Pharmacognosy - Medicinal Plants*, IntechOpen: DOI: 10.5772/intechopen.82860. Available from: https://www.intechopen.com/books/pharmacognosy-medicinal-plants/natural-products-in-drug-discovery

Ali, Houghton and Soumyanath. 2006. "α-Amylase inhibitory activity of some Malaysian plants used to treat diabetes; with particular reference to *Phyllanthus amarus.*" *Journal of Ethnopharmacology,* 107: 449–455.

American Diabetes Association. 2014. "Diagnosis and classification of diabetes mellitus." *Diabetes Care,* 37(Supplement 1): S81–S90.

Aroda Vanita, Stephen Bain, Bertrand Cariou, Milivoj Piletič, Ludger Rose, Mads Axelsen, Everton Rowe and Hans DeVries. 2017. "Efficacy and safety of once-weekly semaglutide versus once-daily insulin glargine as add-on to metformin (with or without sulfonylureas) in insulin-naive patients with type 2 diabetes (SUSTAIN 4): a randomised, open-label, parallel-group, multicentre, multinational, phase 3a trial." *The Lancet Diabetes & Endocrinology*, 5(5): 355–366.

Bassuk Shari and Manson JoAnn. 2005. "Epidemiological evidence for the role of physical activity in reducing risk of type 2 diabetes and cardiovascular disease." *Journal of Applied Physiology*, 99(3): 1193–1204.

Bell, Richard and Hye, Robert. 1993. "Animal models of diabetes mellitus: Physiology and pathology." *Journal of Surgical Research,* 35(40): 453–460.

Bharti, Krishnan, and Kumar A. 2018. "Antidiabetic phytoconstituents and their mode of action on metabolic pathways." *Therapeutic Advances in Endocrinology and Metabolism,* 9(3): 81—100.

Broadhurst, Polansky and Anderson. 2000. "Insulin-like biological activity of culinary and medicinal plant aqueous extracts *in-vitro.*" *Journal of Agriculture and Food Chemistry,* 48: 849–852.

Chao and Huang. 2003. "Bitter gourd (*Momordica charantia*) extract activates peroxisome proliferator-activated receptors and upregulates the expression of the acyl CoA oxidase gene in H4IIEC3 hepatoma cells." *Journal of Biomedical Science,* 10: 782–791.

Chattopadhyay, Ranbiranjan and Bandyopadhyay. 2005. "Effect of Azadirachta indica leaf extract on serum lipid profile changes in normal and streptozotocin induced diabetic rats." *African Journal of Biomedical Research*, 8(2): 101–104.

Colberg Sheri, Sigal Ronald , Fernhall Bo, Regensteiner Judith , Blissmer Bryan, Rubin Richard, Chasan-Taber Lisa, Albright Ann and Braun Barry. 2010. "Exercise and type 2 diabetes: the American College of Sports Medicine and the American Diabetes Association: joint position statement." *Diabetes Care,* 33(12): e147–e167.

De Souza Claudio, Araujo Eliana, Prada, Saad Mario, Boschero Antonio and Velloso Licio. 2005. "Short-term inhibition of peroxisome proliferator-activated receptor-γ coactivator-1α expression reverses diet-induced diabetes mellitus and hepatic steatosis in mice." *Diabetologia,* 48: 1860–1871.

Din Ndong, Dibong Siegfried, Mpondo, Priso, Kwin, Ngoye. 2011. "Inventory and identification of plants used in the treatment of diabetes in Douala Town (Cameroon)." *European Journal of Medicinal Plants,* 1: 60–73.

Ekor Martins. 2013. "The growing use of herbal medicines: issues relating to adverse reactions and challenges in monitoring safety." *Frontiers in Pharmacology,* 4: 177–178.

Gholap and Kar. 2004. "Hypoglycaemic effects of some plant extracts are possibly mediated through inhibition in corticosteroid concentration. *Pharmazie,* 59: 876–878.

Godfrey Richard and Marlene Julien. 2005. "Urbanisation and Health." *Clinical Medicine,* 5(2): 137–141.

Han, Myoung Sook, Dae Young Jung, Morel, Caroline, Lakhani, Saquib., Kim, Jason. K., Flavell, Richard, and Davis Roger. 2013. "JNK expression by macrophages promotes obesity-induced insulin resistance and inflammation." *Science,* 339: 1–9.

Hannan, Marenah, Ali, Rokeya, Flatt, Abdel-Wahab.2006. "*Ocimum sanctum* leaf extracts stimulate insulin secretion from perfused pancreas, isolated islets and clonal pancreatic beta-cells." *Journal of Endocrinology,* 189(2): 127–136.

Hussain, Gauahar, Rizvi, Saadat Ali, Singhal, Shelly, Zubair, Mohammed and Ahmad, Ibrahim. 2013. Serum levels of TNF-α in peripheral neuropathy patients and its correlation with nerve conduction velocity in type 2 diabetes mellitus. *Diabetes & Metabolic Syndrome: Clinical Research & Reviews*, 7(4): 238–242.

Ibezim, Akachukwu, Obi, Bonaventure, Oforkansi, Martha, Mbah, Chika and Nwodo, Ngozi Justina. 2018. "Discovery of Trypanocidal Bioactive Leads by Docking Study, Molecular Dynamic Simulation and In Vivo Screening." *Chemistry Select,* 3(8): 2386–2389.

International Diabetes Federation Atlas Map, 9th Edition.

International Diabetes Federation. 2020.https://idf.org/our-network/regions-members /africa/welcome.html. Retrieved on 8th May 2020.

Jadhav Mahesh and Puchchakayala Goverdhan. 2012. "Hypoglycemic and anti-diabetic activity of flavonoids: boswellic acid, ellagic acid, quercetin, rutin on streptozotocin-nicotinamide induced type 2 diabetic rats." *International Journal of Pharmacy and Pharmaceutical Sciences,* 4(2): 251–256.

Juliana Chan, Nam Cho, Naoko Tajima and Jonathan Shaw. 2014. "Diabetes in the Western Pacific Region—Past, Present and Future." *IDF Atlas,* 103(2): 244–255.

Kar, Choudhary and Bandyopadhyay. 2003. "Comparative evaluation of hypoglycaemic activity of some Indian medicinal plants in alloxan diabetic rats." *Journal of Ethnopharmacology,* 84: 105–108.

Keter Lucia Kipkoech and Mutiso Patrick Chalo. 2012. "Ethnobotanical studies of medicinal plants used by traditional health practitioners in the management of diabetes in lower eastern province, Kenya." *Journal of Ethnopharmacology,* 139: 74–80.

Kirkwood Leigh, Al-Dujaili, Abdullah and Drummond Sean. 2007. "Effects of advice on dietary intake and/or physical activity on body composition, blood lipids and insulin resistance following a low-fat, sucrose-containing, high-carbohydrate, energy-restricted diet." *International Journal of Food Sciences and Nutrition,* 58(5): 383—397.

Kumari and Augusti K.2007. "Lipid lowering effect of S-methyl cysteine sulfoxide from *Allium cepa* Linn in high cholesterol diet fed rats." *Journal of Ethnopharmacology,* 109: 367–371.

Lemus, García, Delvillar and Knop G. 1999. "Hypoglycaemic activity of four plants used in Chilean popular medicine." *Phytotherapy Research,* 13(2): 91–94.

Lenzen, Sigurd. 2008. "The mechanisms of alloxan-and streptozotocin-induced diabetes." *Diabetologia*, 51(2): 216–226.

Lorke, Dietrich.1983. "A New Approach to Practical Acute Toxicity Testing." *Archives of Toxicology,* 54: 275–287.

Mahop Tonye Marcelin and Mayet M. 2007. “Enroute to biopiracy? Ethnobotanical research on antidiabetic medicinal plants in the Eastern Cape Province, South Africa.” *African Journal of Biotechnology,* 6: 2945–2952.

Merlin, Thomas, Richard and George, J. 2005. “Anaemia in diabetes: An emerging-complication of microvascular disease.” *Current Diabetes Reviews,* 1: 107–126.

Metzger, Brian R and Coustan, Donald R., and Organizing Committee. 1998. “Summary and recommendations of the fourth international workshop-conference on gestational diabetes mellitus”. *Diabetes Care,* 21: B161.

Mohammed Aminu, Mohammed Auwal Ibrahim and Md Shahidul Islam. 2014. “Shahidul Islam. African Medicinal Plants with Anti-diabetic Potentials: A Review.” *Planta Medica,* 80: 354–377.

Moshi Mainen and Mbwambo H. 2002. “Experience of Tanzanian traditional healers in the management of non-insulin dependent diabetes mellitus.” *Pharmaceutical Biology,* 40: 552–560.

Nam and Choi. 2008. “Effect of butanol fraction from *Cassia tora* L. seeds on glycemic control and insulin secretion in diabetic rats.” *Nutrition Research and Practices,* 2: 240–246.

Narkhede, Mahesh, Ajimire, Wagh, Mohan, and Shivashanmugam T. 2011. “In vitro antidiabetic activity of Caesalpina digyna (R.) methanol root extract.” *Asian Journal of Plant Science and Research*, 1(2): 101–106.

N’guessa, Kouassi and Kouadio K. 2009. “Ethnobotanical study of plants used to treat diabetes, in traditional medicine, by Abbey and Krobou people of Agboville (Côte-d’Ivoire).” *American Journal of Scientific Research*, 4: 45–58.

Odoh, Uchenna Estella and Ezugwu Christopher Obodoike. 2005. “Chromatographic And Anti-diabetic Diabetic Studies On Root Extract of *Acanthus montanus.* (Acanthaceae) *International Journal of Current Research,* 5(12): 3719–3722.

Onyekere Peculiar Feenna, Odoh Uchenna Estella and Ezugwu Christopher Obodoike. 2020. “Phytcohemical Analysis and Anti-diabetic Activity of Leaf Extract of *Psydrax horizontalis* Schum. & Thonn (Rubiaceae).” *Pharmacognosy Journal,* 12(1): 95–102.

Onyekere Peculiar Feenna, Onyeke Blessing Ugonne, Udodeme Helen Ogechukwu, Anosike Chibueze. 2017. “Comparative Anti-diabetic Activities of Methanol and n-hexane Extracts of Anthocleista vogelii (Gentianaceae) Stem bark in Normoglycemic and Alloxan-Induced Diabetic Rats.” *ARC Journal of Pharmaceutical Sciences,* 3(2): 1–8.

Osadebe Patience, Uzor Philip, Omeje Edwin, Agbo Mathias, Obonga Wilfred .2014. Hypoglycemic activity of the extract and fractions of *Anthocleista vogelii* (Planch) Stem Bark.” *Tropical Journal of Pharmaceutical Research,* 13(9): 1437–1443.

Pinto Mda, Kwon, Apostolidis, Lajolo, Genovese and Shetty K. 2009. “Potential of *Ginkgo biloba* L.leaves in the management of hyperglycemia and hypertension using *in vitro* models.” *Bioresource and Technology,* 100(24): 6599–6609.

Rajasekhar, Visakhapatnam, Kasetti, B., Kondeti, K. and Chippada, R. 2010 Antihyperglycemic and antihyperlipidemic activities of methanol:water (4:1) fraction isolated from aqueous extract of Syzygium alternifolium seeds in streptozotocin induced diabetic rats. *Food and Chemical Toxicology,* 48(4): 1078–1084.

Rees, Aled. D and Alcolado, J.C. Animal models of diabetes mellitus.2005. *Diabetic Medicine*, 22(4): 359–370.

RERUP, C. C. 2005. "Drugs producing diabetes through damage to the insulin secreting cells." *Pharmacology Reviews,* 22: 485–578.

Rutebemberwa Elizeus, Lubega Muhamadi, Katureebe Sheila K, Oundo Abanga, Kiweewa Francis, Mukanga David. 2013. "Use of traditional medicine for the treatment of diabetes in Eastern Uganda: a qualitative exploration of reasons for choice." *BMC International Health Human Rights,* 13: 2–7.

Samuel, Varman, and Shulman Gerald. 2016. "The pathogenesis of insulin resistance: integrating signaling pathways and substrate flux." *The Journal of Clinical Investigation,* 126(1): 12–22.

Schnedl, Wolfgang, Feber, Sarah, Johnson John and Newgard Christopher. 1994. "Streptozotocin transport and cytotoxicity. Specific enhancement in GLUT2 expressing cells". *Diabetes,* 43(11): 1326–1333.

Sharma, Kumar Vivek, Suresh Kumar, Hiltesh Jayantibhai Patel and Shivakumar Hugar. 2010. "Hypoglycemic activity of *Ficus glomerata* in alloxan induced diabetic rats." *International Journal of Pharmaceutical Sciences Review and Research,* 1(2): 18–22.

Singh,Pandey and Srivastava S. 2003. "Chemistry and medicinal properties of Tinospora cordifolia (Guduchi)." *Indian Journal of Pharmacology,* 35: 83–91.

Sofowora, Abayomi E. 2008."Medicinal plants and Traditional Medicine in Africa." 3rd edition. Spectrum Books Limited, Spectrum House, Ring Road Ibadan, Nigeria.

Srinivasan Krishnamoorthy and Ramarao, P. 2007. "Animal model in type 2 diabetes research: An overview." *Indian Journal of Medical Research,* 12: 451–472.

Trease and Evans William Charles. 1996. "Deterioration of stored Drugs Pharmacognosy." Braillar Tiriden Company, pp. 117–120.

Ueda, Kawanishi and Moriyasu M. 2004. "Effects of ellagic acid and 2-(2,3,6-trihydroxy-4-carboxyphenyl) ellagic acid on sorbitol accumulation *in vitro* and *in vivo.*" *Biology and Pharmacy Bulletin,* 27: 1384–1387.

Uzor Philip, Idah Emmanuel and Okoye Theophine. 2015. "Antidiabetic activity and phytoconstituents of Combretum dolichopetalum leaf." *Journal of Experimental and Applied Animal Sciences,* 1(3): 388–395.

Van de Venter, Roux, Bungu. 2008. "Antidiabetic screening and scoring of 11 plants traditionally used in South Africa." *Journal of Ethnopharmacology,* 119(1): 81–86.

Werfalli Mohammed, Engel Mark, Alfred Musekiwa, Kengne Andre, and Naomi Levitt. 2015. "The prevalence of type 2 diabetes among older people in Africa: a systematic review." *The Lancet Diabetes & Endocrinology*, 4(1): 72–84.

Whiting David, Guariguata Leonor, Weil Clifford and Shaw, John. 2011. IDF diabetes atlas: global estimates of the prevalence of diabetes for 2011 and 2030. *Diabetes Research and Clinical Practice,* 94 (3): 311–321.

WHO. 1985. "Study group on diabetes mellitus." Technical report series No. 727, World Health Organization, Geneva.

WHO. 2010. Diabetes mellitus. Available at http://www.who.int/diabetesactiononline/diabetes/ en/2.

Wild Stefan, Roglic Goran, Green, Sicree and King H. 2004. "Global prevalence of diabetes: estimates for the year 2000 and projections for 2030". *Diabetes Care,* 27(5):1047–1053.

Yoshikawa M, Nishida N, Shimoda H, Takada M, Kawahara Y, Matsuda H and Yakugaku Zasshi. 2001. "Polyphenol constituents from *Salacia* species: quantitative analysis of mangiferin with alphaglucosidase and aldose reductase inhibitory activities." *Yakugaku Zasshi,* 121: 371–378.

Yu, Hung, Chen WC and Cheng JT. 2003. "Antihyperglycemic effect of andrographolide in streptozotocin induced diabetic rats." *Planta Medica,* 69: 1075–1079.

Zhang, Fu, Gao. 2013. "Curcumin and diabetes: a systematic review." *Evidence Based Complementary and Alternative Medicine,* 2(17): 636–653.

Chapter 4

Malaria Control in Ghana

Past, Present, and Future Perspectives

Ama Pokuaa Fenny and Patricia Ohenewaa Akuffo-Henaku

Malaria is one of the diseases that have persisted and affected humanity for centuries. In the mid-nineteenth century, malaria was endemic in most countries and territories of the world, affecting about 90 percent of the world's population and stretching as far north as the Arctic Circle (Roll Back Malaria 2008). The disease is caused by five protozoan species, namely: Plasmodium falciparum, P. vivax, P. malariae, P. ovale, and P. knowlesi. The deadliest of these is P. falciparum which is predominant in sub-Saharan Africa (SSA) (Frimpong et al., 2018). Almost 85 percent of all malaria cases globally were in nineteen countries (India and eighteen African countries: Nigeria, Democratic Republic of the Congo, Uganda, Mozambique, Côte d'Ivoire, Niger, Burkina Faso, Mali, Angola, United Republic of Tanzania, Ghana, Cameroon, Rwanda, Benin, Malawi, Kenya, Guinea, and Burundi) (World Malaria Report, 2019). Most malaria cases in 2018 were in the World Health Organization (WHO) African Region (213 million or 93 percent), followed by the WHO Southeast Asian Region with 3.4 percent of the cases and the WHO Eastern Mediterranean Region with 2.1 percent (World Malaria Report, 2019).

Malaria control efforts began in 1945 but gained momentum a decade later when the 8th World Health Assembly launched the Global Malaria Eradication campaign for all malaria-endemic countries with the exception of countries in SSA. The program primarily used dichloro-diphenyl-trichloroethane (DDT) as a vector control tool together with malaria case management. In all, 37 of the 143 countries that were endemic in 1950 became free of malaria by 1978, of which 27 were in Europe or the Americas (Roll Back Malaria, 2008). These efforts had a positive impact on malaria mortality and morbidity in almost all targeted countries. However, some of the countries were unsuccessful in interrupting transmission. Therefore, by 1973, it was concluded that in some countries a "time-limited eradication program was impracticable" and strategies were shifted into long-term integrated malaria control programs. Consequently, the Global Malaria Eradication campaign was abandoned and little attention was paid to malaria control over the subsequent years. Despite the end of the official WHO campaign, some countries have successfully eliminated malaria since that period, including Tunisia in 1979, the Maldives in 1984, and the United Arab Emirates in 2007 (Roll Back Malaria 2008).

In the year 2000, member states of the United Nations unanimously agreed on a set of goals with indicators to be achieved by the year 2015 (WHO, 2020). Among these was the fight against malaria and other diseases. The results of the malaria control efforts showed that the number of malaria cases fell from an estimated 262 million globally in 2000 (range: 205–316 million) to 214 million in 2015 (range: 149–303 million), a decline of 18 percent. Globally, the number of malaria deaths fell from an estimated 839,000 in 2000 (range: 653,000–1.1 million) to 438,000 in 2015 (range: 236,000–635,000), a decline of 48 percent.

In 2019, the following six countries accounted for more than half of all malaria cases worldwide: Nigeria (25 percent), the Democratic Republic of the Congo (12 percent), Uganda (5 percent), and Côte d'Ivoire, Mozambique, and Niger (4 percent each) (World Malaria Report, 2019). Regarding the causes of malaria in these countries, Plasmodium falciparum is the most prevalent malaria parasite in the WHO African Region, accounting for 99.7 percent of estimated malaria cases in 2018. Between 2015 and 2018, only thirty-one countries where malaria is still endemic reduced case incidence significantly and were on track to reduce incidence by 40 percent or more by 2020 (World Malaria Report, 2019).

The Institute for Health Metrics and Evaluation reported that in 2017, malaria ranked first as the disease that caused the most deaths and second among those that led to premature deaths in Ghana ("Ghana" undated). Ghana also happens to have the world's fifth worst malaria burden (WHO, 2017). In a recent study looking at the economic burden of malaria on private sector businesses, it emerged that businesses in Ghana lost about $6.58 million to malaria in 2014, 90 percent of which were direct costs. Between 2012 and 2014, a total of 3,913 workdays were lost by businesses, and an average of 0.5 percent of annual corporate returns were spent on treatment of malaria in employees and their dependents, 0.3 percent on prevention, and 0.5 percent on other health-related corporate social responsibilities (Nonvignon et al., 2016). Again, business leaders affirmed that malaria influenced their businesses' productivity, employee attendance, and output and expenditures.

Most business leaders in this survey (93 percent) expressed the importance of private sector investment in malaria control (Nonvignon et al., 2016).

This chapter looks at efforts to control malaria in Ghana and examines past efforts, current challenges, and future perspectives. Sections discussed cover the history, research agenda, and progress made before and after the National Malaria Control Programme (NMCP). More so, this chapter provides a review of the role of societal and cultural practices in mitigating efforts to control or eradicate malaria in Ghana.

GHANA MALARIA CONTROL EFFORTS

Historical Context

Ghana commenced its fight against malaria as far back as the 1950s. The purpose of this multifaceted intervention was to reduce the disease's burden to the point where it ceases to be a public health challenge. The interventions implemented were residual insecticide application against adult mosquitoes, mass chemoprophylaxis with Pyrimethamine medicated salt, and improvement of the drainage system. However, malaria persisted as the country's leading cause of morbidity (Ghana Health Service, 2017). In 2018, notable increases were recorded of malaria cases in Ghana. These accounted for an 8 percent (0.5 million more cases) globally.

In the quest to control malaria, many different initiatives, programs, and clinical mechanisms have been introduced over the years (2000–2008; 2008–2015). Some of these initiatives are the Roll Back Malaria Initiative, distribution and use of long-lasting insecticide treated nets (ITNs) by children and pregnant women, chemoprevention in pregnant women and children under five years, international and domestic funding, investment in malaria research intend to scale-up prevention, diagnosis and treatments, use of artemisinin-based combination therapies (ACTs), and Rapid Diagnostic Tests (RDTs). Between 2002 and 2004, Ghana adopted ACT as the first-line antimalarial therapy for uncomplicated malaria. Intermittent Preventive Treatment during Pregnancy (IPTp) with sulfadoxine-pyrimethamine (SP) was adopted as the national policy between 2003 and 2004 and was implemented by the Reproductive Health Division in collaboration with the National Malaria Control Programme.

In 2003, international support for malaria control increased sharply. Ghana benefited from a succession of Global Fund grants—the launch of the US President's Malaria Initiative (PMI) in 2007, a significant additional support from the U.K. Department for International Development (DFID), the United Nations Children's Fund (UNICEF), the World Bank, and the governments of Japan, China, and Cuba (US President's Malaria Initiative, 2018).

Beginning in 2005, Indoor Residual Spraying was implemented on a district-wide scale by the AngloGold Ashanti Mining Company (AGA) in Obuasi in the Ashanti region with additional districts in the north of the country receiving Indoor Residual Spray (IRS) supported first by PMI and then by the Global Fund. The availability of unprecedented external resources encouraged the NMCP to pursue an aggressive scale-up of proven malaria control methods from 2008 to present. Considering the marked interregional and urban/rural difference in malaria burden, the NMCP, in collaboration with major malaria partners, namely the Global Fund and PMI, are moving away from the de facto one-size-fits-all approach to programming malaria control interventions which has characterized the past decades. The 2011 Multiple Indicator Cluster Survey (MICS), the PMI-supported Ghana Urban Malaria Study in April 2013, the 2014 Demographic Health Survey (DHS), and the 2016 Malaria Indicator Survey (MIS) indicate that, malaria prevalence tends to be lower in urban areas (11 percent) than in rural areas (28 percent) (US President's Malaria Initiative, 2018). This further proves the burden differentials in urban and rural settings in Ghana.

Recent Malaria Control and Case Management Interventions

According to the US President's Malaria Initiative (PMI) report for 2018, the last twenty years in Ghana has evidenced consistently improved malaria control methods, increased resources for malaria prevention and control, and promptly adopted revised international technical standards. Moving forward, efforts are being made to tailor malaria control and case management interventions based on specific regional circumstances (USAID, 2018). According to the same report, in 2013, the national malaria strategy was reviewed with support from the Roll Back Malaria Partnership and partners, which resulted in the report of the Malaria Program Review and an Aide Memoire that was signed by the Minister of Health and development partners in January 2014 (US President's Malaria Initiative, 2018).

Based on the recommendations from the Malaria Program Review and new and emerging interventions at the global level, the NMCP developed the National Malaria Control Strategic Plan for 2014–2020, which was finalized in August 2014. PMI provided support in the development of the strategic plan (USAID, 2018). The goal of the plan was to reduce malaria morbidity and mortality by 75 percent by 2020 by engaging in the following activities:

- protecting at least 80 percent of the population at risk with effective malaria prevention interventions by 2020;
- providing correct diagnosis to all suspected malaria cases and prompt and effective treatment to 100 percent of confirmed malaria cases in accordance with treatment guidelines by 2020;

- strengthening and maintaining the capacity of program management, partnership, and coordination to achieve malaria programmatic objectives at all levels of the health care system by 2020;
- strengthening the systems for surveillance and Monitoring and Evaluation (M&E) in order to ensure timely availability of quality, consistent and relevant malaria data at all levels by 2020;
- increasing the awareness and knowledge of the entire population on malaria prevention and control to improve uptake and correct use of all interventions by 2020.

Additionally, in 2009, a revised Integrated Vector Control Strategy was released and a National Malaria Vector Control Oversight Committee (MaVCOC) was established with PMI support. This committee's mandate was to ensure safe and effective implementation and management of malaria vector control operations. This committee also serves as the technical advisory body on vector control to the NMCP and the Malaria Inter-Agency Coordinating Committee (MICC) (USAID 2018).

In 2014, MaVCOC reported a revised standard operating procedure for Indoor Residual Spraying. From 2008 to 2015, the MOH sponsored the Cuban Labiofam company to conduct larviciding, beginning with a pilot in central Accra and expanding to central urban districts of Kumasi and Sunyani. Larviciding was not considered a stand-alone intervention, but instead, part of NMCP's integrated vector management and was conducted in areas where breeding sites were few, fixed, and findable. As the number of unbiased studies on its efficacy or effectiveness in Africa is limited, larviciding in Ghana was also conducted with the intention of generating data on its impact. By the beginning of 2016, however, these activities had been suspended due to financial constraints before a formal evaluation of impact (USAID, 2018).

The Ghana Epidemiological Report (2014) recommended that a national schools parasite sampling protocol be developed as an important "Monitoring & Evaluation" collaboration between the NMCP and its research partners. Additional data generation was required as part of the Demographic Health Survey in 2014 which meant the National Malaria Control Programme had to work closely with partners involved in designing and funding the DHS 2014 to ensure that an RDT biomarker was included during this national household survey. Also, the report detailed that NMCP needed to harness any future research or intervention evaluation data likely to be collected by research and implementing partners in Ghana for future risk modeling and mapping work. Carrying out a more detailed mapping of employer locations, malaria risks, and district profiles were identified as a potentially useful advocacy tool to increase specific engagement of the private sector in district-level control (Ghana Epidemiological Report, 2014).

Launching the Malaria Vaccine Trial in Ghana

After decades of extensive research, the pre-erythrocytic stage vaccine (RTS,S) was licensed and expected to undergo further testing in malaria endemic areas before possible approval for immunization. Currently, together with RTS,S, only twenty candidate vaccines are undergoing clinical trials (Frimpong, Kusi, Ofori and Ndifon, 2018). Prior to the launch of the vaccine, a communication strategy was adopted. This was to bridge any communication gap that may undermine the effectiveness of the vaccine implementation. The strategy sought to address the identification and definition of key audiences to be targeted, the development of appropriate messages and the channels to communicate the benefits and risks of the vaccine to all stakeholders, including decision-makers at family, community, district, regional, and national levels.

The strategy addressed promotion of the acceptance of the malaria vaccine, and urged continued use of bed nets, indoor residual spraying, and other effective interventions recommended by public health officials. It also stressed the provision of clear information at the appropriate time on who should and should not be vaccinated. Additionally, the reasons, places, time, and frequency of getting the vaccine would be addressed. Healthcare providers, vaccinators, and communicators would be guided on how to successfully communicate with their target audience about the MVIP and malaria vaccination and be provided timely and accurate information to tackle rumors and other crisis situations (Advocacy, Communication and Social Mobilization Committee of the Ghana EPI, 2019). A study on an endemic country's perspective on the malaria vaccine development buttressed the essence of enforcing public education on the nature and correct use of vaccines because this has an influence on the progress expected to be marked in the fight against malaria (Koram and Gyan, 2010).

The launch of the malaria vaccine pilot in Ghana in April 2019 marked an important step in Ghana's fight against malaria. Stakeholders acknowledged that this effort and commitment on the part of Ghana's Ministry of Health would ultimately save the lives of many children under the age of two years and improve child health and malaria control. In addition, the invention of new solutions is potentially promising tools in this global fight. The vaccine pilot program includes areas of Brong Ahafo (now Ahafo, Bono and East Bono regions), Central and Volta (now Oti and Volta) regions and some districts in the Upper East region in Ghana. Within these regions, some districts are receiving the vaccine, while others are expected to receive it later. The remaining districts and regions are continuing to benefit from other malaria control measures implemented nationwide (Malaria Vaccine Pilot Launched in Ghana, 2020). This pilot program is aimed at producing evidence and lessons to inform the WHO policy recommendations on the broader use of the

RTS,S malaria vaccine. It aims to achieve declines in child mortality, vaccine uptake (including whether parents bring their children on time for the four required doses), and vaccine safety in the context of routine use (Malaria Vaccine Pilot Launched in Ghana, 2020).

In a news report by Citi News Room, the director general of the Ghana Health Service debunked all fears and rumors to the effect that the vaccine was being tested in Africa for racial and financial reasons. According to him, the attempt to sensitize citizens could have been more widespread spanning the entire country. He admitted that the implementation took place in seven of Ghana's sixteen regions, namely: Bono, Ahafo, Oti, Volta, Bono East, and Central regions and hinted that the preliminary clinical trials had been conducted on fifty military personnel from the United States and Belgium in malaria-endemic countries. At the third phase of the trial, Ghana was involved. The director general added emphatically that the vaccine was not introduced to replace the existing National Malaria Campaign Program (Adogla-Bessa, 2019).

In an interview on the same subject with the immediate past deputy minister of health, the minister said, "In the beginning you'll always have this kind of resistance, this skepticism. When they started with polio, measles vaccines it was the same but now all those vaccines have been accepted . . . They should understand that it is not clinical trials that are being done now. It is the proper roll out phase. The reason why Ghana was chosen is because in Africa, our FDA if not the best it is one of the best in ensuring that products that come out are of the highest quality in terms of the analysis, they make . . . There is nothing to fear." This was in counterresponse to some news that had gone viral on social media to discourage the public from accepting the vaccines (Nyabor, 2019).

Role of Societal Norms and Cultural Values in NMC Interventions

This section provides details on some of the societal norms and cultural values that may have undermined the progress of malaria interventions. In Ghana, the issue of societal norms and culture certainly comes to play in the success of malaria intervention strategies. Sharma and Mehrotra state that "for successful malaria control, whether today or tomorrow, people's participation is absolutely essential, and in the future, much will depend on the community-will" (Sharma and Mehrotra, 1986). Various factors influence the choice of methods of control appropriate for a specific region. These may span from an understanding of deforestation and population movement, the role of the community, local perceptions of malaria and its causes, treatment-seeking behavior, and people's perceptions of the efficacy of a preventive measure.

Some researchers developed a framework with a set of variables believed to be applicable in disease control programs such as malaria control (Heggenhougen, Hackethal and Vivek, 2003). However, very often, the people in the community are not involved in the decision-making process. Yet, community members do not only contribute to vector control and broad epidemiological surveillance for keeping local malaria incidence under control, but they are essential for the success of such work. It is strongly recommended that outsiders be willing to listen to and help meet the needs expressed by the community, even when these needs are ancillary to the focus of the outside public health implementers, and, if public health efforts to control infectious diseases can also be combined with an income-producing side project, so much the better (Heggenhougen, Hackethal and Vivek, 2003). Competing political ideologies can also contribute to the success or failure of community-based disease control programs (Heggenhougen, Hackethal and Vivek, 2003, 134).

The main reasons for the failure of health education in malaria control programs at the community level in many countries include low education of the audience, poor housing, lack of physical and social resources, and apathy. Secondly, population groups have accepted malaria as part of their lives and would rather have their poverty and poor living conditions addressed. Furthermore, people have difficulty in understanding the complexities of malaria etiology and epidemiology. Finally, existing control methods have often been formulated without enough knowledge of the target population and the situations in which they live (Heggenhougen, Hackethal and Vivek, 2003).

To mitigate these hindrances, behavioral research can be integrated into malaria control programs to reduce any behavioral and social blockades that may exist (Heggenhougen, Hackethal and Vivek, 2003). A study conducted in Kintampo to ascertain the level of knowledge people had on malaria vaccines showed that knowledge was widespread, yet limited to injectable vaccines and oral vaccines such as the Oral Polio Vaccine (OPV). Many respondents in the study wished their children to be vaccinated for all the known diseases covered by the Expanded Programme of Immunization (EPI). Comparatively, a greater number of respondents preferred vaccines to drugs for malaria control with the assumption that the vaccine is highly efficacious. Beliefs and cultural practices that could serve as hindrances to the acceptance of a malaria vaccine were not identified (Febir et al., 2013).

In the quest to look into the risk behaviors, practices, and attitudes that could be associated with malaria in rural Tanzania, researchers discovered that livelihoods and shared resources and social and special cultural events had major influences. With respect to their livelihoods and resources, participants reported that their rice fields were far from their homes and pastoralists grazed their cattle on their farms. This informed their decision to settle in farming plots (shambas) during the rainy season, where protection from mosquitoes is impossible. Hence, sleeping arrangements, that is, the use of mattress and mosquito nets seemed to be a challenge to protection against mosquito bites, although, some participants reported otherwise. Daily tasks such as collection of fire wood and fetching water, which had to be done at dawn or dusk, potentially raised the risk of exposure (Dunn, Le Mare and Makungu, 2011).

On the other hand, the findings indicated how social events take on particular salience in malaria-related risk and bed net use. The social and cultural gatherings the people engaged in, besides being gendered, evidently required that both men and women stay outdoors late thereby, increasing the risk of mosquito bites. As an example, the study reported that people who slept under bed nets at funerals were perceived as witches, proud, unsympathetic and disregarded tradition (Dunn, Le Mare and Makungu, 2011).

A study undertaken in parts of South Eastern Nigeria found that awareness of malaria as a public health problem was high (89.8 percent), whereas, awareness about a potential malaria vaccine was not high (48.2 percent). Up to 88.2 percent of respondents showed positive perception toward the vaccine, of which 65.2 percent had strong positive perception. The study found a high level of intent to comply with the prospective malaria vaccine among the study group (95.6 percent positive). Significant association was established between caregivers' perception and intent to comply with the prospective malaria vaccine ($\chi2 = 144.52$; $p < 0.0001$). A majority (86.6 percent) strongly agreed that the vaccine is not against their cultural belief. Many of the caregivers in Southeastern Nigeria were receptive of the use of the malaria vaccine when developed. This is very encouraging for the malaria vaccine implementation program in the area. The study identified factors such as high literacy level and awareness about malaria to be influential in the caregivers' stance. The need to deepen and continue public health education, information and communication on contemporary health issues such as malaria control and vaccinations were highlighted as the gateway to unhindered implementation, compliance, and acceptance considering the control and elimination of malaria (Chukwuocha et al., 2018).

In another study, a systematic review of articles was conducted on studies addressing the challenges faced during the implementation phase of malaria vaccination programs and randomized trials conducted in sub-Saharan Africa which reports proposed solutions to the challenges identified. Findings indicate an overall positive reaction toward the new malaria vaccine. The main challenges to vaccine acceptance identified were inadequate community engagement due to lack of information about the vaccine, fear of the vaccine's side effects, inefficient delivery of vaccination services to children, and suboptimal quality of the health services. The main themes that emerged from the proposed solutions consisted of the use of dynamic communication models and trusted sources for delivery of vaccine-related health information to the communities, community engagement at both national and district levels and, implementation of the new vaccine services alongside the existing health services already delivered (Dimala et al., 2018).

It was identified in a similar study that malaria was the commonest health issue among children (Meñaca et al., 2014). Though the use of treated bed nets was considered an effective prevention tool by participants of the study, they agreed that there was no single prevention tool for malaria. Vaccines were noted as highly valued in the communities and the main incentive for sending children to Child Welfare Clinics. While communities accepted the idea of minor vaccine side effects such as general body discomfort, swelling and high body temperature, other side effects considered more serious, such as paralysis, deterred families from taking children for vaccination, especially during vaccination campaigns. The study identified some factors that could facilitate the introduction of a licensed malaria vaccine. They include the need to build on the generally positive attitude toward vaccines in the communities, an understanding that malaria prevention requires a comprehensive approach, the availability of well-established programs to deliver new vaccines, the need to increase and improve communication around childhood vaccination, and the identification of flexible, active health communication structures, and processes to disseminate information (Meñaca et al., 2014). Similar trends are observed in Ghana.

Researchers have discovered that in Kassena-Nankana East and West Districts, many of the people were aware of the benefits of insecticide-treated nets. However, nonuse of the treated nets was because of factors such as poverty, high room occupancy, excessive heat, and the belief that treated nets could not provide absolute protection against malaria. Therefore, many people also used traditional strategies, such as the drinking of herbal concoctions, wearing of long cloths, and consulting ancestors to control malaria. Hence, most people combine both orthodox and traditional remedies for their suspected malaria attacks (Azabre, Teye and Yaro, 2013).

In summary, it is evident that societal and cultural values have the potential to delay the progress of work on malaria eradication and, in some cases, render interventions ineffective in both Ghanaian and other contexts. Thus, there is the need to go beyond simply identifying these factors by additionally managing them and adjusting interventions to fit different contexts.

Behavioral Change and Social Interventions

In ensuring that disease interventions work, the behavior, perceptions, and attitudes of the people whom the interventions are directed at cannot be overlooked. Social marketing communication plays an important role in the prevention of diseases, of which malaria is no exception. Social marketing communications efforts directed at promoting the use of ITNs, however, face serious challenges. Social marketing communication is an integral element of public health interventions designed to influence social norms or change the behavior of individuals, families, and communities (Smith et al., 2005 as cited in Tweneboah-Koduah, Braimah and Otuo, 2012). Behavior change communications can be considered as a set of organized communication interventions and processes aimed at influencing social and community norms which promote individual behavioral change or positive behavior maintenance for a better quality of life (Chen, 2006 as cited in Tweneboah-Koduah, Braimah and Otuo 2012).

In a study by Tweneboah-Kodua et al. (2012), it was clear from the interviews that most of the institutions involved in social marketing communications do not use models when planning their interventions. However, it is necessary to acknowledge the role that the understanding of behavioral change plays in the enhancement, potential impact, and effectiveness of any intervention. Although the majority of the views on whether the objectives of the communication strategies achieved were affirmative, there were opposing views to the effect that communication strategies could ensure ownership of ITNs but not necessarily its use (Tweneboah-Kodua et al., 2012).

In Ghana, ITNs are distributed for free on National Immunization Day for children under five and for pregnant women. It is also sold at a meager price by health workers and volunteers. In spite of this, the problem of malaria still persists as there are cultural and socioeconomic barriers. Some of such factors include poor sanitation, occupation (particularly for people who work at night), poverty, poor housing, and education. It was also discovered that 56.3 percent of the participants did not use mosquito nets. The reasons given for not using mosquito nets included not having money, the weather being hot, the assumption that it was meant for children only, working at night, not knowing how to use it, and the use of mosquito sprays. These findings reveal an underlying problem of poor communication in malaria transmission and use of treated nets. Thus, there is little to zero behavior change toward preventing malaria infections (Onyeji, 2008).

Thus, it is necessary to acknowledge that addressing the communication gap is not enough. Rather, other external influencers such as poverty must be considered. In a similar study on the prevalence and management of malaria in Ghana, particularly in the Volta Region, researchers concluded that malaria reduction strategies ought to be incorporated into Ghana's Poverty Reduction Strategy. They anticipate that with a considerable reduction in poverty levels, households and communities would become increasingly responsible for the improvement of their health status and quality of life (Mba and Aboh, 2007).

In order to be well positioned in the country's efforts to control malaria, a communication strategy was put together for the malaria vaccine implementation. This strategy was to ensure accurate understanding of the potential pros and cons associated with immunization against malaria across various audiences, and to mobilize the population for immunization against malaria (Advocacy, Communication and Social Mobilization Committee of the Ghana EPI 2019). The 2016 MIS showed that while 66 percent of the population has access to an ITN, only 42 percent of the population slept under an ITN the night before the survey. There is a significant difference between ITN access and ITN use in both the 2014 and 2016 surveys. Both ITN access and use have increased slightly since 2014 (Ghana National Malaria Control Programme [NMCP], Ghana Health Service [GHS], and ICF, 2018).

The PMI in their 2019 report looked at key determinants of use of ITNs among people with access. The report shows that in Ghana the use-to-access ratio was 0.40 for the wealthy and 0.81 for the poor. The human-centered design was also applied as a means to identify facilitators and obstacles to ITN use and to create messages to increase demand for ITNs from retail outlets. Ghana was also noted for using school dramas successfully for several years; students were given scripts and school performances are held for the community (U.S. President's Malaria Initiative, 2019).

CONCLUSION

In the 2019 Malaria Report by the WHO, it is envisioned that by 2030, malaria incidence and mortality rates will be reduced by at least 90 percent. Additionally, at least thirty-five countries would have eliminated malaria and reestablishment of malaria in all countries that are malaria-free would have been prevented.

Sub-Saharan Africa stands out, as population growth is noticeably higher than elsewhere, though it is decreasing over time, leading to a slow increase in health spending per capita growth rate (Chang et al., 2019). It is noteworthy that reducing the burden of malaria will immensely contribute to or benefit from progress made toward the SDGs (goals 1–13 and goals 15–17). For instance, continued investments in health and malaria will result in the enhancement of human capital which increases productivity and growth. In the same vein, it is reported that a 10 percent reduction in malaria has been associated with a 0.3 percent rise in annual GDP (World Malaria Report 2019). Again, at the household level, reducing malaria will increase financial protection as household income and earnings will not be lost to the costs of seeking care (World Malaria Report 2019). Malaria control should not be a campaign, it should be a policy, a long-term program. It cannot be accomplished or maintained by spasmodic effort. It requires the adoption of a practicable program, the reasonable continuity of which will be sustained for a long term of years (Karunamoorthi, 2011). Ghana's National Malaria Control Programme is one of such practicable programs that has been implemented for years.

Lessons learned in Ghana during the introduction of new vaccines against diseases such as hepatitis B, rotavirus, and pneumococcus highlight the necessity for timely preparation, including the development of effective communication and training plans well in advance of introduction, and implementation of the plans at the appropriate time (Advocacy, Communication and Social Mobilization Committee of the Ghana EPI, 2019). Evidently, the country has made progress in controlling malaria largely through securing funds from international donors and setting-up various supervisory committees to oversee progress of work. Among the challenges facing the future of effective control include a more rational basis for stratified intervention delivery, better planning information, and an ability to generate sufficient evidence to demonstrate impact and value for money (National Malaria Control Program, 2013). In the 2017 annual report from the National Malaria Control Programme, there were indications that challenges similar to those listed above have been addressed through intensified mass media communication, community sensitization, behavior change activities, partnerships with key health sector suppliers, research, surveillance and monitoring, and evaluation activities (Ghana Health Service, 2018).

As a recommendation, Awine et al. (2017) suggest that ultimately, the opportunity for interaction between malaria control experts and modelers will create a platform for information sharing, presenting a unique platform for the development of more practically focused models for guiding malaria control activities in Ghana. For programs to succeed, it is proposed that not only should communities be involved in both planning and implementation but (as part of the overall approach) there must also be a willingness to address community expressed priority needs even when these are not directly related to the control of malaria. Additionally, the potential of culture and societal norms to facilitate or stall the progress of interventions can be addressed with adequate and rigorous communication and behavioral change strategies that are tailored to fit different cultural settings.

REFERENCES

Adogla-Bessa, Delali. 2019. "Education on Malaria Vaccine Could Have Been Better - Health Service Admits". Citinewsroom - Comprehensive News in Ghana, Current Affairs, Business News, Headlines, Ghana Sports, Entertainment, Politics,

Articles, Opinions, Viral Content. https://citinewsroom.com/2019/05/education-on-malaria-vaccine-could-have-been-better-health-service-admits/.
Advocacy, Communication and Social Mobilization Committee of the Ghana EPI. 2019. "Malaria Vaccine Implementation Program: Communication Strategy for Ghana". https://www.myghanalinks.com/images/pdf/malaria-vaccine-implementation-strategy.pdf.
Alonso, Pedro L., Graham Brown, Myriam Arevalo-Herrera, Fred Binka, Chetan Chitnis, Frank Collins, Ogobara K. Doumbo, et al. 2011. "A research agenda to underpin malaria eradication." *PLoS Medicine*, 8(1): e1000406.
Awine, Timothy, Malm, Keziah, Bart-Plange, Constance and Sheetal. 2017. "Towards malaria control and elimination in Ghana: challenges and decision-making tools to guide planning." *Global Health Action*, 10(1): 1381471.
Azabre, Bismark Atiayure, Joseph Kofi Teye, and Joseph Awetori Yaro. 2013. "Malaria Control Strategies in the Kassena-Nankana East and West Districts of Ghana". *Ghana Journal of Geography,* 5: 108–117.
Chang, Angela Y., Krycia Cowling, Angela E. Micah, Abigail Chapin, Catherine S. Chen, Gloria Ikirezi, Nafis Sadat, et al. 2019. "Past, present, and future of global health financing: a review of development assistance, government, out-of-pocket, and other private spending on health for 195 countries, 1995–2050." *The Lancet*, 393(10187): 2233–2260.
Chukwuocha, Uchechukwu M., Peter C. Okorie, Gregory N. Iwuoha, Sally N. Ibe, Ikechukwu N. Dozie, and Bertram E. Nwoke. 2018. "Awareness, Perceptions and Intent to Comply with The Prospective Malaria Vaccine in Parts of South Eastern Nigeria". *Malaria Journal,* 17: 1
Dimala, Christian Akem, Belmond Tse Kika, Benjamin Momo Kadia, and Hannah Blencowe. 2018. "Current Challenges and Proposed Solutions to The Effective Implementation of the RTS, S/AS01 Malaria Vaccine Program in Sub-Saharan Africa: A Systematic Review". *PLos One*, 13: 12.
Dunn, Christine E., Ann Le Mare, and Christina Makungu. 2011. "Malaria Risk Behaviours, Socio-Cultural Practices and Rural Livelihoods in Southern Tanzania: Implications for Bed net Usage". *Social Science & Medicine,* 72 (3): 408–417.
Febir, Lawrence G, Kwaku P Asante, Dan-Bright S Dzorgbo, Kojo A Senah, Timothy S Letsa, and Seth Owusu-Agyei. 2013. "Community Perceptions of a Malaria Vaccine in the Kintampo Districts of Ghana". *Malaria Journal,* 12 (1): 139. doi:10.1186/1475-2875-12-156.
Frimpong, Augustina, Kwadwo Asamoah Kusi, Michael Fokuo Ofori, and Wilfred Ndifon. 2018. "Novel strategies for malaria vaccine design." *Frontiers in Immunology,* 9: 2769.
"Ghana". undated. Institute for Health Metrics and E"Towards malaria control and elimination in Ghana: challenges and decision-making tools to guide planning valuation. Accessed April 10. http://www.healthdata.org/ghana.
Ghana Health Service. 2018. "2017 ANNUAL REPORT NATIONAL MALARIA CONTROL PROGRAMME". https://www.google.com/url?sa=t&rct=j&q=&esrc=s&source=web&cd=&cad=rja&uact=8&ved=2ahUKEwilhqTN78fpAhXN8uAKHd4NDSgQFjAEegQIBhAB&url=http%3A%2F%2Fwww.ccmghana.n

et%2Findex.php%2Fstrategic-plans-reports%253Fdownload%253D200%3Anmcp2017&usg=AOvVaw0_NaWIjk75wIojGLVfYQfF

Ghana National Malaria Control Program (NMCP), Ghana Health Service (GHS), and ICF. 2018. "Ghana Malaria Indicator Trends: Outputs from a DHS Program Workshop". In, 6. Accra, Ghana and Rockville, Maryland, USA.

Ghanahealthservice.org. 2017. National Malaria Control Programme | Ghana Health Service. [online] Available at: <https://www.ghanahealthservice.org/ghssubcategory.php?cid=4&scid=41> [Accessed 31 March 2020].

Heggenhougen, H. Kristian, Veronica Hackethal, and Pramila Vivek. 2003. *The Behavioural and Social Aspects of Malaria and Its Control: An Introduction and Annotated Bibliography*. No.TDR/STR/SEB/VOL/03.1. Geneva: World Health Organization.

Karunamoorthi, K. 2011. "Vector Control: A Cornerstone in the Malaria Elimination Campaign." *Clinical Microbiology and Infection*, 17(11): 1608–1616.

Koram, Kwadwo A., and Ben A. Gyan. 2010. "Malaria Vaccine Development: An Endemic Country Perspective". *Human Vaccines,* 6 (1): 15.

Malaria, Roll Back. "The Global Malaria Action Plan." Roll Back Malaria partnership. 2008.

"Malaria Vaccine Pilot Launched in Ghana". 2020. WHO | Regional Office for Africa. https://www.afro.who.int/news/malaria-vaccine-pilot-launched-ghana.

Mba, Chuks J., and Irene K. Aboh. 2007. "Prevalence and Management of Malaria in Ghana: A Case Study of Volta Region". Bioline.Org.Br. http://www.bioline.org.br/pdf?ep07007.

Meñaca, Arantza, Harry Tagbor, Rose Adjei, Constance Bart-Plange, Yvette Collymore, Antoinette Ba-Nguz, Kelsey Mertes, and Allison Bingham. 2014. "Factors Likely to Affect Community Acceptance of a Malaria Vaccine in Two Districts of Ghana: A Qualitative Study". *PLos One*, 9(10): e109707. doi:10.1371/journal.pone.0109707.

National Malaria Control Programme (NMCP). 2017. "Ghana Malaria Control Programme Periodic Bulletin Issue 9", 2017. https://www.ghanahealthservice.org/downloads/2017-1st_Quarter_Bulletin.pdf.

National Malaria Control Program. 2013. "An Epidemiological Profile of Malaria and Its Control in Ghana." National Malaria Control Program.

Nonvignon, Justice, Genevieve Cecilia Aryeetey, Keziah L. Malm, Samuel Agyei Agyemang, Vivian N. A. Aubyn, Nana Yaw Peprah, Constance N. Bart-Plange, and Moses Aikins. 2016. "Economic Burden of Malaria on Businesses in Ghana: A Case for Private Sector Investment in Malaria Control". *Malaria Journal*, 15(1). doi:10.1186/s12936-016-1506-0.

Nyabor, Jonas. 2019. " Malaria vaccines safe; Ghanaians not going to be used for trials – Alexander Abban". Citinewsroom - Comprehensive News in Ghana, Current Affairs, Business News, Headlines, Ghana Sports, Entertainment, Politics, Articles, Opinions, Viral Content.https://citinewsroom.com/2019/05/malaria-vaccines-safe-ghanaians-not-going-to-be-used-for-trials-alexander-abban/

Onyeji, Adaku. 2008. "Malaria Knowledge, Beliefs, and Behavior in Ghana and Its Effect on the Implementation of National Malaria Prevention Initiatives. https://nmfonline.org/wp-content/uploads/2016/02/2008-Ghana-Onyeji-A.pdf

Pierre-Louis, Anne-Maryse, Jumana Qamruddin, Isabel Espinosa, and Shilpa Challa. 2010. "The malaria control success story." Yes Africa Can: 417.

Romore, Idda, Ali Mohamed Ali, Innocent Semali, Hassan Mshinda, Marcel Tanner, and Salim Abdulla. 2015. "Assessment of Parental Perception of Malaria Vaccine in Tanzania". *Malaria Journal,* 14 (1). doi:10.1186/s12936-015-0889-7.

The Implementation of National Malaria Prevention Initiatives". Presentation.

Tweneboah-Koduah, Ernest Yaw, Mahama Braimah, and Priscilla Ntriwaa Otuo. 2012. "Behavioral Change Communications on Malaria Prevention in Ghana". *Health Marketing Quarterly,* 29 (2): 130–145. doi:10.1080/07359683.2012.678257.

USAID. 2018. "PRESIDENT'S MALARIA INITIATIVE GHANA Malaria Operational Plan FY 2018". https://www.pmi.gov/docs/default-source/default-document-library/malaria-operational-plans/fy-2018/fy-2018-ghana-malaria-operational-plan.pdf?sfvrsn=5.

US President's Malaria Initiative. 2018."Nigeria Country Profile". https://www. pmi.gov/docs/default-source/default-document-library/country-profiles/nigeria_ profile. pdf? sfvrsn= 18.

U.S. President's Malaria Initiative. 2019. "Social and Behaviour Change for Insecticide-Treated Nets". https://www.pmi.gov/docs/default-source/default-document-library/tools-curricula/pmi-vectorworks-social-and-behavior-change-for-insecticide-treated-nets-2019-toolkit.pdf

World Malaria Report 2015. World Health Organization. 2016. "World Malaria Report World Health Organization". 2015. World Health Organization. https://www.who.int/malaria/publications/world-malaria-report-2015/wmr2015 keypoints _eng.pdf.

World Health Organization 2018. World Malaria Report 2017. World Health Organization, Geneva.

World Health Organization 2019. World Malaria Report 2019. World Health Organization, Geneva.

World Health Organization. 2015. Global Technical Strategy For Malaria 2016–2030. World Health Organization.

World Health Organization, Roll Back Malaria Partnership. "High Burden to High Impact. A Targeted Malaria Response". https://www.who.int/publications-detail/high-burden-to-high-impact-a-targeted-malaria-response

"WHO Millennium Development Goals (Mdgs)". 2020. Who.Int. https://www.who.int/topics/millennium_development_goals/about/en/.

Chapter 5

Intimate Partner Violence as a Silent Killer

Analyzing Domestic Violence as a Health Hazard in Uganda

Proscovia Namuli

Violence claims people's lives every day in the world (FRA, 2014; WHO, 2014). Up to 2.5 percent of global death is as a result of self-directed, interpersonal, and collective violence (WHO, 2014). The World Health Organization (WHO) defines violence as "the intentional use of physical force, power, threatened or actual, against oneself, or against a group or community that either results in or has high likelihood of resulting in injury, death, psychological harm, mal-development or deprivation" (WHO, 2014, p. 2).

Intimate partner violence (IPV) is the most common form of violence experienced by women (Gracia & Merlo, 2016). IPV is defined as "any behavior within an intimate relationship that causes physical, psychological or sexual harm to those in the relationship" (WHO, 2012, p. 1). Although both men and women can be victims of IPV, women suffer more violence than men (Benebo et al., 2018; Uganda Bureau of Statistics [UBOS], 2013). Women are at risk of being injured, assaulted, raped, or even murdered by their intimate partners than by any other person (Ellsberg & Heise, 2005).

Globally one in three women experience physical or sexual IPV in their lifetime (Bourey et al., 2015). Up to 54 percent of women in Uganda experience IPV in their lifetime (Ogland et al., 2014). This is not only much higher than 35.6 percent of women who experience IPV worldwide (WHO, 2013) but also higher than 30 percent of men in Uganda who suffer spousal violence (UBOS, 2013). This chapter focuses on IPV against women in Uganda. It analyses the causes of IPV and its health consequences.

IPV is not only a human right violation facet but also a severe public health issue which is associated with physical, reproductive, and mental health effects (Benebo et al., 2018; Bourey et al., 2015; Ellsberg & Heise, 2005; Gracia & Merlo, 2016; Kouyoumdjian et al., 2013; USAID, 2008). It does not only affect the victims but also other individuals. Examples include unborn babies who may lose their lives, and children and other family members who witness the abuse can be affected psychologically due to fear and stress (Benebo et al., 2018; Cools & Kotsadam, 2017; USAID, 2008; GTZ, 2009). IPV is common in many societies. However, it goes unrecognized and unreported (Patra et al., 2018; USAID, 2008). In Uganda, women and girls represent the largest part of the population. Currently, Uganda's population comprises 17,573,818 women and 17,060,832 men (UBOS, 2016). It is therefore vital to include women in all spheres of development, and this may partly contribute to sustainable socioeconomic transformation. Violence against women hinders their full participation in development activities and this may result in slowed development (GTZ, 2009; UBOS, 2016; Uganda Vision, 2040). To address the objective of this chapter, the following questions were asked: What are the causes of intimate partner violence in Uganda? What are the health effects of intimate partner violence in Uganda?

This chapter is organized in five sections. The current section is the introduction. The next section reviews the literature on the causes and health effects associated with IPV around the world. The third section presents the methodology that was used and the fourth part presents the findings. The last section presents the conclusions and recommendations.

LITERATURE REVIEW

Causes of Intimate Partner Violence (IPV)

There is no "one fit for all" or, no single factor that can fully explain the occurrence of IPV against women. Although violence against women (VAW) is a global problem, its causes are not universal, they vary from place to place (Benebo et al., 2018; Ellsberg & Heise, 2005; GTZ, 2009). IPV causes can be attributed to demographic, socioeconomic, sociocultural, and lifestyle-related factors (Karamagi et al., 2006). They are not only complex but also interconnected (GTZ, 2009). Various researchers use the ecological framework to understand the interconnection between IPV causes (Ellsberg & Heise, 2005; Heise, 2011; WHO, 2005).

Justification of violence against women by their husbands has been documented as one of the IPV causes. This often stems from gender norms; for example, social norms that distinguish roles and responsibilities between men and women (Benebo et al., 2018; Ellsberg & Heise, 2005; Heise, 2011; Hindin et al., 2008). Gender disparities and ideologies of male superiority, toughness, and dominance features that are associated with men may enhance men to use physical force against women (Benebo et al., 2018; Bourey et al., 2015; Ellsberg & Heise, 2005; Jewkes, 2002).

It has also been documented that intimate partner violence is more common and severe in poor communities (Ellsberg & Heise, 2005; Jewkes, 2002). Men living in poverty are more likely to abuse their wives (Jewkes, 2002). This is because men who are unemployed and of low socioeconomic status are likely to be stressed which may trigger them to be violent toward their family members (Jewkes, 2002; McCloskey et al., 2016; USAID, 2008; Umubyeyi et al., 2014; WHO, 2012).

Previous studies have revealed that women living with unemployed men are more likely to suffer violence from them (McCloskey et al., 2016). Similarly, women who have fewer resources are at risk of being abused than those with more resources (Cools and Kotsadam, 2017; WHO, 2012).

Additionally, children who were exposed to parental violence are likely to be perpetrators and victims of IPV in their relationships as adults (Heise, 2011; Hindin et al., 2008). This creates an intergenerational cycle of IPV (Heise, 2011; Jewkes, 2002; McCloskey et al., 2016; WHO, 2012).

Violence also tends to be high among women who have no education and lower among women with education (Abramsky et al., 2011; Hindin et al., 2008; Kishor & Johnson, 2004; USAID, 2008). The use of alcohol and drugs has also been linked to IPV (Abramsky et al., 2011; Ellsberg & Heise, 2005; Heise, 2011; Hindin et al., 2008; Jewkes, 2002; Kishor & Johnson, 2004).

Consequences of Intimate Partner Violence (IPV)

The occurrence of IPV results not only in various diseases. It also causes disabilities and death in addition to a number of health and social effects (Black, 2011; Makayoto et al., 2013; Patra et al., 2018; WHO, 2014). IPV is associated with a number of health-related conditions, which may include drug and alcohol abuse, severe pain, pregnancy complications, unwanted pregnancies, abortion, low birth weight, premature birth, sexually transmitted infections (STIs), HIV/AIDS, mental health, depression, and suicide (Benebo et al., 2018; Black, 2011; Ellsberg & Heise, 2005; Patra et al., 2018; WHO, 2005; WHO, 2013).

Over the past years, there has been a growing body of literature that associates IPV with women's vulnerability to HIV/AIDS and STIs (Durevall, 2014; Jewkes et al., 2010; McCloskey et al., 2016; Wagman et al., 2015; WHO, 2013). Various studies reveal that women who experience IPV are at a high risk of acquiring HIV. This is partly because of their likelihood to suffer forced sexual intercourse (Karamagi et al., 2006; Silverman et al., 2007; WHO, 2013).

IPV has also been linked to various reproductive health conditions such as unwanted/unintended pregnancies, induced abortion, miscarriages, and low birth weight (Black, 2011; Rahman et al, 2012; WHO, 2005). The high rate of reproductive health conditions among IPV victims can be attached to sexual coercion, isolation, fear, chronic stress, and limited access to family planning methods due to lack of approval from the victim's husbands (Black, 2011; Singh et al., 2009; WHO, 2013).

Research identifies that women who experience IPV are likely to suffer from mental health disorders, especially depression and post-traumatic stress disorder (Black, 2011; Ellsberg & Heise, 2005). Women who suffer traumatic stress are also at a higher risk of committing suicide (Ellsberg et al., 2008; WHO, 2013; Pulerwitz et al., 2015). In the same vein, IPV in its extreme form can lead to death (Patra et al., 2018). Globally, between 40 percent and more than 70 percent of homicides are as a result of violence. In South Africa, it was revealed that up to 41 percent of all homicides are due to intimate femicide (Ellsberg & Heise, 2005; Pulerwitz et al., 2015; WHO, 2014).

METHODOLOGY

Information was extracted from both qualitative and quantitative data sources. The study relied on existing literature. There was no primary data involved. Information was extracted from survey reports, academic articles and journals, among others. Documents published between January 2000 and 2018 were used to capture current information and also to find out the variances in IPV over time. A total of forty-seven documents drawn from different websites, for example, Web of Science, UN Women, Bio Med Centre (BMC), Reproductive Health, Lancet Global Health, World Bank, Uganda Bureau of Statistics (UBOS), Feminist Economics, International Journal of Humanities and Social Science, and Google scholar, were reviewed and used. The key words used to search for information were intimate partner violence, effects of IPV, IPV causes, and domestic violence against women. Only documents written in English were reviewed; no translations were involved. The inclusion criteria prioritized papers that had research objectives/questions close to the research in question.

Since the study relied on already existing information, this might have led to the missing out of firsthand information that would have been captured from primary sources. On the contrary, the fact that there is a large body of secondary data available that could be underutilized provided the opportunity to utilize the available information.

FINDINGS

The findings of the study are mainly based on the three most current Uganda demographic and health surveys (UDHS) (i.e., 2006, 2011 and 2016 UDHS). This is because these three reports have the most recent nationally representative information about the status of IPV in Uganda. Additionally, community-based surveys and other studies that have been carried out in Uganda were employed. Since most community-based studies do not represent the whole population in the country, whenever such studies are used, details of the study location and population are given.

The Republic of Uganda is a landlocked country located in East Africa. The 2014 national population and housing census revealed that the country has a total population of 34.6 million persons (UBOS, 2016). Uganda still experiences inequalities between men and women, especially in areas of education and employment (ICRW & UNFPA, 2009; Ogland et al., 2014; UBOS, 2017; UBOS & ICF, 2018). Despite the fact that 80 percent of women in the country participate in the country's labor force, the majority (75 percent) of them are in the agriculture sector and most of them work on family-owned fields where in most cases they do not receive any monetary compensation (Ogland et al., 2014; ICRW & UNFPA, 2009).

The country considers a number of international conventions and resolutions that emphasize equality in opportunities and access to human rights for all people (Uganda Vision, 2040). Uganda has also established various policies and frameworks that aim at preventing and responding to gender-based violence (GBV) (UBOS & ICF, 2018, p. 314). Additionally, there are various community-based interventions in the country that have been implemented in an attempt to curb domestic violence against women. These include safe homes and respect for everyone which was implemented in Rakai district in Central Uganda by Rakai Health Program between 2005 and 2009 (Wagman et al., 2015). Start, Awareness, Support, Actions (SASA) that was implemented in central Uganda (Abramsky et al., 2014) is one of such interventions. However, some of the existing customary laws and practices, especially regarding marriage, make national policies and frameworks difficult to be implemented and achieved (UBOS & ICF, 2018; Uganda Vision, 2040). This is because some gender norms and social structures make women vulnerable to spousal violence (Ellsberg & Heise, 2005; USAID, 2008).

Many people in Uganda, both men and women, still suffer domestic violence (Karamagi et al., 2006; Kaye et al., 2006a; UBOS, 2013). However, women experience more spousal violence than men (UBOS, 2013). Most violence suffered by women in Uganda is perpetrated by their current partners. For example, 56 percent of women in the 2016 UDHS reported that they had suffered physical abuse from their current spouses which is much higher than 29 percent by their former partners (UBOS & ICF, 2018).

CAUSES OF INTIMATE PARTNER VIOLENCE (IPV) IN UGANDA

Power Imbalance

Patriarchal ideologies that give men excessive power over women increase the likelihood of IPV against women in Uganda (Ogland et al., 2014). According to UBOS (2013), the major cause of domestic violence is power imbalances between partners. This is backed by the prevalence of IPV due to differences in education levels between partners (Ogland et al., 2014).

Research identifies that IPV against women decreases with an increase in the level of education for both partners in Uganda (Karamagi et al., 2006; Koenig et al., 2003; UBOS & ICF, 2018). Educated men are less likely to abuse their wives as compared to uneducated men. Similarly, educated women experience less spousal abuse than their counterparts who have no education (Koenig et al., 2003; UBOS & ICF, 2018). The 2016 UDHS documented that 61 percent of women with uneducated husbands had experienced violence which was much higher than 46 percent of those with husbands who had attained secondary education or higher (UBOS & ICF, 2018). A study carried out in Rakai district revealed that 44.7 percent (2674) of women who had only attained up to seven years of schooling had suffered IPV which was much higher than 25.6 percent (1,533) of women with more than seven years of education (Kouyoumdjian et al., 2013). This could partly be due to the fact that educated women are more protected by community and family members (Koenig et al., 2003). Educated women are also anticipated to have the ability to challenge various traditional norms about sex roles (Jewkes, 2002). Furthermore, it has been shown that empowerment such as education reduces the risk of abuse among women (Karamagi et al., 2006). Additionally, women who are economically independent have the ability to leave violent relationships because they can afford to live on their own (Jewkes, 2002).

Justification of Wife Beating

Intimate partner violence is more severe in societies where wife beating is justifiable (Koenig et al., 2003). Wife beating is among the most common form of physical violence in Uganda (UBO, 2013). Some men and women in Uganda justify wife beating in cases where she "offends" the husband

(Kouyoumdjian et al., 2013). Forty-five percent of women in the 2011 UDHS indicated that a man has a right to beat his wife in cases when she neglects the children. Thirty-seven percent of women in the same survey agreed to wife beating in cases when the woman goes somewhere without telling the husband. Women in Uganda seem to agree to wife beating more than men. For example, in 2006 UDHS, it was identified that 70.2 percent of women in the survey justified wife beating in at least one or more specified circumstances/reasons, which was much higher than justification by men at 60.2 percent. The attitude has changed tremendously in recent years. For example, the overall percentage for both men and women who justify wife beating decreased from 60.2 percent for men in 2006 to 43.7 percent in 2011 and from 70.2 percent for women in 2006 to 58.3 percent in 2011 (UBOS, 2013). Similar trends were reported by Karamagi et al. (2006) who reported that women agreed to wife beating more than men in Mbale district. Koenig et al. (2003) revealed that 16 percent men and 28 percent women reported that wife beating was justifiable. They further reported that more women (27 percent) and less men (22 percent) believed that it was justifiable to beat a woman in cases where she starts using family planning methods without a man's consent.

The Absence of Community Sanctions, Neighbor Involvement, and Family Support

Intimate partner violence is alleged to be high among women living in communities where there are no sanctions and community/family support. A study carried out in three countries including Uganda indicate that, in Uganda, the majority of the abused women do not seek help from formal and informal structures partly because of the cost involved in seeking assistance (ICRW & UNFPA, 2009). It was identified that a woman spends an average of $5 out of pocket expenditure on abuse. Seeking police intervention was reported to be the most expensive way of seeking for help, and women reported to having spent up to $10 when it came to seeking help from police (ICRW & UNFPA, 2009). Some women do not seek for help because they consider spousal violence a private matter and they feel ashamed to share their experience (Karamagi et al., 2006; Kitara et al., 2012).

Additionally, the 2016 UDHS indicates that only a few (i.e., 13 percent of women), who experience sexual violence, and 31 percent of those who experience physical violence seek for assistance. The report further documents that married women are more likely to seek help in cases of abuse than the unmarried; it revealed that only 24 percent of women who were never married reported to having sought help in case of abuse much lower than 33 percent of those who were married (UBOS & ICF, 2018).

Poverty and Its Associated Stress

Poverty has been identified as one of the major causes of IPV in Uganda (Kinyanda et al., 2016; UBOS, 2013). Men who do not have enough socio-economic resources are likely to use force or violence against their wives. This is because they want to show their dominance in the relationship and express their masculine authority (Ogland, et al., 2014). The 2016 UDHS revealed that an increase in wealth registered a decrease in IPV. For example, 60 percent of women in the lowest wealth quintile had experienced violence in 2016 which was much higher than 44 percent of those in the highest wealth quintile (UBOS & ICF, 2018). Karamagi et al. (2006) also report in Mbale district in Eastern Uganda that 55 percent (102) of women who belonged to the poorest class had experienced spousal violence. This was higher than 52 percent (64) of those who were considered less poor. The reasons for these trends could be the fact that women with fewer/lesser resources often depend on their husbands for economic/financial support and this reduces their ability to leave violent relationships (Ogland et al., 2014).

Alcohol and Drug Abuse

Alcohol abuse has for long been associated with IPV (Annan & Brier, 2010; Koenig et al., 2003; Makayoto et al., 2013). This is not different in Uganda where studies have revealed a relationship between both the husband and wife's drinking behaviors and IPV. It has been reported that (84 percent) of women with husbands who often get drunk have experienced IPV. This is much higher as compared to 42 percent of those with husbands who never got drunk and 45 percent of those who do not drink at all (UBOS & ICF, 2018). Furthermore, the majority 56.2 percent (3136) of women in Rakai community with partners using alcohol had experienced violence, which was much higher than 43.8 percent (2,440) of women whose husbands were not using alcohol (Kouyoumdjian et al., 2013). Similarly, Kinyanda et al. (2016) report that in Eastern Uganda, IPV was much higher among women who use alcohol than those who were nondrinkers. Some of the reasons that increase abuse among those women whose husbands use alcohol could be the fact that alcohol users may neglect their marital responsibility (Makayoto et al., 2013). Makayoto et al. (2013) has also documented that alcohol use has been linked to having multiple partners and this can trigger jealousy hence violence. Some men intentionally take alcohol to gain strength to abuse their wives (Makayoto et al., 2013). Additionally, intoxication from drug and alcohol use can trigger violence (UBOS & ICF, 2018). Jewkes (2002) has documented that excessive consumption of alcohol by women makes them cross gender boundaries and this may cause men to use physical force to control them.

It has also been identified that a person who drinks alcohol is likely to lose self-control and judgment, which in turn may cause violence (Jewkes, 2002; WHO, 2012; McCloskey et al., 2016).

Childhood Exposure to Violence

Research shows that in Uganda, women and men who were violated during childhood by parents are more likely to experience violence in their adult lives than those who were not abused. The UDHS (2016) reports that 68 percent of women who were abused by their parents during childhood had experienced IPV, which was much higher than 49 percent of those who did not suffer childhood abuse (UBOS & ICF, 2018).

HEALTH CONSEQUENCES OF IPV IN UGANDA

IPV results in various health consequences that do not affect the well-being of only the victims but also their household members and communities at large (ICRW & UNFPA, 2009). It results in injuries, reproductive health conditions, and depression (Annan & Brier, 2010).

Low Birth Weight, Abortion, and Maternal Death

Violence against women during pregnancy has been related to adverse pregnancy outcomes such as abortions, low birth weight, and preterm labor (ICRW & UNFPA, 2009; Kaye et al., 2006b; Makayoto et al., 2013). For example, a study carried out in Mulago hospital antenatal clinic in Uganda among 612 pregnant women from May 2004 to July 2005 identified that women who were exposed to physical and/or sexual violence were more likely to suffer pregnancy-related complications. These complications included hypertension, anemia, and low birth weight infants. Additionally, women who were exposed to violence during pregnancy were likely to experience antepartum hospitalization (maternal ill-health after giving birth) (Kaye et al., 2006b). The effects of violence during pregnancy among women can be both direct and indirect (Benebo et al., 2018; Kaye et al., 2006b). The direct effect could be in the form of abdominal trauma that may result in abortion, death of the infant, preterm labor, and giving birth to a preterm infant. The indirect effects of sexual and physical violence during pregnancy can cause stress and isolation. However, low birth weight has also been associated with other factors such as inadequate access to health care, malnutrition, smoking, drug abuse, alcohol abuse, among others (Kaye et al., 2006b).

Unintended Pregnancies

Intimate partner violence victims are likely to get unwanted pregnancies partly because some women in abusive relationships live in fear and have less ability to suggest the use of family planning methods such as condoms (Kouyoumdjian et al., 2013). A case in point is a woman respondent in Mbale district in Eastern Uganda who asserted that "men never allow us to use condoms, if we suggest they beat us" (Karamagi et al., 2006. p.7).

This partly results in getting unwanted/unintended pregnancies, hence increasing the likelihood of carrying out an abortion which puts women and infants lives at health risk. Similarly, Kaye et al. (2006a) indicate that, globally, 38 percent of pregnancies are unintended and 22 percent of the unwanted pregnancies are aborted/terminated. Abortion put women's lives at a risk of acquiring various infections and/or may result in death. A study conducted in Mulago hospital in Uganda, from September 2003 to June 2004 among 955 women, indicates that abortion was one of the major causes of maternal morbidity and mortality (Kaye et al., 2006a). Kaye et al. (2006a) assert that in Uganda, abortion causes between 15 percent and 30 percent of maternal deaths. They further report that 47 percent of women who were physically abused during pregnancy carried out an abortion (Kaye et al., 2006a).

HIV and IPV

Studies have documented a link between HIV and IPV (Karamagi et al., 2006; Koenig et al., 2003; Kouyoumdjian et al., 2013). Victims of IPV may have limited ability to negotiate for HIV prevention measures (Karamagi et al., 2006). Koenig et al. (2003) report that women are also abused when they ask their husbands to use HIV preventive measures. A study carried out in Rakai district of Uganda between 2000 and 2009 among 10,252 women aged between 15 and 49 years reports that women who had experienced violence frequently were at high risk of having HIV infection more than their counterparts who reported less/no abuse (Kouyoumdjian et al., 2013). From focus group discussions in Mbale district, it was identified that men normally react violently in cases where women went for HIV testing, shared their HIV test results, and/or ask them to use condoms. Men were abusive in such situations partly because they perceived the acts to be an evidence of "prostitution." They believed that a woman will only go for HIV test if she was a "prostitute" (Karamagi et al., 2006). For instance, a woman during a focus group discussion asserted that "he can ask me why I went for a (HIV) test and call me a prostitute and beat me" (Karamagi et al., 2006; p. 7).

Injuries

Women in Uganda who experience violence from their intimate partners are likely to sustain injuries such as cuts, bruises/aches, eye injuries, sprains, dislocations, burns, deep wounds, broken bones, broken teeth among others (Koenig et al., 2003; UBOS, 2013; UBOS & ICF, 2018). The 2016 UDHS indicates that 39 percent of women who had experienced IPV had sustained some form of injuries. The occurrence of injuries among women in Uganda has increased over the last ten years (i.e., from 37 percent in 2006 to 39 percent in 2016) (UBOS & ICF, 2018).

Mental Health, Suicide, and Alcoholism

Data from a cross-sectional survey in rural areas of two districts (Amuria and Katakwi) in eastern Uganda carried out among 1,560 respondents revealed that a number of women who had experienced physical IPV had ever thought of or attempted suicide. Additionally, some of those who had suffered sexual IPV had high chances of resorting to heavy drinking (alcoholism) and they were also likely to suffer major depression disorder than their counterparts who did not experience any violence (Kinyanda et al., 2016).

CONCLUSIONS

This study has established that IPV is a common life threat which is normally under-recognized. It is related to power imbalances, education, poverty, justification of wife beating, childhood abuse, alcohol abuse, and the absence of community sanctions. The study has registered numerous health risk factors experienced by bartered women and these include low birth weight, unintended pregnancies, abortion, HIV, mental disorders, physical injuries, and suicide.

In an attempt to curb domestic violence against women, Uganda has developed various policies and frameworks that aim at preventing and responding to gender-based violence. These include the 2007 Uganda Gender Policy, the 2008 National Action Plan on women, the 2008 National Action Plan on the United Nations Security Council Resolution 1325, 1820 and Goma Declaration, among others (UBOS & ICF, 2018, p.314; Uganda Vision 2040).

This study had some limitations. These include the reliance on secondary data that might have led to a missing out on more accurate information. Secondly, it is documented that underreporting of results is possible for studies conducted on a sensitive topic like the occurrence of partner violence. The underreporting could be due to conflict of interest for the researcher or other causes and this may affect the results of the studies using such literature (Speizer, 2010).

RECOMMENDATIONS

Results from surveys like demographic health surveys should be disseminated to the general public. This can be done through media sources like radios, televisions (TV), newspapers. Again, the results can also be put on notice boards of local government and of religious institutions (churches/mosques).

Corruption especially among authorities where women are supposed to report cases of abuse should be eliminated to make it easy for women and men to report cases of abuse instead of suffering in silence. Corruption can be reduced by improving the remuneration of police officers, establishing dismissal laws from service in case of bribery and developing anti-corruption policies in the country. Additionally, women and men should also be informed about their right to justice.

Intimate partner violence against men is also on the rise and this calls for further research and more interventions. The effects of violence affect not only individuals but also families, communities, and countries at large. There is the need to join hands and curb partner violence against both women and men.

REFERENCES

Abramsky, Tanya, Karen Devries, Ligia Kiss, Janet Nakuti, Nambusi Kyegombe, Elizabeth Starmann, Bonnie Cundill, Leilani Francisco, Dan Kaye, Tina Musuya, Lori Michau, and Charlotte Watta. 2014. "Findings from the SASA! Study: a cluster randomized controlled trial to assess the impact of a community mobilization intervention to prevent violence against women and reduce HIV risk in Kampala, Uganda." *BMC Medicine* 12(122): 1741–7015.

Abramsky, Tanya, Watts, Charlotte H., Garcia-Moreno, Claudia, Devries, Karen, Kiss, Ligia, Ellsberg, Mary, Jansen, Henrica A. F. M., and Heise, Lori. 2011. "What factors are associated with recent intimate partner violence? Findings from the WHO multi-country study on women's health and domestic violence." *BMC Public Health* 11(109): 1471–2458.

Annan, Jeannie, and Brier Moriah. 2010. "The risk of return: Intimate partner violence in Northern Uganda's armed conflict." *Social Science & Medicine,* 70(1): 152–159.

Benebo, Faith Owunari, Schumann Barbara, and Vaezghasemi Masoud. 2018. "Intimate partner violence against women in Nigeria: A multilevel study investigating the effect of women's status and community norms." *BMC Women's Health*, 18: 136.

Black, C. Michele. 2011. "Intimate partner violence and adverse health consequences: Implications for clinicians." *American Journal of Lifestyle Medicine, 5*: 428.

Bourey, Christine, Whitney Williams, Bernstein Elizabeth Erin, and Stephenson Rob. 2015. "Systematic review of structural interventions for intimate partner violence in low- and middle income countries: Organizing evidence for prevention." *BMC Public Health*, 15: 1165.

Cools, Sara, and Kotsadam Andreas. 2017. "Resources and intimate partner violence in SubSaharan Africa." *World Development, 95*: 211–230.

Deutsche Gesellshaft fur Technische Zusammenarbeit (GTZ). 2009. "Violence against Women: Violence against women—A gross violation of human rights that hinders development." GTZ. Eschborn/Germany.

Durevall, Dick, and Lindskog Annika. 2014. "Intimate partner violence and HIV in ten sub-Saharan African countries: What do the Demographic and Health Surveys tell us?" *Lancet Global Health, 3*(1): e34–e43.

Ellsberg, Mary Carroll, and Heise Lori. 2005. *Researching Violence Against Women: A Practical Guide for Researchers and Activists*. Washington DC, United States: World Health Organization, PATH.

Ellsberg, Mary, Henrica A. F. M. Jansen, Lori Heise, Charlotte H. Watts, and Claudia Garcia-Moreno. 2008. "Intimate Partner Violence and Women's physical and mental health in the WHO multi-country study on Women's health and domestic violence: an observational study." *The Lancet 371*(9619): 1165–1172.

European Union Agency for Fundamental Rights (FRA). 2014. "Violence Against women: an EU – Wide Survey, main results." *Vienna: European Union Agency for Fundamental Rights.*

Gracia, Enrique, and Merlo Juan. 2016. "Intimate partner violence against women and the Nordic paradox." *Social Science & Medicine 157*: 27–30.

Heise, Lori L. 2011. "What Works to Prevent Partner Violence? An Evidence Overview. Working Paper." *STRIVE Research Consortium, London School of Hygiene and Tropical Medicine, London.*

Hindin, J. Michelle, Kishor Sunita, and Ansara L. Donna. 2008. "Intimate partner violence among couples in 10 DHS countries: predictors and health outcomes." *DHS Analytical Studies. Calverton ,Maryland, USA: Macro International Inc. (18).*

International Centre for Research on women (ICRW) and United National Population Fund (UNFPA). 2009. "Intimate Partner Violence High Costs to Households and Communities." *International Center for Research on Women (ICRW) and United Nations Population Fund (UNFPA).*

Jewkes, Rachel. 2002. "Intimate partner violence: Causes and prevention." *The Lancet* 359(9315): 1423–1429.

Jewkes, K. Rachel, Kristin Dunkle, Mzikazi Nduna, and Nwabisa Shai. 2010. "Intimate partner violence, relationship power inequality, and incidence of HIV infection in young women in South Africa: a cohort study." *The Lancet, 376*(9734): 41–48.

Karamagi, AS Charles, Tumwine K. James, Thorkild Tylleskar, and Kristian Heggenhougen. 2006. "Intimate partner violence against women in eastern Uganda: implications for HIV prevention." *BMC Public Health,* 6:284.

Kaye, K. Dan, Mirembe M. Florence, Bantebya Grace, Annika Johansson, and Anna Mia Ekstrom. 2006a. "Domestic violence risk factor for unwanted pregnancy and induced arbortion in Mulago Hospital, Kampala, Uganda." *Tropical Medicine and International Health,* 11(1): 90–101.

Kaye, K. Dan, Mirembe M. Florence, Bantebya Grace, Johansson Annika, and Ekstrom Anna Mia. 2006b. "Domestic Violence during pregnancy and risk of low birthweight and mental complications: a prospective cohort study at Mulago Hospital, Uganda." *Tropical Medicine and International Health 10*: 1576–1584.

Kinyanda, Eugene, Weiss A. Helen, Mungherera Margaret, Onyango-Mangen Patrick, Ngabirano Emmanuel, Kajungu Rehema, Kagugube Johnson, Muhwezi Wilson, Muron Julius, and Vikram Patel. 2016. "Intimate partner violence as seen in post-conflict eastern Uganda: prevalence, risk factors and mental health consequences." *BMC International Health and Human Rights, 16*(5).

Kishor, Sunita, and Kiersten Johnson. 2004. "Profiling domestic violence: a multi-country study." *MEASURE DHS+ ORC Macro.*

Kitara, D. L., Odongkara, B. M., Anywar, D. A., Atim, P., Amone, C., and Komakech, D. 2012. "Domestic violence in Gulu, Northern Uganda." *East and Central African Journal of Surgery, 17*(1): 29–36.

Koenig, A. Michael, Tom Lutalo, Feng Zhao, Fred Nalugoda, Fred Wabwire-Mangen, Noah Kiwanuka, Jennifer Wagman, David Serwadda, Maria Wawer and Ron Gray. 2003. "Domestic violence in rural Uganda: evidence from a community-based study." *Bulletin of the World Health Organization, 81*: 53–60.

Kouyoumdjian, G. Fiona, Calzavaraa, M. Liviana, Bondy, Susan J., O'Campo Patricia, Serwadda, David., Nalugoda, Fred, Kagaayi, Joseph, Kigozi, Godfrey, Wawer, Maria, and Gray, Ron. 2013. "Intimate partner violence is associated with incident HIV infection in women in Uganda." *AIDS, 27*(8), 1331–1338.

Makayoto, A. Lyndah, Omolo Jared, Kamweya M. Abel, Harder S. Valarie, and Mutai Joseph. 2013. "Prevalence and Associated Factors of Intimate Partner Violence Among Pregnant Women Attending Kisumu District Hospital, Kenya." *Maternal Child Health Journal*, 17:441–447.

McCloskey, Ann Laura, Boonzaier, Steinbrenner, Floretta, Young, Sheila, and Hunter, Theresa. 2016. "Determinants of intimate partner violence in Sub-Saharan Africa: A review of prevention and intervention programs." *Partner Abuse* 7: 277–315.

Ogland, G., Emmanuelle, Xu Xiaohe, Bartkowski John P. and Ogland Curtis P. 2014. "Intimate partner violence against married women in Uganda." *Journal of family violence 29*(8): 869–879.

Patra, P., Prakash Jyoti, Patra B. and Khanna Puneet. 2018. "Intimate partner violence: Wounds are deeper." *Indian Journal of Psychiatry* 60(4): 494–498.

Pulerwitz, Julie, Wang Hui, Jennifer Arney, and Lisa Mueller Scott. 2015. "Changing gender norms and reducing HIV and violence risk among workers and students in China." *Journal of Health Communication 20* (8), 869–878.

Rahman, Mosfequr, Sasagawa Toshiyuki, Fujii Ryota, Tomizawa Hideki, and Makinoda Satoru. 2012. "Intimate partner violence and uninted pregnancy among Bangladeshi women." *Journal of Interpersonal Violence* 27(15): 2999–3015.

Silverman, JG., Gupta J, Decker MR., Kapur N., Raj A. 2007. "Intimate partner violence and unwanted pregnancy, miscarriage, induced arbortion, and still birth among a national sample of Bangladeshi women." *BJOG: Gynaecology 114*(10): 1246–1252.

Singh, Susheela, Wulf Deirdre, Hussain Rubina, Bankole Akinrinola, and Sedgh Gilda. 2009. "Abortion Worldwide: A decade of uneven progress". *Guttmacher Institute.*

Speizer, S. Ilene. 2010. "Intimate partner violence attitudes and experience among women and men in Uganda." *Journal of Interpersonal Violence 25*(7): 1224–1241

Uganda Bureau of Statistics. 2013. "*Uganda Facts and Figures on Gender.*" Uganda Bureau of Statistics, Statistics House plot 9 Colville Street, P.O Box 7186, Kampala, Uganda.

Uganda Bureau of Statistics. 2016. "The National Population and Housing Census 2014 Main Report." Kampala, Uganda.

Uganda Bureau of Statistics. 2017. *Women and Men in Uganda Facts and Figures 2016*. Kampala, Uganda: UBOS, and Rockville, Maryland, USA: UBOS and ICF.

Uganda Bureau of Statistics (UBOS) and ICF. 2018. *Uganda Demographic and Health Survey 2016*. Kampala, Uganda and Rockville, Maryland, USA: UBOS and ICF.

Uganda Bureau of Statistics (UBOS) and ICF. 2018. *Uganda Demographic and Health Survey 2016*. Kampala, Uganda and Rockville, Maryland, USA: UBOS and ICF.

Uganda Vision 2040. Accessed July 18, 2018 http://npa.ug/wp-content/themes/npa theme/documents/vision2040.pdf.

United States Agency for International Development. 2008. *Gender-based violence in sub-Saharan Africa: A review of Demographic and Health survey findings and their use in National planning*. United States Agency for International Development.

Wagman, A. Jennifer, Gray, Ronald H, Campbell, Jacquelyn C., Thoma, Marie., Ndyanabo, Anthony, Joseph., Ssekasanvu, Fred Nalugoda, Kagaayi, Joseph., Nakigozi, Gertrude, Serwadda, David., and Brahmbhatt, Heena. 2015. "Effectiveness of an integrated intimate partner violence and HIV prevention intervention in Rakai, Uganda: Analysis of an intervention in an existing cluster randomised cohort." *Lancet: Global Health 3*: e23–e33.

World Health Organization. 2005. *WHO Multi-Country study on women's health and domestic violence against women: initial results on prevalence, health outcomes and women's response*. Geneva: World Health Organization.

World Health Organization. 2012. *Understanding and addressing violence against women: Intimate partner violence*. Geneva: World Health Organization.

World Health Organization. 2013. *Global and regional estimates of violence against women: prevalence and health effects of intimate partner violence and non-partner sexual violence*. Geneva: World Health Organization.

World Health Organization. 2014. *Global status report on violence prevention*. Geneva: World Health Organization.

Chapter 6

Caring for the Aged

Africa's Next Health Challenge

Emmanuel Ashiedu Codjoe

The healthcare status of every society is inextricably linked to its future prosperity. This relationship remains an essential part of the construction of the Human Development Index (HDI). It is undoubtedly the case that Africa's healthcare situation mirrors its economic challenges. Many assessments by the World Health Organization (WHO) show that the state of healthcare in Africa remains the worst in the world.[1] Significantly, the region accounts for 24 percent of global disease burden in human and financial cost (International Finance Corporation, 2016). These are manifested in various ways. For instance, the region accounts for almost half of the world's under-five mortality and this is compounded by the many public health crises brought on by diseases, such as HIV/AIDS, malaria, and in recent times the Ebola and COVID-19 pandemics. In addition, other noncommunicable and chronic diseases, such as diabetes, hypertension, and coronary heart disease have in recent decades began to put a strain on the already fragile healthcare systems.

Despite these challenges, it is worth acknowledging the fact that over the past century or so, the region's system of healthcare provision has evolved from one that was largely dominated by traditional medical practice to one that is now dominated by orthodox western medical systems (Anyinam, 1987; Baronov, 2008). In the last five decades, investments in public health interventions in areas such as child health, malnutrition, maternal health, and primary healthcare have resulted in relatively substantial progress in the fight against preventable childhood illnesses such as polio and measles. Other diseases in the wider population, such as river blindness, have been eliminated as a public health problem. Leprosy is close to elimination while guinea worm control efforts have resulted in a 97 percent reduction in cases since 1986 across the sub-Saharan African region. The overall impact has been an increase in life expectancy (World Health Organization, 2014).

Nevertheless, the challenges confronted by the continent in healthcare provision for the wider population remains daunting. One important area that has not received a lot of attention in terms of public health interventions and investment in healthcare systems is that of care for the aged. This is in stark contrast with the efforts put into improving child health, maternal health, or other public health interventions. In a way, it is easy to understand why attention to caring for the aged has been minimal. The population in Africa is relatively younger compared to the situation in other regions of the world. Indeed, the need to improve child and maternal health as well as reduce mortality at all levels can be justified based on the need to increase life expectancy on the continent, which remains the lowest globally (United Nations, 2019a). Because of sustained investments in primary health, among others, life expectancy on the continent has risen over the years resulting in a gradual though small increase in the proportion of the population who are aged. Looking ahead, it is obvious that the next frontier in healthcare challenge for African countries will be how to provide good and efficient healthcare for the aged. As noted by Parmar et al. (2014), access to appropriate healthcare remains a major concern for the majority of the aging population in SSA. This chapter, therefore, explores some of the pertinent issues involving the care for the aged.

DEFINING THE AGED

The subject matter of care for the aged raises the fundamental question: who are the aged? How old should a person be to be described as aged? While it may seem obvious who the aged are, the answer may not be so straightforward. It is, however, worth noting that the notion of *aged* or *elderly* has both bio-physiological, emotional, psychological as well as sociological dimensions (Johnson, 1976; Roebuck, 1979; Dziechciaż and Filip, 2014). Each one of these dimensions would denote a separate definition of what constitutes aged. Despite these differential aspects of aging, many developed countries use the chronological age of 65 years as a definition of "elderly" or an older person. But, like many Westernized concepts, this does not adapt well to the situation in Africa (WHO, 2002). In the African context, the use of chronological age may not be relevant because other biological and social factors come to play (Cohen and Menken, 2006). Nevertheless, there is a wide acceptance of the chronological age of 60 years as the cut of point in the definition of the aged or the elderly in Africa (WHO, 2002; Velkof and Kowal, 2006; United Nations Economic Commission for Africa, 2007). Therefore, this chapter defines the aged as adult persons in the population aged 60 years or more. Furthermore, we shall be using the terms *aged*, *older people*, and *elderly* interchangeably, mindful of the nuances that might exist in different contexts with the usage of any of these terms.

CONTEXTUALIZING THE AGED IN THE AFRICAN POPULATION DYNAMICS

Africa's population currently accounts for about 16 percent of the world's population and the present structure of the population shows a youth bulge: the majority are under the age of 40 (United Nations, 2019a). Ritchie and Roser (2020) note that globally the African region has the lowest median age, which, according to the United Nations (2019b), has been the result of recent reductions in fertility. As a result of this phenomenon, the working age population (25–64 years) is growing faster than in other age groups, thereby providing an opportunity for accelerated economic growth, known as the demographic dividend. Indeed, projections by the United Nations (*ibid*) show that the African region could account for more than half of the growth of the world's population between 2019 and 2050. Current estimates also indicate that its relatively young population structure is expected to double in the next thirty years.

While this population increase holds great potential for the region, it is worth bearing in mind the sobering situation that the continent is host to the largest number of Least Developed Countries (LDCs) in the world; thirty-four of the fifty-four African countries are classified as LDCs (UNCTAD, 2019). Evidently, the continued rapid population growth presents challenges for the attainment of sustainable development (and more generally the sustainable development goals) by many of the countries in the region. This is especially so considering the constraints on the region's resources brought about by a combination of a growing population and the desire to exploit these resources to achieve rapid growth and development. Beyond the constraints imposed by the rapidly growing population on sustainable development, Bloom et al. (2010) and Kwankye (2013) also point out the various effects on several aspects of society by the age structure of a population. They argue that the age structure has a range of effects on society such as on economic growth rates, labor force participation, educational and healthcare services, and housing markets.

Although in Africa the age structure is predominantly youthful, this structure is, nonetheless, undergoing gradual change. An observation by Cohen and Menken (2006) shows that while older people made up a relatively small fraction of the total population from the latter half of the twentieth century to the first decade of the twenty-first century, the numbers of older people on the continent were expected to increase rapidly. Further to the observation by

Cohen and Menken, Velkov and Kowal (2006) argue that the small increase in the proportion of the population over the age of 59 years in sub-Saharan Africa masks a large increase in the number of people in this age group. Moreover, the current evidence from United Nations population estimates shows that the number of older people is growing more rapidly in sub-Saharan Africa. Nevertheless, the projected growth of the proportion of the older population will be relatively slower compared to other areas in the world. Significantly, in 2010, an estimated 43 million people aged 60 years and older were in sub-Saharan Africa and this was projected to reach 67 million by 2025 and 163 million by 2050 (WHO, 2014; United Nations, 2019b). Based on recent data, the proportion of the aged in Africa is 3.5 percent, although across the various subregions on the continent there are some variations. In West Africa and Middle Africa, this proportion is 2.8 percent, in Eastern Africa it is 2.9 percent, and 2.3 percent and 5.7 percent in Southern Africa and Northern Africa, respectively (United Nations, 2019b).[2] Significantly, there is a strong and positive correlation between the proportion of the aged in the population and the respective life expectancy across countries and subregions.[3]

These statistics do not reveal the trends within each of the subregions. Nevertheless, broadly speaking, the northern and southern regions of the continent are aging faster than the rest of the subregion. Thus, in many of the countries, older persons comprise under 5 percent of the overall population, while in a few others the proportion of older persons was much greater (i.e., over 10 percent).[4] Despite these trends in Africa, the UN (2019a) shows that persons aged 65 and above make up the world's fastest-growing age group, and it is anticipated that in the decades ahead the percentage of older persons around the world will increase. In view of this, Ritchie and Roser (*ibid*) have argued that many countries across the world are going through an important demographic transition: from young to increasingly aging populations. A contributory factor to this pattern has been the increase in life expectancy at birth for the world's population. This reached 72.6 years in 2019 representing an improvement of more than 8 years since 1990. The projections show that this is likely to increase to about 77.1 years in 2050 globally. The greatest gains in life expectancy were in sub-Saharan Africa, where improvements in survival added nearly 12 years to the average length of life since 1990, reaching 63.2 years in 2019 and expected to be 69.5 years by 2050 (United Nations, *ibid*).

Further analysis of recent United Nations population data shows that there is significant variation in life expectancy at birth across the subregions. Table 7.1 depicts trends in life expectancy and the proportion of the population older than 64 years for Africa and for the various subregions. The subregions with the lowest life expectancy rates are Middle and Western Africa, where the average person born in 2019 is expected to live up to about 58 years. In contrast, life expectancy is higher in Northern Africa, which is 72.6 years. In Southern and Eastern Africa, the life expectancy is on average over 63 years.

Undoubtedly, if this trend continues over the next few decades, the rise in life expectancy across Africa should translate into an increase in the proportion of adults over 64 years in the population. This would manifest in a rising number of older people in the population across all the subregions. Indeed, the relationship between increased life expectancy and aging can be seen in the second part of table 6.1. This shows that in the next decade, all the subregions will have a significant proportion of the aged in their population.

Although this is not depicted in table 6.1, another aspect of the elderly population is that women outnumber men owing to their longer average life expectancy. In 2019, women comprised 55 percent of those aged 65 years and above and 61 percent of those aged 80 years and above, globally (United Nations, 2019a). In Africa, the existing data show that there are slightly more women than men owing, in large part, to the difference in life expectancy among them. At the same time, older men and women in Africa with little to no access to pensions and other sources of income experience economic and social hardships, the majority of whom are thus unable to access basic social and health services.

What is obviously clear is that an increasing number of older persons in the general population presents a range of challenges to governments and the wider society. An important challenge will be the increased demand for primary healthcare and long-term care for the aged, especially so because life expectancy on the continent is improving. The fundamental question then is how to care for the aged and what challenges lie ahead.

CARING FOR THE AGED

We have noted earlier that aging poses many challenges to societies particularly those related to the provision of good healthcare. The aged usually lose their independence because they are no longer able to look after themselves. Besides, in the case of the very old, most lose their ability to live independently because of limited mobility, frailty, or other physical or mental health problems. Many therefore require some form of long-term care, which can include home nursing, community care and assisted living, residential care and long stays in hospitals (WHO Africa Region Office fact sheet on Ageing, 2020).

Significantly, several African countries have incorporated the ethos of the Madrid International Plan of Action on Ageing (MIPAA) and the African Union Policy Framework and Plan of Action on Ageing (PFPA) into their

Table 6.1 Trends in Life Expectancy and Proportion of the Population Older than 64 Years for Africa and Various Subregions

	Life Expectancy at Birth (years)				
	2019	*1995–2000*	*2005–2010*	*2015–2020*	*2025–2030*
Africa	63.2	52.3	60.3	62.7	65.4
Eastern Africa	64.8	49.2	56.1	64.2	67.3
Middle Africa	59.9	48.6	53.9	59.4	62.2
Southern Africa	63.8	58.2	54.0	63.3	65.8
Western Africa	57.9	48.4	52.6	57.3	60.5
Northern Africa	72.6	66.5	69.8	72.3	74.1
	Percentage of Population Aged 65+				
	2000	*2010*	*2020*	*2030*	*2050*
Africa	3.4	3.3	3.5	4.0	5.8
Eastern Africa	2.9	2.7	2.9	3.3	5.2
Middle Africa	3.0	2.8	2.8	3.0	4.0
Southern Africa	4.4	4.7	5.4	6.5	10.1
Western Africa	2.9	2.8	2.8	3.0	4.2
Northern Africa	4.6	5.0	5.8	7.4	11.2

Source: World Population Prospects (2019), Volume II: Demographic Profiles.

policy framework. The MIPAA and PFPA capture the need to cater for the health needs and well-being of the aged. To this end, the African Union adopted a protocol on the rights of older people at the 26th Ordinary Session on 31 January 2016 in Addis Ababa, Ethiopia.[5] Unfortunately, progress at implementation has been uneven and patchy across countries, with varying levels of mainstreaming and policy development within countries (African Union, 2015).

Although it is apparent that African governments generally recognize the challenge of population aging and the need to cater for their needs, the healthcare needs for the aged are worlds apart compared to those for children and young adults. This is further complicated by the presence of an already overburdened healthcare delivery system in nearly all African countries. Moreover, the forecasted increase in the number of aged persons in African countries means that these countries must begin to focus attention and efforts on providing age-appropriate preventive healthcare and medical needs of the elderly population.

Traditionally, within the African context, there is pride in the belief that older people as well as the young are well-cared for within family groups (Seeley et al., 1993; Brown, 1999; Foster, 2000). However, over the past three decades, many African societies have experienced dramatic social and economic transformation resulting in significant changes in family structure. The rapid rate of urbanization has also meant the reliance on traditional extended family systems to care for the young and old who are frail and vulnerable can no longer be guaranteed. And as succinctly argued by Gysels et al. (2011), the capacity of the traditional extended family structure to provide care has changed permanently. Moreover, they note that it is also a myth that the extended family structure is endowed with inexhaustible resources to withstand crisis, especially relating to healthcare for the elderly.

Concerning the well-being of the aged, Aboderin (2005) notes that, in Africa, this presents significant health challenges. Lifestyle changes associated with modernization and urbanization have resulted in a gradual shift away from communicable and infectious diseases to noncommunicable diseases in many parts of the continent. Additionally, the World Health Organization (2018) notes that the age cohorts for which the services are least available on the continent are the adolescents and the elderly. Sadly, of the two age cohorts, it is the elderly who possess a relatively higher disease burden. This is not a surprise given that aging populations have an increased prevalence of chronic diseases, physical disabilities, mental illnesses, and other comorbidities (Boutayeb and Boutayeb, 2005).

THE HEALTHCARE NEEDS OF THE AGED

As people live longer, their healthcare needs also increase. This is so because they live with long-term medical conditions such as arthritis, blindness, hypertension, diabetes, disabilities, heart disease, and stroke (Ayernor, 2012; Jaul and Barron, 2017). While some of these conditions may be caused by lifestyle choices or conditions such as increased sedentariness, smoking and alcohol abuse, others are the result of and compounded by the processes of aging (Thorogood et al., 2007; Acosta et al., 2010; Westaway, 2010; National Institutes of Health, 2011; World Health Organization, 2014; Mugisha et al., 2016). Given the complexities involved in the health conditions of the aged, the provision of good healthcare services for them must involve careful planning and coordination by many actors. In the main, this would involve the state, non-state actors, such as charities and nongovernmental organizations (NGOs), and critically families.

It is worthy to emphasize that prior to the adoption by the African Union of the protocol on older people in Africa, many African countries had put in place national policies or legislation on aging or for the aged. These countries include Tunisia, Egypt, Ghana, Kenya, Mozambique, South Sudan, South Africa, Ethiopia, Madagascar, Malawi, Uganda, Tanzania, and Zimbabwe (UNFPA and HelpAge International, 2011; Geng, 2019; Saka et al., 2019).[6] Despite the presence of these policies and legislations, there is the persistent problem of implementation of national policies as well as the existence of inequalities in access to services, particularly healthcare. Thus, in Africa, many older persons do not have universal and equal access to healthcare services. These inequalities are not surprising, however. As observed by Marmot and Wilkinson (2005), in general health inequalities are usually the product not only of unequal access to healthcare services but also of social and economic inequality.

One contributory factor to such inequalities has been the skewed pattern of investment in the provision of healthcare services across the continent. We previously observed that in Africa investment in healthcare provision for the population has tended to be concentrated on the children and women. To buttress this point, an assessment by the World Health Organization (2018) for the African region shows that most countries have only been able to make available 36 percent of the essential services needed by their population to attain good health and well-being. The report further notes that the situation is even worse for the elderly where a large proportion of countries do not have any services to cater for their healthcare needs. It is apparent that the situation over the years across the continent has not improved. A few years back, the World Health Organization (2014) pointed out that health systems had not made adequate provision for older people and were not prepared to respond to their needs.

But this picture of the general state of healthcare provision for the aged masks individual exceptions in a few countries since 2002. For example, in Ghana, Cameroon, Nigeria, Namibia, Morocco, and Egypt, there are policies and programs on equal and affordable access to primary and secondary healthcare which explicitly include older persons and promote their access to health facilities. In other countries, such as Kenya, South Africa, and Mozambique, older persons' healthcare has been mainstreamed into general health policy (UNFPA and HelpAge International, *ibid*).

Nevertheless, the situation concerning the overall state of preparedness and state of healthcare services' provision across the continent requires urgent action. In fact, the urgency to improve the provision of essential healthcare services for the general population and especially for the aged cannot be overemphasized. In addition, considering the population dynamics highlighted earlier, there is no need to overstate the importance for countries in the region to focus energies and attention toward the healthcare needs of the aged. This is because the medical conditions that afflict the aged are mostly chronic in nature, incurable, and invariably result in disabilities and degenerative disorders. But, sadly, the aged lack access to the needed services.

In thinking of how countries must respond to this situation, we are guided by Cohen and Menken's (2006) observation that the policy response to the health and disability needs of the aged cannot be uniform across countries or regions. This is because the living conditions of the elderly and the nature of the problems they face differ considerably within and across countries. Notwithstanding the heterogeneous nature of the state of affairs, we believe there are many generalizations that can be made regarding the healthcare needs for the aged. And as recently suggested by the World Health Organization (2018) concerning the availability of essential healthcare services, there are some cohort-specific services which every country's health sector must proactively plan to ensure their provision. Therefore, in respect of the healthcare services and care for the aged, it will be important to provide specific and necessary interventions—at the societal and medical levels—to address their healthcare needs.

SOCIETAL INTERVENTIONS

At the societal level it is critical to the well-being—socially and mentally—of the aged for the society to assist them achieve the maximum possible functioning in everyday life and for them to gain the highest possible level of welfare, thereby improving their health-related quality of life (Murphy, 2018; Westway and Maluka, *ibid*). For this to be achieved, a wide array of social factors must be considered. These, for example, include how to address the empty nest syndrome and thus assist the aged deal with the challenge of isolation, how to support the aged when they go without any physical support in their daily activities, and how to overcome maltreatment toward the elderly, especially gender-related discrimination toward older women. Others issues include how to overcome the limited knowledge on food and nutritional requirements that minimize risk factors associated with old age, how to help them deal with psycho-emotional concerns (mental stress, difficulty in keeping themselves occupied), and financial constraints that are the result of reduced income upon retirement or the lack of adequate pensions.

Remarkably, the United Nations Economic Commission for Africa's report on the state of older people in 2007 indicated a high level of awareness by several African governments to the needs of the aged. Countries such as South Africa, Mauritius, and Tunisia were recognized as having some of the best practices in dealing with the challenge of aging. In South Africa, an old age grant is provided monthly to elderly citizens without other means of regular income support. Likewise, Botswana, Lesotho, Mauritius, and Namibia provide similar grants to their elderly. In all these countries, the grants were found to substantially reduce poverty rates among older persons. These examples are, however, in contrast to the general situation on the continent. In recognition of the need to do more, the Economic Commission for Africa in conjunction with HelpAge International and other international agencies urged governments to put in place appropriate policies to ensure older people were not left behind in efforts to achieve the Sustainable Development Goals (UNECA, 2019).

Governments' actions are therefore crucial in how society responds to the needs of the aged. In an age of hyperglobalization and increased migration, many of the aged are going to be confronted with isolation and possible desolation. In the absence of formal structures to provide home visits and home care for the aged, especially those who are frail, the social welfare departments in countries will have to develop innovative ways to engage younger members within neighborhoods to be visiting elderly people who are alone or isolated due to physical disabilities. Ultimately, the objective of such programs and interventions will be to achieve sustained, not marginalized, levels of physical and social functioning for the aged within the society. An aged person with an active life, even if a reduced rate, will inevitably have a balanced, mentally stable lifestyle.

MEDICAL INTERVENTIONS

Perhaps, the most critical interventions in caring for the aged is at the clinical level. The aged population will require essential healthcare services to monitor their health status and ensure early and effective interventions to maintain a generally healthy state of well-being. Nevertheless, as noted by Saka et al. (*ibid*), the current policies to promote access to health care for older people in sub-Saharan Africa are not encouraging. Moreover, Parmar et al. (*ibid*) have also observed the increased vulnerability of older people in relation to illness and healthcare expenditures. However, as sign of progress and in contrast to the general case in the region, countries such as Senegal, Ghana, and South Africa have implemented Social Health Protection (SHP) programs—Plan Sesame in Senegal, National Health Insurance Scheme in Ghana, and National Health Insurance in South Africa—that specifically target older people. Under these programs, older people have access to free healthcare or are exempted from paying health insurance premiums (Parmar et al., 2014; Saka et al., *ibid*).

In general, however, most older people on the continent lack or have inadequate health insurance coverage for older. This will ultimately limit their access to healthcare. To overcome some of these challenges, we note Murphy's (*ibid*) argument regarding care for the aged. He has suggested the need to provide lifetime health promotion, ensure universal and equal access to healthcare services, provide training for care and health staff to attend effectively to the health needs of the aged and in particular those living with HIV/AIDS, mental health issues and disabilities. In addition, considering the levels of inactivity that many older persons suffer, it will be pertinent to invest in physiotherapy care to assist and enable the aged overcome physical inactivity, which may be caused by chronic diseases, such as diabetes, stroke as well as other degenerative disorders.

What types of medical intervention can be put in place to address the healthcare needs of the aged? We are guided by three recommendations by the World Health Organization (2018) concerning essential services for the elderly. These are instituting systems to ensure annual screening and medical examination for the aged, providing social support services, and the provision of clinical and rehabilitative services.

About the first, which is ensuring annual screening and medical examinations, governments can fully integrate elderly care into a national universal primary healthcare system. This way, the care of the elderly will be given the same treatment accorded to children and women, especially pregnant women. Persons who turn sixty can easily walk into any primary healthcare provider and undergo these examinations. Considering the operating environments of most healthcare institutions, it will be essential that dedicated units for older people are set up. This will make it easier and less stressful for the elderly to access such services. The universal component of this provision means it must be free at the point of service.

The provision of social support services is important in the care of older persons, particularly those who are not too ill to be in hospital but need care in one form or another. But this requires both physical infrastructure as well as personnel to cater for the care needs of the aged. The aim of providing social support services is to augment the societal interventions discussed earlier. However, the social support service envisioned is the establishment of day care for the elderly as well as care homes to take care of very ill persons. The day care centers will help in addressing some of the problems of isolation, loneliness, boredom, and mental stress which older persons experience.

The final piece of the medical interventions is the clinical and rehabilitative services. Unfortunately, in many countries, the health systems are unprepared and underfunded to respond to the healthcare needs of the aged. Many reports by the World Health Organization show that healthcare facilities focusing on elderly people are lacking, infrastructure is inappropriate, and health professionals are not well trained in old age care. As summarized by the World Health Organization (2014), there is a lack of healthcare services specifically catering for older people, inappropriate infrastructure, and inadequate geriatric medicine and gerontology.

In that regard, government investment in scaling up existing facilities and reorienting medical staff toward the needs of the aged is vital. Besides, focus of clinical and rehabilitative services must as a matter of priority be geared toward prevention and self-care. As the adage goes, prevention is better, but also cheaper, than a cure. The clinical conditions that old persons present are much difficult to handle when health facilities are lacking in the expertise and resources to handle, and invariably the consequences for the aged are dire.

Finally, it is worth emphasizing that these three approaches—instituting systems to ensure annual screening and medical examination for the aged, providing social support services, and providing clinical and rehabilitative services—must not be regarded as stand-alone measures, but as part of a well-integrated and coordinated set of health interventions to address the needs of the aged in society.

CHALLENGES IN HEALTHCARE PROVISION FOR THE AGED

Our discussions so far point to the need for a reinvigoration of existing healthcare systems to recognize and address the needs of the aged. Critical in all these is how to ensure equitable access to essential health and care providers, medicines, and health diagnostics. But the unanswered question is who pays for the costs? It is worth mentioning that many who are old in Africa are also very poor. Sadly, healthcare costs are very high and for persons who are typically not working or enjoying comfortable pensions the costs of care and medication can induce further trauma. This is because the medical conditions faced by the aged are chronic and ultimately result in disabilities. Therefore, the medical costs become long term and tend to escalate with time due to the higher than normal rates of inflation in the cost of healthcare services.

Additionally, governments across the continent must invest in more systematic and proactive management of chronic diseases with the objective of improving health outcomes. It should not be the norm where medical personnel regard the process of aging as a form of illness for which the aged must become accustomed to being unwell all the time. The goal of the clinical and rehabilitative system must be to improve health outcomes, reduce inappropriate use of hospitals, and address in a significant manner the health inequalities faced by the aged.

Finally, governments across the continent must invest in developing systems to acquire appropriate and timely aging-related data. This will help in the development of well-targeted policies and programs to address the healthcare and well-being needs of the aged.

CONCLUSIONS

The population in Africa is gradually experiencing the demographic transition seen elsewhere in the world. Eventually, the number of older persons in the population will be such that it will be impossible to ignore their health needs.

Consequently, there will be an increased demand for primary healthcare and long-term care. This will require a larger and better trained workforce and the need to make the lived environments more age-friendly.

Furthermore, governments must invest in and scale-up existing healthcare infrastructure and enhance the standards and quality of training in health training institutions. Additionally, other support systems such as housing, transportation, water and sanitation, which are currently inadequate to meet the basic needs of a growing aging population must be expanded.

Finally, governments must ensure that in their efforts to achieve economic development they must be guided by the sustainable development goals, so that truly no one is left behind, especially the aged in our societies.

NOTES

1. This is based on several issues of the African Regional Health Report published by the WHO.

2. There is a slight complication regarding the presentation of statistics on the aged in this chapter. Whilst we use the chronological cut off age of 60 years or above to define the elderly, the available statistics on population structure are based on standardized age cohorts. Hence, we make approximations regarding the aged in Africa using the cut off age of 65 and over. This surely underestimates the actual proportion of the aged in the African context.

3. Using data from the United Nations Population Prospects 2019, part of which is presented in table 7.1 in the main text, we find a strong positive correlation between life expectancy and the proportion of the aged in the population for various years and across the subregions and countries.

4. A fuller analysis of the population trends in Africa is outside the scope of the chapter.

5. The full title of the protocol is Protocol to the African Charter on Human and Peoples' Rights on the Rights of Older People in Africa.

6. Below are a few examples of national policies on the elderly as well as legislation addressing the needs of the elderly in selected countries in Africa.

National Policies:

Ghana: National Ageing Policy "Ageing with Security and Dignity" and Implementation Action Plan 2010
Kenya: National Policy on Older Persons and Ageing 2009
Mozambique: National Policy on Older Persons 2002; National Plan for Older People 2006–2010
South Africa: South Africa Older Persons' Policy 2006
Uganda: National Policy for Older Persons 2009
Tunisia: Decennial Plan to care about the Elderly 2003
Tanzania: National Ageing Policy 2003

Legislation:
Madagascar: Law no 2008/030 Protection of Older People's Rights 2008
South Africa: Older Persons Act 2006

REFERENCES

Acosta, Daisy, Ruth Rottbeck, Juana G. Rodríguez, Loida M. González, Mary R. Almánzar, Susana N. Minaya, Maria del C Ortiz, Cleusa P. Ferri and Martin J. Prince. 2010. "The prevalence and social patterning of chronic diseases among older people in a population undergoing health transition. A 10/66 group cross-sectional population-based survey in the Dominican Republic." *BMC Public Health* 10(344). https://doi.org/10.1186/1471-2458-10-344

African Union 2015. The African Union and HelpAge urge member states to promote the rights of older people in Africa. https://au.int/en/newsevents/28087/african-union-and-helpage-urge-member-states-promote-rights-older-people-africa

Anyinam, Charles. 1987. "Traditional medical practice in contemporary Ghana: A dying or growing "profession"?" *Canadian Journal of African Studies* 21(3): 315–36.

Ayernor, P. K. 2012. "Diseases of ageing in Ghana." *Ghana Medical Journal* 46(Supplement 2): 18–22.

Baronov, David. 2008. *The African transformation of western medicine and the dynamics of global cultural exchange*. Philadelphia: Temple University Press.

Bloom, David E., David Canning and Günther Fink. 2010. "Implications of population ageing for economic growth." *Oxford Review of Economic Policy* 26(4): 583–612.

Boutayeb Abdesslam and Saber Boutayeb. 2005. "The burden of non-communicable diseases in developing countries." *International Journal for Equity in Health* 4(2). doi:10.1186/1475-9276-4-2.

Brown, Malcolm J. 1999. "The plight of rural elderly in South Africa: A case for a community development cadre?" *Community Development Journal* 34(2): 143–150.

Cohen B. and J. Menken (editors). 2006. *Aging in Sub-Saharan Africa: Recommendation for furthering research.* Washington, DC: National Academies Press, USA.

Dziechciaż, Malgorzata and Rafal Filip. 2014. "Biological psychological and social determinants of old age: Bio-psycho-social aspects of human aging." *Annals of Agricultural and Environmental Health* 21(21): 832–838.

Foster, G. 2000. "The capacity of the extended family safety net for orphans in Africa." *Psychology, Health and Medicine* 5(1): 55–62.

Geng, Peter Garang. 2019. *Protection of rights of older persons in South Sudan: Towards enactment of legislative framework.* Sudan: The Sudd Institute.

Gysels, Marjolein., Christopher Pell, Lianne Straus and Robert Pool. 2011. "End of life care in Sub-Saharan Africa: A systematic review of the qualitative literature." *BMC Palliative Care* 10(6). https://doi.org/10.1186/1472-684X-10-6

International Finance Corporation. 2016. *The business of health in Africa: Partnering with the private sector to improve people's lives*. Washington DC: International Finance Corporation.

Jaul, Efraim and Jeremy Barron. 2017. "Age-related diseases and clinical and public health implications for the 85 years old and over population." *Frontiers in Public Health* 5(335) doi: 10.3389/fpubh.2017.00335.

Johnson, M. 1976. "Is 65+ old?" *Social Policy*. (Nov/Dec): 9–12.

Kwankye, Stephen Owusu. 2013. "Growing old in Ghana: Health and economic implications." *Postgraduate Medical Journal* 2(2) 88–97.

Marmot, Michael and Richard, G. Wilkinson (editors). 2005. *Social determinants of health, Second Edition*. Oxford University Press.

Mugisha, Joseph O., Enid J. Schatz, M. Randell, Madeleine Kuteesa, Monica Kuteesa, Paul Kowal, Joel Negin, and Janet Seeley. 2016. "Chronic disease, risk factors and disability in adults aged 50 and above living with and without HIV: Findings from the wellbeing of older people study in Uganda." *Global Health Action* 9(1), 31098. DOI: 10.3402/gha.v9.31098.

Murphy, Michael. 2018. "Ageing in Sub-Saharan Africa in the context of global development: The multiple indicator survey project (MISA)." United Nations Department for Economics and Social Affairs (UNDESA). https://www.un.org/development/desa/dspd/wp-content/uploads/sites/22/2019/06/population-ageing-project.pdf

National Institutes of Health. 2011. "Global health and ageing." NIH Publication no. 11-7737.

Parmar, Divya, Gemma Williams, Fahdi Dkhimi, Alfred Ndiaye, Felix Ankomah Asante, Daniel Kojo Arhinful and Philipa Mladovsky. 2014. "Enrolment of older people in social health protection programs in West Africa—Does social exclusion play a part?" *Social Science and Medicine* 119 (2014): 36–44.

Ritchie, Hannah and Max Roser. 2020. "Age structure." Published online at OurWorldInData.org. Retrieved from: 'https://ourworldindata.org/age-structure' [16/04/2020].

Roebuck Janet. 1979. "When does 'old age begin?': The evolution of the English definition." *Journal of Social History*, 12(3): 416–28.

Saka, Sule, Frasia Oosthuizen, and Manimbulu Nlooto. 2019. "National policies and older people's healthcare in Sub-Saharan Africa: A scoping review." *Annals of Global Health* 85(1): 91, 1–7. DOI: https://doi.org/10.5334/aogh.2401.

Seeley, J., E. Kajura, C. Bachengana, M. Okongo, U. Wagner and D. Mulder. 1993. "The extended family and support for people with AIDS in a rural population in south west Uganda: A safety net with holes?" *AIDS Care: Psychological and Socio-medical Aspects of AIDS/HIV* 5(1): 117-122.

Thorogood, Margaret, Myles D. Connor, Gillian Lewando Hundt and Stephen M. Tollman. 2007. "Understanding and managing hypertension in an African sub-district: A multidisciplinary approach." *Scandinavian Journal of Public Health* 35(Supplement 69): 52–59.

UNCTAD. 2019. *The Least Developed Countries report 2019*. New York: United Nations.

UNFPA and HelpAge International. 2011. *Overview of available policies and legislation, data and research, and institutional arrangements relating to older persons - progress since Madrid.* New York: United Nations Population Fund.

United Nations. 2019a. "World population prospects 2019: Highlights." United Nations Department for Economic and Social Affairs.

United Nations. 2019b. "World population prospects 2019: Volume II demographic profiles." United Nations for Economic and Social Affairs.

United Nations Economic Commission for Africa. 2007. *The state of older people in Africa—2007: Regional review and appraisal of the Madrid International Plan of Action on Ageing.* Addis Ababa: UNECA.

United Nations Economic Commission for Africa (2019). United Nations Economic Commission for Africa Press Issue *on Inclusion of older people in SDGs crucial for Africa's development* https://www.uneca.org/stories/inclusion-older-people-sdgs-crucial-africa%E2%80%99s-development [Retrieved 28/04/2020]

Velkoff, Victoria A., and Paul R. Kowal. 2006. "Aging in Sub-Saharan Africa: The changing demography of the region." In *Aging in Sub-Saharan Africa: Recommendation for furthering research*, edited by Barney Cohen and Jane Menken, 55—91. Washington, DC: National Academies Press (USA).

Westaway, Margaret S., and Constance S. Maluka. 2004. "Impact of chronic diseases on the health-related quality of life of South Africans." *South African Medical Journal* 94(12): 937.

Westway, Margaret S. 2010. "Effects of ageing, chronic disease and co-morbidity on the health and well-being of older residents of Greater Tshwane." *South African Medical Journal* 100(1): 35–36.

World Health Organisation. 2002. "Proposed working definition of an older person in Africa for the Minimum Data Set for Ageing in Africa Project." Geneva: WHO.

World Health Organization. 2018. *The State of Health of the WHO African Region: An analysis of the status of health, health services and health systems in the context of the Sustainable Development Goals.* Brazzaville, Congo: WHO.

World Health Organization. 2020. WHO Factsheet on Aging. https://www.afro.who.int/health-topics/ageing, Retrieved on 21/04/2020.

World Health Organization. 2014. *The African Regional Health Report: The health of the people, what works.* Geneva: World Health Organization.

Chapter 7

Ghana's National Health Insurance Authority and Provision of Quality Healthcare Services

Some Reflections on the Provider Payment Reforms within the National Health Insurance Scheme

Francis-Xavier Andoh-Adjei

HEALTH CARE FINANCING, INCLUDING INSURANCE IN GHANA

Historical Background to Healthcare Financing in Ghana

Healthcare financing in Ghana started in the 1880s during which period persons who accessed curative healthcare services were made to pay fees for the services they used (Ministry of Health, 2015). When Ghana attained independence in 1957, however, the user fees were abolished but later in 1971, some minimal fees were introduced as partial cost recovery measure to ensure uninterrupted service provision at the health facilities (Appiah-Denkyira and Preker, 2007). Between 1969 and 1972, the government of Ghana initiated moves to introduce a social health insurance scheme to provide financial risk protection against the cost of healthcare services for the citizens. This initiative was, however, curtailed with the overthrow of the government in 1972.

Between the mid-1970s and early 1980s, Ghana experienced economic downturn, a situation that compelled the country to heed to the advice and support of the World Bank (WB) and the International Monetary Fund (IMF) to adopt Economic Recovery Program (ERP) in 1983. The government agreed to remove subsidies on social services, including those on healthcare services as part of the conditions to qualify for the ERP package. In 1985, the

Hospital Fees Regulation, 1985 (L.I. 1313) which sought to raise the user fees charged at government health facilities was introduced in order to generate more income to pay for at least 15 percent of the Ministry of Health's total recurrent expenditure (Vogel, 1988). The user fees were used to purchase equipment and medicines but this was inadequate as more financial resources were needed to cover the total cost of service provision.

With an average per capita income of US$390 at the time, and a daily minimum wage of less than US$1, a large proportion of the population could not afford to pay their medical bills. The user fees, which became known as "cash and carry" system, generated a number of debates in the country with a section of the public arguing that it denied the sick from accessing needed healthcare services, thereby, contributing to preventable deaths among the population. They therefore advocated its withdrawal from the health delivery system in Ghana.

The Genesis of Health Insurance in Ghana

While the government was considering feasible solutions to address the problem of financial access to healthcare services, communities also started mobilizing themselves to respond to their health needs in their own ways. In 1992, the first Community-Based Health Insurance Scheme (CBHIS) was established by the Nkoranza community with support from the Catholic Church to mobilize financial resources to pay for their healthcare costs (Agyepong and Adjei, 2008). The initiative inspired other communities such as Techiman and Damango to adopt the same method for implementation in their respective areas.

In 1998, the government also designed a social health insurance scheme for piloting in the eastern region with the ultimate aim of replicating it nationwide but the initiative could not go beyond the pilot stage (Agyepong and Adjei, 2008). This attempted initiative, nonetheless, raised awareness about the need for some form of social health protection to cater for health care in times of need. Consequently, by 2003, about 159 voluntary health insurance schemes had been established in sixty-seven districts across the country (Atim, 1999; International Labour Organization, 2005). These community initiatives were, however, not coordinated nor regulated by any legal framework and membership was strictly based on members' contribution and, therefore, the poor and needy who could not make the required contributions were left out of the safety net (Andoh-Adjei , 2019).

Health Insurance as a Political Agenda

In the run-up to elections 2000, the issue of healthcare financing became politically topical with the then opposition New Patriotic Party (NPP) promising to establish a National Health Insurance Scheme for the population if voted into power (Agyepong and Adjei, 2008). The NPP eventually won the elections and in keeping with its promise, the NPP-led government established the National Health Insurance Scheme (NHIS) through the National Health Insurance Act, 2003 (Act 650) in 2003. This was to provide financial access to health care for all citizens and legal residents in Ghana. The law made provision for the establishment of three health insurance schemes: District Mutual Health Insurance Scheme (DMHIS), Private Mutual Health Insurance Scheme (PMHIS), and Private Commercial Health Insurance Scheme (PCHIS) (Government of Ghana, 2003; Government of Ghana, 2012). It provided for a basic benefit package that covers close to 95 percent of diseases that afflict the population. It also established a National Health Insurance Fund (NHIF) to be financed through earmarked tax to provide consistent and sustainable funding to the scheme.

Sources of funding include a 2.5 percent Value-Added Tax (VAT), 2.5 percentage points of 18.5 percent employees' Social Security Contributions to the Pension Fund, government of Ghana annual budgetary allocations proposed and approved by parliament to the NHIF; accruals from investments of surplus funds held in the NHIF by the NHIA; grants, gifts, and donations made to the NHIF; and graduated membership contributions paid by members in the informal sector (Government of Ghana, 2003). The Act 650 has since 2012 been replaced with a new National Health Insurance Act 2012 (Act 852) as part of the continuous reforms of the health insurance policy. The NHIF has contributed immensely toward health financing in Ghana since its establishment.

The NHIS, however, started facing financial sustainability challenges from 2009 partly due to inefficiencies in the provider payment system. With only about 34 percent of the projected national population covered by the NHIS in 2010, it was observed that service utilization rates, especially outpatients services, had been increasing. For instance, Outpatient Department OPD utilization increased from 597,859 in 2005 to 16,931,263 in 2010 while claims payment to service providers increased from GH¢7.60 million in 2005 to GH¢394.27 million in 2010 (NHIA, 2010). Thus, growth in utilization translated into growth in claims expenditure and whereas one may acknowledge that the growth in service utilization may be due to the yearly growth in membership and the removal of financial barrier to accessing healthcare service, it was not certain whether this phenomenon was a genuine one and that it was not partly due to moral hazard. Whichever reason one may conjecture, the fact still remained that the yearly increase in utilization and claims expenditure, particularly outpatient (OPD) claims, posed challenges for cost containment and sustainability of the NHIS. Managers of the scheme, therefore, decided to introduce reforms into the provider payment system to address the inefficiencies identified.

PROVIDER PAYMENT REFORMS WITHIN THE NATIONAL HEALTH INSURANCE SCHEME

The Need for Provider Payment Reforms in Countries' Health Systems

Reforms in health system financing, including provider payment reforms worldwide, are driven by the need to improve efficiency in the provision and use of healthcare services. In the United States of America (USA), Medicare introduced payment reforms on the back of escalating health expenditure (Grabowski, Afendulis, and McGuire, 2011). In Hungary, payment reforms were introduced in 2008 to improve efficiency in the allocation of scarce healthcare resources (Nagy and Brandtmuller, 2008). In Sweden, provider payment at the primary care level is directed by patients' choice of primary care provider and a predetermined amount per registered patient is paid to the provider (Anell, Glenngard, and Merkur, 2012).

Key provider payment methods applied in countries' health systems include fee-for-service (FFS), diagnosis-related-groupings (DRG) and capitation payments, among others. Under FFS payment method, healthcare providers are reimbursed based on the item of service they provide and their income is aligned to the quantity of service that they provide (Rudmik, Wranik, and Rudisill-Michaelsen, 2014). It is aassociated with supplier-induced demand (Barnum, Kutzin and Saxeniam, 1995) and it is described by some experts as reward for "volume and intensity rather than value," and "inflationary and ineffective in containing cost" (Econex, 2010). This is because it creates incentives to increase service provision and pushes the financial risk to the payer only. FFS is used in countries such as Belgium, Germany, and Japan (Park et al., 2007), as well as in many low- and middle-income countries, including Ghana. On realizing the negative incentives that FFS payment creates, many countries have adopted moves toward DRG payment in their countries' health system (Mathauer and Wittenbecher, 2013). DRG was initially designed as a quality and utilization-monitoring tool (Averill et al., 2003). It aligns diagnosis and treatment to cost. Under DRG, providers are paid predetermined rate for services they provide based on illness episode. It has strong incentive to induce efficiency and cost-containment (Park et al., 2007). The advantages of DRG are that it offers incentives for providers to give patients a more severe diagnosis to attract a higher reimbursement (Agyepong et al., 2014). Hence, many countries combine it with other forms of payment methods, such as capitation payment at the primary care level. Under capitation payment system, providers are paid agreed sum of money per listed patient for a period of time, usually one year, to provide predetermined services for them. Experts in provider payment systems agree that capitation payment helps to eliminate supplier-induced demand that is normally associated with fee-for-service payment (Rudmik, Wranik, and Rudisill-Michaelsen, 2014; Rosen, 1989) but also caution that unless the capitated rate is risk-adjusted, at least by age and sex, providers may pay less attention to perceived risk groups on their list (Park et al., 2007; Randall and McGuire, 1986).

Acknowledging that each provider payment method has its own strengths and weaknesses, countries have been reforming their provider payment systems to improve efficiency in healthcare delivery (Ginsburg, 2013; Qingyue, 2005). One characteristic of such reform is the adoption of mixed payment methods, leveraging their strengths and minimizing their weaknesses to ensure cost-efficiency and quality improvement in their health systems (Rosenthal, 2008).

Provider Payment Methods and Payment Reforms under the NHIS

Regulation 37(2) of the Legislative Instrument, 2004 (L.I. 1809), mandates the National Health Insurance Authority (NHIA) to develop uniform provider payment mechanisms (PPM) to pay its credentialed healthcare providers for services that they render to active members of the NHIS (NHIA, 2010). The L.I. 1809 particularly mentioned capitation and fee-for-service payments as the key provider payment methods, but also stated that "others as determined by the NHIA" may be used for reimbursement under the NHIS. At the inception of its operations in 2005, the NHIA adopted FFS payment method to pay its credentialed providers. Later in 2008, the Ghana version of DRG which became known as Ghana-Diagnosis-Related Grouping (G-DRG) system was introduced with the view to containing the escalating cost that was being experienced under the FFS payment method. The G-DRG method was implemented nationwide and at all levels of care. It is currently used to pay for both outpatients (OPD) and inpatients (IPD) services while FFS is used to pay for medicines.

The switch from FFS to G-DRG was done without any study to understand the underlying causes of the effects of FFS. Likewise, the G-DRG was introduced without any pilot, neither was it subjected to prospective evaluation to assess its likely impact in relation to the cost-containment objective for which it was introduced. Consequently, the G-DRG was later observed to have rather contributed further to cost escalation. A joint assessment of the Ghana Health Sector Programme of Work by the Ministry of Health, its agencies and partners in 2012 revealed that since its introduction, the NHIS has led to an increase in utilization of OPD services across all the regions. The assessment team noted that only 34 percent of the projected national population were active members of the NHIS but the OPD per capita had doubled with 80 percent of total outpatients being NHIS-insured members. They, therefore, raised concerns that the high proportion of OPD attendance could either be a reflection of frivolous use of services by NHIS members or a reflection of high NHIS membership among those in need of services. They concluded that a positive answer to those concerns poses potential financial risk to NHIS (Ministry of Health-Ghana, 2013).

Capitation as Provider Payment Method for Primary Care

Under capitation payment, providers are paid agreed sum of money per insured member for a period of time, usually one year, to provide predetermined services for registered members. Two types of capitation systems may be identified: list capitation system and geographic capitation system (Jegers et al., 2002). The list capitation payment ties the aggregate income of the provider to the number of patients enrolled to him/her while geographic capitation payment ties reimbursement to the population living within a particular geographical area. Capitation payment is expected to promote efficient use of resources by controlling prices and volumes of services provided. Payers of healthcare services have the benefit of knowing their budgets in advance under capitation payment, while providers pay attention to health education to keep their enrolees healthy in order to reduce utilization of curative services to save cost. It addresses the issue of supplier-induced demand associated with fee-for-service payment (Rudmik, Wranik, and Rudisill-Michaelsen, 2014; Rosen, 1989).

Many countries in the world, including the Scandinavian countries, the United Kingdom (UK), and Thailand apply capitation payment but with variations (Scott et al., 2011; Waters et al., 2004). The UK applies full risk-adjustment formula for calculating the capitated rate, Denmark adjusts its capitated rate by age and sex while capitation rate in Thailand is determined by government and has no risk-adjustment formula. Many countries in Central Europe and the Baltic states use capitation adjusted for age and sex to pay for primary care (Szende and Mogyorosy, 2004). On realizing that the FFS and the DRG payments could not help control the observed escalating growth in utilization and claims expenditures, the NHIA decided to introduce capitation payment for primary care services but unlike other countries, the capitated rate in Ghana was not risk-adjusted. Besides, unlike other countries where the capitation is organized around general practitioners (GPs), the model in Ghana was organized around institutional providers, be they public or private.

The Politics and Politicization of Capitation Payment Policy in Ghana

The introduction of capitation payment for primary care was met with resistance from healthcare provider professional associations (acting on behalf of their members) and some civil society organizations on the grounds that capitation payment would have adverse effects on healthcare delivery. The Society of Private Medical and Dental Practitioners (SPMDP), in a press release, communicated to the public that they had suspended provision of services to NHIS members because they believe that the capitation payment system was "*detrimental to quality of health care provision and a major threat to the survival of private health facilities*" (The Ghanaian Times newspaper of 02/01/2012). The Pharmaceutical Society of Ghana was also reported to have sued the NHIA over capitation payment on the grounds that it "*poses grave danger to patients given among other factors the recognition it (capitation payment) gives to persons outside the pharmacy profession*" (The Daily Guide newspaper of 23/01/2012). The *Daily Guide* newspaper of 25/01/2012, again, reported a statement attributed to a civil society group, the Ashanti Development Union (ADU), to the effect that "*since the implementation of the (capitation) policy in the region started hospital attendance has gone down considerably*," a situation that suggested perceived poor quality of care on the part of health insurance subscribers in the region following the introduction of the capitation payment policy.

The leadership of the faith-based provider groups was, however, supportive of the capitation payment policy. The executive director of Christian Health Association of Ghana (CHAG) was reported to have stated that "*our pledged support (for capitation payment) is premised on the belief that the pilot has the vibrant objective to promote efficiency of health facilities, (...) and also ensure cost containment for payers as well as ensuring financial sustainability of the health facilities without compromising quality of care*" (The Ghanaian Times Newspaper of 27/01/2012). Capitation payment, thus, became a public and political economy discourse in Ghana, with proponents rationalizing its importance and usefulness for healthcare delivery in Ghana; and opponents calling for its withdrawal. This was an interesting public discourse because while economic theory has it that the way providers are paid can influence their behavior negatively to provide less quantity and quality of service, studies have shown that capitation payment, and indeed, all other provider payment methods, have both positive and negative effects on healthcare delivery and that the way each of them is designed and implemented determines how much benefits health systems can derive from them (Andoh-Adjei et al., 2016).

However, besides the technical reasoning was the political debate which sought to question why the Ashanti region was selected for the pilot. Incidentally, the Ashanti region, from the political point of view, is the so-called stronghold of the then opposition party, NPP, and as was reflected in the responses of a survey in the region, the choice of the region for the pilot was perceived to be politically motivated. A study of provider-patient trust relationship revealed that notwithstanding respondents' high trust in their preferred primary care providers (PPP) and in the NHIS under the capitation payment and their positive perception about the attributes of capitation, they nonetheless exhibited negative attitude toward capitation payment. About 58 percent had the feeling that implementation of capitation payment in the Ashanti region was politically motivated while 65 percent perceived capitation payment as causing frustration to the insured patients at the health facilities. Another 49 percent indicated that capitation contributes to deaths in the implementing region (Andoh-Adjei et al., 2016). Thus, one key question that generated debate around the choice of the capitation pilot area was "why Ashanti Region?" Without necessarily defending the choice of Ashanti Region for the pilot, one may want to reason out that the region serves as a relatively good sample for such an endeavor for reasons which include, but not limited to the following:

i. it had the highest number of schemes and the highest number of active card-bearing members,
ii. the region is relatively compact and is strategically located in the heart of Ghana which makes it more convenient for close supervision and coordination of the pilot,
iii. it has all three levels of communities, namely urban, peri-urban, and rural districts,
iv. it has a good mix of providers in terms of type, level, and ownership which makes it convenient for comparative analysis, and
v. it has equally a good mix of people with diverse cultural backgrounds considering the fact that culture influences the health-seeking behavior of people.

Thus, though it might not have been politically sound to pilot the policy in that region to potentially avoid its politicization, technically it was not a bad idea to have piloted the policy in that region. That notwithstanding, in the year 2017, a new management team and governing body appointed by the NPP-led government took over affairs of the NHIS and suspended the capitation payment policy that had been on pilot implementation since 2012. The suspension was to allow the new management some time to review the policy and make the necessary decision on the way forward. However, for nearly four years since the suspension, it is not known whether the policy will be reintroduced or completely abolished.

Some Reflections on the Capitation Payment Policy in Ghana

Evidence from the literature shows that misunderstanding between providers and reformers of payment systems tends to slow down the reform process and that such reforms require the intense involvement of all stakeholders, both in the preparation, and implementation of the reform in order to achieve the intended objective (Nagy and Brandtmuller, 2008).

As Ghanaians wait for a policy statement on the way forward, it will be useful to reflect on the capitation payment policy in relation to

i. its relevance within the Ghana health system and the NHIS,
ii. its effectiveness in achieving the objectives which motivated its introduction,
iii. its impact or effects on utilization, claims expenditure and membership growth, and
iv. its sustainability in terms of its acceptance by stakeholders should it be reintroduced and scaled-up across the country.

Such reflections will not only bring some technical perspectives to the debate but will also provide inputs to guide policy makers in making a sound decision on whether or not to reintroduce the policy and scale it up across the country. These reflections are based on an evaluation study of the provider payment reforms of the NHIS (Andoh-Adjei FX, 2019). The study applied a mixed method approach: a narrative review of the literature on the effects of capitation payment, database review of membership, utilization and claims expenditure, and a survey of insured members and NHIS-credentialed providers on their attitude toward the payment method. The study was cross-sectional using a nonequivalent pretest and posttest control group design which, according to Creswell (2014), is a popular approach to quasi-experiments where both the intervention and control groups are selected without random assignment. The dataset used for the utilization and cost analysis contains district-level information on healthcare utilization for OPD and IPD from the National Health Insurance Authority's database, while data on the demographic and socioeconomic factors were obtained from records of the Ghana Statistical Service (GSS) (Ghana Statistical Service, 2012). In total, data from all the fifty-two districts in three regions were used for analysis. Descriptive analysis was performed to examine trends in both OPD and IPD utilization and cost in the intervention region (i.e., Ashanti) and the two control regions (Central and Volta) over a five-year period, 2010–2014. A generalized linear regression model was performed to determine differences in OPD utilization and claims expenditure between the intervention region and the two control regions before and after implementation of the capitation payment system in the Ashanti region. In addition, difference-in-difference analysis (DID) was performed to estimate the effect of capitation payment policy on utilization and claims expenditure. With regard to the membership data, a trend analysis within and among the three regions to determine trends in new enrolment, renewal, and overall growth rates over a five-year period was done. The independent-samples *t*-test was performed to compare the sample means of growth rates between the intervention region (Ashanti) and the two control regions (Volta and Central). Having determined differences between the sample means of the intervention and control regions to assess the significance level, the effect size was calculated to determine how substantive the findings were. With regard to the perception study, a principal component analysis (PCA) was performed to transform the set of statements for assessing quality of care into five uncorrelated components of dignity and respect, confidentiality, service quality, communication, and accommodation/cleanliness. The factor scores obtained from this analysis were used to estimate mean perception score for each respondent.

RELEVANCE

The relevance of any policy intervention may be judged from the extent to which the objectives of such policy are consistent with beneficiaries' requirements and country needs (The International Bank for Reconstruction and Development/The World Bank, 2009). The relevance of capitation payment in Ghana may, therefore, be judged by the problem it sought to address in the context of the NHIS and the health delivery system. Indeed, countries all over the world face challenges with funding their healthcare systems (The Internation Bank for Reconstruction/The World Bank, 2005); and as they strive to attain universal health coverage, they pay critical attention to ways of improving the income levels of the health system while reducing inefficiencies in the application of scarce healthcare resources.

Thus, a two-pronged approach is applied: revenue-side and expenditure-side interventions. On the revenue side, many low- and middle-income countries have resorted to new and innovative approaches, with (social) health insurance becoming the new paradigm (Preker et al., 2013). However, since no country in the world has unlimited funds to meet their health sector expenditures, policy makers complement the revenue-side interventions with expenditure side interventions. One such expenditure-side intervention is the reform of the provider payment systems (Jegers et al., 2002) which is intended to influence provider behavior in terms of efficient application of resources in healthcare delivery (Randall and McGuire, 1986). As noted in earlier sections, at the inception of the NHIS, the NHIA adopted fee-for-service payment system to reimburse NHIS-credentialed healthcare providers. This provided natural incentives for provider-induced demand for services, resulting in unexpected increases in utilization and claims expenditures of the NHIA. It was this trend that prompted the NHIA to initiate reforms of the provider payment system in 2008, by implementing a Ghanaian version of the DRG payment method which could also not help address the problem effectively.

Therefore, after careful consideration of the challenges facing the NHIS, the NHIA committed to address the challenges by continuing the provider payment reforms by introducing capitation payment for primary care as additional payment method to improve its purchasing arrangement with credentialed providers. The introduction of capitation payment at the time was, therefore, a decision in the right direction. Addressing the design defects such as implementing two baskets of capitated services alongside the DRG at the outpatients' department; the implementation challenges identified during the pilot period; and reintroducing it will be a good intervention to contribute to addressing the potential financial sustainability challenge that faces the NHIS.

EFFECTIVENESS

Effectiveness, in this context, is a measure of the extent to which the objectives of the capitation payment policy was achieved during the pilot implementation period. A key objective for the introduction of capitation payment under Ghana's National Health Insurance Scheme was to hold down growth in total healthcare expenditure by controlling outpatients' utilization and related expenditure. Findings of a study on utilization and cost under the capitation payment policy (Andoh-Adjei et al., 2018) revealed that growth in outpatient utilization and claims expenditure increased in the pre-capitation period in all three regions but slowed in post-capitation period in the intervention region. A linear regression analysis showed that there were significant differences in outpatient utilization (p = 0.0029) and claims expenditure (p = 0.0003) between the intervention and the control regions before implementation of the capitation payment. However, only claims expenditure showed significant difference (p = 0.0361) between the intervention and control regions after the introduction of capitation payment. A difference-in-differences analysis, however, showed that capitation payment had a significant negative effect on utilization only, in the Ashanti region (p<0.007). This suggests that implementation of capitation payment to control utilization yielded some positive results for the NHIA. On the expenditure side, a generalized linear regression model showed significant difference in claims expenditure between the intervention and control regions in the pre-capitation period, 2010–2011, F (2, 49) = 9.65, p = 0.0003 and post-capitation period, 2013–2013; F (2, 49) = 3.56, p = 0.0361. The result of a difference-in-differences analysis showed that capitation payment had a negative effect on both outpatients utilization and related claims expenditure in the intervention region. The effect was, however, significant on outpatient utilization only (p<0.007) (Andoh-Adjei, FX et al., 2018). Thus, the analysis suggests that the expected positive effect achieved in the intervention region was not significant, plausibly, partly due to the relatively short period of time the study covered (2012–2014) and the removal of some services from the basket of capitated package. That notwithstanding, the findings were consistent with those in other studies that showed that capitation payment is associated with slower growth of healthcare expenditures on services that seem profitable under fee-for-service (Mills et al., 2000). The findings also corroborate a study on capitation payment for primary outpatient services in Zhuhai, China, which found a positive effect in controlling costs of healthcare services (Sun et al., 2016). In the China study, the OPD cost increased rapidly over two years before the implementation of the capitation payment system but increased at a much lower rate after the implementation, just as the Ghana study revealed that capitation payment had some positive effect in 2012 which was the first year of implementation after which utilization and costs started to increase again but at a slower rate (Andoh-Adjei FX et al., 2018). Besides the short period that the study covered, the capitation payment could have achieved a much better effect but for some design defects of the policy, one being the implementation of the G-DRG alongside the capitation payment at the OPD. The managers of the scheme designed two baskets of services for outpatient care under the capitation payment policy; one being primary outpatients services and the other being "non-primary outpatients services." The non-primary outpatient services were paid by DRG and since the DRG was applied alongside capitation payment at the general OPD, it is plausible that potentially primary outpatient services may have been shifted to the "non-primary outpatients" services as found in the literature (Glazier et al., 2009).

On the basis of the study upon which these reflections are made, it could be concluded that the capitation payment policy was potentially effective and that its optimum effectiveness could adequately be achieved over a longer period of implementation after addressing the design defects and implementation challenges experienced during the pilot period (Andoh-Adjei, FX 2019).

IMPACT

Impact in the context of Ghana's capitation payment policy may be assessed from the positive and negative effects of the policy on NHIA's operations, either directly or indirectly, intended or unintended. An impact assessment of the capitation payment policy should reflect the cost-containment objectives as well as concerns raised by stakeholders regarding the perceived negative effects that motivated various groups to rise against its introduction. On the cost-containment objective, as noted under effectiveness, the capitation payment policy made some positive impact as it contributed to the slowed growth in utilization and cost, albeit the impact on cost reduction was not significant compared to that of the control regions. At the onset of the capitation pilot implementation, the NHIA indicated that the capitation payment was being piloted for one year, after which it would be rolled out in all regions. However, the pilot implementation continued after the one year without any explanation to the public, a situation that engendered various reactions from residents in the pilot region, including providers, politicians and civil society groups. Some of the issues they raised about the capitation payment policy include, among others, falling NHIS-membership enrolment and renewal rates in the region.

A study of the effect of capitation payment on membership retention (Andoh-Adjei et al., 2018) revealed that all the three regions used for the study experienced negative growth in both the new enrolment and renewal categories at one point or the other within the period 2010–2014. Analysis of both new enrolment and renewal data showed no significant differences in mean growth rates between Ashanti (M = – 13.76, SE 17.68) and Volta (M = 5.48, SE 5.50), p = 0.329; and between Ashanti and Central (M = – 6.47, SE 12.68), p = 0.746. However, capitation payment had some effect in Ashanti compared with Volta (r = 0. 12) and Central (r = 0. 14) but could not be sustained beyond 2012. Responses from in-depth interviews did not also show that capitation payment was a key factor in subscribers' renewal decision. It could, therefore, be argued that other factors as documented in the literature (Fenenga et al., 2014; Jehu-Appiah et al., 2012; Jehu-Appiah et al., 2011; Aryeetey et al., 2013; Atinga, Abiiro, and Kuganab-Lem, 2015) may have contributed significantly to the drop in membership growth rates in the intervention (pilot) region. Put together, the positive impact outweighs the negative impact.

SUSTAINABILITY

The notion of sustainability in project management refers to the ability of project managers to continue the implementation after project funding from donors has ceased (The International Bank for Reconstruction and Development/The World Bank, 2009). In the context of capitation pilot implementation, sustainability may be looked at from the possibility of the pilot migrating into full-scale implementation. Whether or not the capitation pilot will migrate into full-scale implementation also depends on how stakeholders' concerns were addressed during the implementation stage and whether results from the monitoring and evaluation activities point to success. In this reflection, the sustainability of the capitation payment policy is assessed from the attitude of providers and members of the scheme toward the policy; and how they perceive the quality of care during the pilot stage. Assessing the sustainability from this dimension stems from the fact that the onset of capitation implementation in the Ashanti region was characterized by policy debate between the leadership of the Association of Private Medical and Dental Practitioners and civil society groups on the one hand, and leadership of NHIA and policy makers on the other hand.

The debate was centered on the perceived negative effects of capitation payment on NHIS membership retention and healthcare delivery under the capitation payment dispensation. Regarding the concern raised about the negative effect of capitation payment on membership retention, results of analysis of the membership data suggest that capitation payment policy had a negative effect on membership growth in the first year of implementation only but could not be sustained beyond the first year. Responses from individual in-depth interviews on capitation-specific questions also indicated that capitation payment is not a key factor in membership enrolment and retention decision making (Andoh-Adjei et al., 2018). Respondents, however, expressed their opinions, both positive and negative, about the capitation payment policy and the implementation process. On the positive side, some respondents mentioned that the choice of one preferred primary care provider (PPP) was a good innovation to improve quality of care in the health delivery system. On the other hand, some respondents harbored negative perception about the policy. Others with balanced opinion about capitation payment indicated that capitation payment was good but needed to be improved. Judging from the responses from respondents, one may say that a few respondents were positive about capitation. Their appreciation of the fact that capitation is a good innovation is, however, good for the debate on the capitation payment policy. Their analytical thinking that capitation payment offers opportunity for continuity of care speaks to the fact that the communication messages about the positive attributes of capitation made positive impact. It is, however, worth noting the reasons for seeing capitation as a bad policy by many of the respondents. The reason that subscribers who fall sick and attend facilities other than their PPP are refused treatment; co-payments demanded by some healthcare providers; the dispensing of perceived poor-quality medication on the grounds of inadequate capitated rate; and/or delayed reimbursement to providers are some of the issues that have the potential to erode subscribers' confidence in the scheme. The bad perceptions expressed by respondents are also noted by Owusu-Sekyere et al. (2014) in indicating how urgent the need is for the NHIA to address the issues to improve peoples' confidence in the scheme. This is importantly so because the issue of co-payment which, hitherto, has been treated as anecdotal, has been admitted by the Christian Health

Association of Ghana (CHAG) in their 2015 Annual Report as real in the following statement: *"Providers are compelled to do balanced billing to make up for the difference between what the NHIA pays and what it costs them to provide the care, thereby perpetrating out of pocket payments (co-payment) and pushing poor clients into catastrophic health expenditure"* (Christian Health Association of Ghana, Annual Report 2015, p57). It is also important for the NHIA to address itself to this concern because some respondents perceive the capitation payment policy as a good innovation and by addressing their concerns, the NHIA could move those who may be opposed to the capitation payment policy from their negative position to the positive position of those who are sympathetic to the policy.

It is also noteworthy that most of the reasons underlying negative perceptions on capitation are borne out of inadequate information, education and communication to the public, especially the subscribers. The NHIA would, therefore, have to step up its information, education, and communication program to educate the public on the NHIS and the capitation payment policy. In a related study (Andoh-Adjei et al., 2016), it was found that notwithstanding people's negative attitude toward the capitation payment, a majority of survey respondents expressed their willingness to renew their membership card when it expires. It can, therefore, be said that although some respondents had negative perception about the capitation payment policy, capitation payment per se was not a significant factor in their membership enrolment and renewal decision.

Another study on providers and members' perception of quality care delivery under capitation payment (Andoh-Adjei et al., 2018) revealed that in general, a little over half of NHIS card-bearing members who participated in the study expressed positive perception about the quality of care. In terms of individual regions, 53 percent of respondents in Ashanti region where the pilot was implemented perceived quality of care as good compared to 51 percent and 62 percent in the Volta and Central regions, respectively. On the provider side, 86 percent of respondents in Ashanti region perceived quality of care as good compared to 63 percent and 89 percent in Volta and Central regions, respectively. Thus, in general, the study findings showed that both users of healthcare services and their providers have relatively good perception of quality of health care delivered. The finding is consistent with those from similar studies in Ghana (Dixon, Tenkorang, and Luginaah, 2013; Dalinjong and Laar, 2012) and Iraq (Burnham et al., 2011) but at variance with those of other studies from Tanzania (Khamis and Njau, 2014), Korea (Ock et al., 2014), and Ghana (Amo-adjei et al., 2016). While the differences in quality perception between Ghana and Korea may be attributed to the level of development in these two countries, those among different studies from Ghana and between those of Ghana and Tanzania may be attributed to the respective study settings.

One other way of determining providers support or otherwise of the capitation payment policy may be assessed from a study of provider preference for payment method under capitation payment policy (Andoh-Adjei et al., 2019). Among the different type of payment methods used by the NHIA, a majority of healthcare providers preferred to be paid by the Ghana Diagnosis-Related Groupings (G-DRG) method, followed by capitation for all type of services, except for diagnostics. In Ashanti region, looking at the absolute proportions, capitation payment was the preferred payment method for both primary and non-primary outpatients services as well as inpatients services, which is an indication of a positive attitude of Ashanti providers toward the capitation payment method. Thus, from the study results, one may suggest that the initial resistance in the Ashanti region may be attributable to the reported lack of clarity in the minds of providers between the capitation payment and the G-DRG (Aboagye, 2013; Dodoo, 2013) and the perception that the introduction of capitation payment policy in Ashanti was politically motivated (Koduah, Dijk, and Agyepong, 2016; Agyei-Baffour, Oppong, and Boateng, 2013; Atuoye et al., 2016). The trend in Ashanti, therefore, suggests that after resisting its introduction at the initial stage, providers in the region may have later recognized and, therefore, come to terms with the positive attributes of capitation payment method. Providers in the Ashanti region can, thus, be made "captains" of capitation payment policy to help champion the campaign for its reintroduction to scale-up across the country.

On the members' side, a study of provider-member trust relationship showed that 88 percent rated their trust in their provider as (very) high. Eighty-eight percent had no intention to switch provider and a majority (91 percent) would renew their membership when it expires. Notwithstanding some negative experience they had with capitation payment, 81 percent of respondents would recommend to their peers to enroll with the NHIS, with rural dwellers (87 percent; n = 156) being more likely to do so than urban dwellers (76 percent; n = 188). Almost all respondents (92 percent) rated the NHIS as (very) good (Andoh-Adjei, Cornelissen et al., 2016).

CONCLUSION

The NHIS in Ghana was borne out of politics and since its birth, political meanings seem to be read into any move by managers of the scheme to strengthen its operational capacity. Hence, it was not surprising that the introduction of the capitation payment policy attracted debates by politicians, healthcare providers, and civil society organizations. The key issues on the table for debate were the cost-containment objectives advanced by the NHIA and the perceived unintended effects anticipated by healthcare providers and the general public. In concluding the reflection on the subject matter, a summary of the assessment of the policy from four dimensions of monitoring and evaluation framework, namely relevance, effectiveness, impact, and sustainability is presented below.

Relevance: Given the problem of cost-escalation influenced by inefficiencies in the provider payment system at the time, there was the need to introduce reforms into the provider payment systems to secure the long-term financial sustainability of the NHIS; and having noted with evidence that the fee-for-service and the G-DRG could not adequately address the problem on hand, capitation payment which has been found in the literature to have the potential of addressing cost-escalation at the primary care level was, technically, a necessary policy intervention.

Effectiveness: With regard to effectiveness of the policy to achieve its stated objective, even though some modest gains were made in the area of slowed growth in utilization and cost, one can maintain that cost-savings was not significant in the short term. Besides, design and implementation defects compromised the cost-saving objective thereby contributing to the nonoptimal attainment of the objective. Nonetheless, capitation payment policy, from studies, has the potential to contain cost within the NHIS in the long term, if well-designed and efficiently implemented.

Impact: Impact may be seen from two angles: positive and negative, intended and unintended. On the positive side, and as noted earlier, the policy had some positive effect by slowing down growth in utilization and cost, albeit insignificant in the case of cost reduction. However, it gives hope that if the design and implementation defects are addressed, its reintroduction could help make significant positive impact on claim expenditure in the long term. On the anticipated negative impact of capitation payment on membership enrolment and retention, findings from the study referred to in this chapter clearly showed that capitation payment as a policy does not affect (potential) members' enrolment and renewal decision. Therefore, the anticipated negative effect of capitation payment on membership retention could have been a misplaced concern.

Sustainability: Since both providers and members of the scheme have relatively good perception of quality care under the capitation payment policy and the fact that the majority of providers in Ashanti, who were initially opposed to the policy, prefer capitation as payment method for primary care, there is a high potential of support from the Ashanti region to champion the reintroduction of the policy and its nationwide scale-up.

Finally, one may conclude that with more education on the positive attributes of capitation payment method and active involvement of healthcare providers in the (re)-design, development and implementation of the policy, capitation payment could be a viable payment method for primary care services in Ghana's health delivery system.

REFERENCES

Aboagye, AQQ. 2013. "Capitation in Healthcare Financing in Ghana-an Analysis of the Ashanti Region Pilot Study." *East African Medical Journal Medical Journal* 90 (8): 227–84.

Agyei-Baffour, Peter, Regina Oppong, and Daniel Boateng. 2013. "Knowledge, Perceptions and Expectations of Capitation Payment System in a Health Insurance Setting: A Repeated Survey of Clients and Health Providers in Kumasi, Ghana." *BMC Public Health* 13 (13): 1220. https://doi.org/10.1186/1471-2458-13-1220.

Agyepong IA, Aryeetey GC, Nonvignon J, Asenso-Boadi F, Dzikunu H, Antwi E, Ankrah D, Adjei-Acquah C, Esena R, Aikins M and Arhinful DK. 2014. "Advancing the Application of Systems Thinking in Health: Provider Payment and Service Supply Behaviour and Incentives in the Ghana National Health Insurance Scheme - a Systems Approach." *Health Research Policy and Systems / BioMed Central* 12 (1): 35. https://doi.org/10.1186/1478-4505-12-35.

Agyepong, Irene Akua, and Sam Adjei. 2008. "Public Social Policy Development and Implementation: A Case Study of the Ghana National Health Insurance Scheme." *Health Policy Plan* 23 (2): 150–60. https://doi.org/czn002 [pii]\r10.1093/heapol/czn002.

Amo-Adjei, Joshua, Prince Justin Anku, Hannah Fosuah Amo, and Mavis Osei Effah. 2016. "Perception of Quality of Health Delivery and Health Insurance Subscription in Ghana." *BMC Health Services Research*, 1–11. https://doi.org/10.1186/s12913-016-1602-4.

Andoh-Adjei, Francis-Xavier, Dennis Cornelissen, Felix Ankomah Asante, Ernst Spaan, and Koos van der Velden. 2016. "Does Capitation Payment under National Health Insurance Affect Subscribers' Trust in Their Primary Care Provider? A Cross-Sectional Survey of Insurance Subscribers in Ghana." *BMC Health Services Research* 16 (1): 437. https://doi.org/10.1186/s12913-016-1622-0.

Andoh-Adjei, Francis-Xavier, Ernst Spaan, Felix A Asante, Sylvester A Mensah, and Koos Van Der Velden. 2016. "A Narrative Synthesis of Illustrative Evidence on Effects of Capitation Payment for Primary Care: Lessons for Ghana and Other Low/Middle-Income Countries." *Ghana Med J* 50 (504): 207–219. https://doi.org/10.4314/gmj.v50i4.3.

Andoh-Adjei, Francis-Xavier, Renske van der Wal, Eric Nsiah-Boateng, Felix Ankomah Asante, Koos van der Velden, and Ernst Spaan. 2018. "Does a Provider Payment Method Affect Membership Retention in a Health Insurance Scheme? A Mixed Method Study of Ghana's Capitation Payment for Primary Care." *BMC Health Services Research* 18 (1): 52. https://doi.org/10.1186/s12913-018-2859-6.

Andoh-Adjei, F. X., B.Boudwijns, E. Nsiah-Boateng, F. A. Asante, K. van der Velden, and E. Spaan. 2018. "Effects of Capitation Payment on Utilization and Claims Expenditure under National Health Insurance Scheme : A Cross-Sectional Study of Three Regions in Ghana." *Health Economics Review* 8 (17).

Andoh-Adjei, F. X., E. Nsiah-Boateng, F. A. Asante, K. van der Velden, and Spaan E. "Provider Preference for Payment Method under a National Health Insurance Scheme : A Survey of Health Insurance-Credentialed Health Care Providers in Ghana." *Plos One* 14 (9): 1–13.

Andoh-Adjei, F. X., E. Nsiah-Boateng, A. Asante Felix, E. Spaan, and K. van der Velden. 2018. "Perception of Quality Health Care Delivery under Capitation Payment : A Cross-Sectional Survey of Health Insurance Subscribers and Providers in Ghana." *BMC Family Practice* 19 (1): 1–12.

Andoh-Adjei, Francis-Xavier. 2019. "Provider Payment Reforms in Ghana's National Health Insurance Scheme: Monitoring and Evaluation of Capitation as a Provider Payment Mechanism for Primary Outpatient Services." PhD Thesis, Radboud University Medical Centre.

Anell, Anders, Anna H. Glenngard, and Sherry M. Merkur. 2012. "Sweden: Health System Review." http://www.euro.who.int/en/who-we-are/partners/observatory.

Appiah-Denkyira E and Preker A. 2007. "Reaching the Poor in Ghana with National Health Insurance-an Experience from the Districts of the Eastern Region of Ghana." In *Extending Social Protection in Health: Developing Countries' Experiences, Lessons Learnt and Recommendations*, 1–225. ESCHBORN: GTZ GmBH.

Aryeetey, Genevieve C, Caroline Jehu-Appiah, Agnes M Kotoh, Ernst Spaan, Daniel K Arhinful, Rob Baltussen, Sjaak van der Geest, and Irene A Agyepong. 2013. "Community Concepts of Poverty: An Application to Premium Exemptions in Ghana's National Health Insurance Scheme." *Globalization And Health* 9 (1): 12. https://doi.org/10.1186/1744-8603-9-12.

Atim Chris, 1999. "Social Movements and Health Insurance: A Critical Evaluation of Voluntary, Non-Profit Insurance Schemes with Case Studies from Ghana and Cameroon." *Social Science and Medicine* 48 (7): 881–96. https://doi.org/10.1016/S0277-9536(98)00390-6.

Atinga, Roger A, Gilbert Abotisem Abiiro, and Robert Bella Kuganab-Lem. 2015. "Factors Influencing the Decision to Drop out of Health Insurance Enrolment among Urban Slum Dwellers in Ghana." *Tropical Medicine & International Health : TM & IH* 20 (3): 312–21. https://doi.org/10.1111/tmi.12433.

Atuoye, K. N., Vercillo, S., Antabe, R., Galaa, S. Z., and Luginaah, I. 2016. "Financial Sustainability versus Access and Quality in a Challenged Health System: An Examination of the Capitation Policy Debate in Ghana." *Health Policy Plan* 31 (9): 1240–49. https://doi.org/https://doi.org/10.1093/heapol/czw058.

Averill, Richard F, Norbert Goldfield, Jack S. Hughes, Janice Bonazelli, Elizabeth C McCullough, Barbara A Steinbeck, Robert Mullin, et al. 2003. "All Patient Refined Diagnosis Related Rroups (APR-DRGs): Methodology Overview," 1–81. http://www.hcup-us.ahrq.gov/.../APR-DRGsV20MethodologyOverview.

Barnum H.; Kutzin J.; Saxeniam. 1995. "Incentives and Provider Payment Methods." *Internationa Journal of Health Policy and Management* 10: 23–45.

Burnham, Gilbert, Connie Hoe, Yuen Wai Hung, Agron Ferati, Allen Dyer, Thamer Al Hifi, and Rabia Aboud. 2011. "Perceptions and Utilization of Primary Health Care Services in Iraq : Findings from a National Household Survey." *BMC International Health & Human Rights* 11 (15): 1–9.

Creswell, J. W. 2014. *Research Design: Qualitative, Quantitative and Mixed Methods Approaches*. Edited by Knight Vicki. 4th editio. London: SAGE Publications Ltd.

Dalinjong, Philip Ayizem, and Alexander Suuk Laar. 2012. "The National Health Insurance Scheme: Perceptions and Experiences of Health Care Providers and

Clients in Two Districts of Ghana." *Health Economics Review* 2 (1): 13. https://doi.org/10.1186/2191-1991-2-13.

Dixon, Jenna, Eric Y. Tenkorang, and Isaac Luginaah. 2013. "Ghana's National Health Insurance Scheme: A National Level Investigation of Members' Perceptions of Service Provision." *BMC International Health and Human Rights* 13 (1): 35. https://doi.org/10.1186/1472-698X-13-35.

Econex. 2010. "Provider Payment Systems." 6. Health Reform Note. South Africa. www.econex.co.za.

Fenenga, Christine J., Kwasi Boahene, Daniel Arhinful, Tobias Rinke De Wit, and Inge Hutter. 2014. "Do Prevailing Theories Sufficiently Explain Perceptions and Health-Seeking Behavior of Ghanaians?" *International Journal of Health Planning and Management* 29 (1): 26–42. https://doi.org/10.1002/hpm.2159.

Ghana Statistical Service. 2012. "2010 Population and Housing Census." *Seoul, Korea, Various Issues*. Accra. http://www.statsghana.gov.gh/docfiles/2010phc/Census2010_Summary_report_of_final_results.pdf.

Ginsburg, Paul B. 2013. "Analysis & Commentary Achieving Health Care Cost Containment through Provider Payment Reform That Engages Patients and Providers." *Health Affairs* 32 (5): 929–34. https://doi.org/10.1377/hlthaff.2012.1007.

Glazier, Richard H, Julie Klein-Geltink, Alexander Kopp, and Lyn M Sibley. 2009. "Capitation and Enhanced Fee-for-Service Models for Primary Care Reform: A Population-Based Evaluation." *CMAJ : Canadian Medical Association Journal = Journal de l'Association Medicale Canadienne* 180 (11): E72–81.

Government of Ghana. 2003. *National Health Insurance Act, 2003 (Act 650)*. Ghana: Assembly Press.

Government of Ghana. 2012. *National Health Insurance Act, 2012 (Act 852)*. Ghana: Assembly Press.

Grabowski, David C., Christopher C. Afendulis, and Thomas G. McGuire. 2011. "Medicare Prospective Payment and the Volume and Intensity of Skilled Nursing Facility Services." *Journal of Health Economics* 30 (4): 675–84.

International Labour Organization. 2005. "Improving Social Protection for the Poor : Health Insurance in Ghana The Ghana Social Trust Pre-Pilot Project Final Report." *Organization*. Geneva. http://www.ilo.int/public/english/protection/secsoc/downloads/policy/999sp1.pdf.

Jegers, Marc, Katrien Kesteloot, Diana De Graeve and Willem Gilles, 2002. "A Typology for Provider Payment Systems in Health Care." *Health Policy* 60 (3): 255–73. https://doi.org/10.1016/S0168-8510(01)00216-0.

Jehu-Appiah, Caroline, Genevieve Aryeetey, Irene Agyepong, Ernst Spaan, and Rob Baltussen. 2012. "Household Perceptions and Their Implications for Enrolment in the National Health Insurance Scheme in Ghana." *Health Policy and Planning* 27 (3): 222–33. https://doi.org/10.1093/heapol/czr032.

Jehu-Appiah, Caroline, Genevieve Aryeetey, Ernst Spaan, Thomas de Hoop, Irene Agyepong, and Rob Baltussen. 2011. "Equity Aspects of the National Health Insurance Scheme in Ghana: Who Is Enrolling, Who Is Not and Why?" *Social Science and Medicine* 72 (2): 157–65. https://doi.org/10.1016/j.socscimed.2010.10.025.

Joseph Nii Otoe Dodoo. 2013. "A Stakeholder Analysis of the Capitation Pilot under Ghana's National Health Insurance Scheme in Ashanti Region." Thesis. University of Ghana. http://ugspace.ug.edu.gh.

Kate Wilson, Brian Latko, Cheryl Cashin, Alice Garabrant Cees Hesp, Paul Stepne, Herman Bennema, Alvin Marcelo , Oliver Harrison, YoungEun Lee, John C. Langenbrunner. 2013. "Provider Payment Reform and Information Technology Systems: a chicken and egg question for national coverage programs. Joint Learning Network for universal coverage, 2019." Available from http://www .jointlearningnetwot.org.

Khamis, Kudra, and Bernard Njau. 2014. "Patients ' Level of Satisfaction on Quality of Health Care at Mwananyamala Hospital in Dar Es Salaam , Tanzania." *BMC Health Service Research* 14 (400): 1–8.

Koduah, Augustina, Han van Dijk, and Irene Akua Agyepong. 2016. "Technical Analysis, Contestation and Politics in Policy Agenda Setting and Implementation: The Rise and Fall of Primary Care Maternal Services from Ghanas Capitation Policy." *BMC Health Services Research* 16. https://doi.org/http://dx.doi.org/10 .1186/s12913-016-1576-2.

Mathauer, Inke, and Friedrich Wittenbecher. 2013. "Hospital Payment Systems Based on Diagnosis-Related Groups: Experiences in Low- and Middle-Income Countries." *Bulletin of the World Health Organization* 91 (10): 746-756A. https:// doi.org/10.2471/BLT.12.115931.

Mills, Anne, Sara Bennett, Porntep Siriwanarangsun, and Viroj Tangcharoensathien. 2000. "The Response of Providers to Capitation Payment: A Case-Study from Thailand." *Health Policy* 51 (3): 163–80. https://doi.org/10.1016/S0168-8510(00)00059-2.

Ministry of Health. 2015. "Ghana Health Financing Strategy 2015," 1–70.

Ministry of Health-Ghana. 2013. "Joint Holistic Assessment of Ghana's Health Sector Programme of Work, 2012." Accra.

Nagy, Balazs, and Agnes Brandtmuller. n.d. "Implementing Risk Adjusted Capitation Payments with Health Care Reforms in Hungary." *Jounal of Economic Literature*, 147–60.

National Health Insurance Authority (2010). National Health Insurance Authority Annual Report, 2010, pgs. 17, 21-22. www.nhia.gov.gh, Accessed June 5, 2020

Ock, Minsu, Jung-eun Kim, Min-woo Jo, Hyeon-jeong Lee, Hyun Joo Kim, and Jin Yong Lee. 2014. "Perceptions of Primary Care in Korea : A Comparison of Patient and Physician Focus Group Discussions." *BMC Family Practice* 15 (178): 1–14.

Owusu-sekyere, Ebenezer, and Daniel A Bagah. 2014. "Towards a Sustainable Health Care Financing in Ghana : Is the National Health Insurance the Solution ?" *Public Health Research* 4 (5): 185–94. https://doi.org/10.5923/j.phr.20140405.06.

Park, M, T Braun, G Carrin, and D Evans. 2007. "Provider Payments and Cost-Containment: Lessons from OECD Countries." *Organization*, 1–7.

Preker, Alexander S., Marianne E. Linder, Dov Chernichovsky and Onno P. Schellekens, eds. 2013. *Scaling up Affordable Health Insurance: Staying the Course*. Washington DC: World Bank: The World Bank. https://doi.org/10.1596 /978-0-8213-8250-9.

Qingyue, Meng. 2005. "Review of Health Care Provider Payment Reforms In," no. March: 1–30.

Randall P. Ellis and Thomas G. McGuire. 1986. "Provider Behaviour under Prospective Reimbursement: Cost Sharing and Supply." *Journal of Health Economics* 5: 129–51.

Rosen, B. 1989. "Professional Reimbursement and Professional Behavior: Emerging Issues and Research Challenges." *Social Science & Medicine* 29 (3): 455–62. https://doi.org/10.1016/0277-9536(89)90294-3.

Rosenthal, MB. 2008. "Beyond Pay for Performance - Emerging Models of Provider Payment Reform." *New England Journal of Medicine* 359 (12): 1197–1200. http://www.nejm.org/doi/full/10.1056/NEJMp0804658.

Rudmik, Luke, Dominika Wranik, and Caroline Rudisill-Michaelsen. 2014. "Physician Payment Methods: A Focus on Quality and Cost Control." *Journal of Otolaryngology - Head & Neck Surgery* 43 (1): 34. https://doi.org/10.1186/s40463-014-0034-6.

Scott, Anthony, Peter Sivey, Ait Ouakrim D, Lisa Willenberg, Lucio Naccarella, John Furler, Doris Young, et al. 2011. "The Effect of Financial Incentives on the Quality of Health Care Provided by Primary Care Physicians (Review)." *Cochrane Database of Systematic Reviews* 9 (9): CD008451. https://doi.org/10.1002/14651858.CD008451.pub2.

Sun, Jing, Xiaotian Zhang, Zou Zhang, Anita K Wagner, Dennis Ross-degnan, and Hans V Hogerzeil. 2016. "Impacts of a New Insurance Benefit with Capitated Provider Payment on Healthcare Utilization , Expenditure and Quality of Medication Prescribing in China." *Tropical Medicine & International Health* 21 (2): 263–74. https://doi.org/10.1111/tmi.12636.

Szende, Agota, and Zsolt Mogyorosy. 2004. "Health Care Provider Payment Mechanisms in the New EU Members of Central Europe and the Baltic States. Current Reforms, Incentives, and Challenges." *European Journal of Health Economics* 5 (3): 259–62. https://doi.org/10.1007/s10198-004-0249-y.

The Internation Bank for Reconstruction/World. 2005. *Spending Wisely. Buying Health Services for the Poor.* Edited by Jonh C. Langenbrunner Alexander S. Preker. Wash: The World Bank. www.worldbank.org.

The International Bank for Reconstruction and Development/The World Bank. 2009. *The Road to Results: Designing and Conducting Effective Development Evaluations.* Edited by Imas Lindaa G. Morra, Rist Ray C. Washington DC: The World Bank. https://doi.org/10.1596/978-0-8213-7891-5.

Vogel, Ronald J. 1988. *Cost Recovery in the Health Care Sector FILE 0PuY.* Available from: www.onlinelibrary.wiley.com/doi/10.1002/hpm.4740060303/pdf.

Waters, Hugh R., Peter Hussey, Hugh R. Peter Hussey, and Hugh R. Waters, and Peter Hussey. 2004. "Pricing Health Services for Purchasers-A Review of Methods and Experiences." *Health Policy* 70 (2): 175–84. https://doi.org/10.1016/j.healthpol.2004.04.012.

Chapter 8

Cultural Negotiation and Invention of Healthcare Strategies among Cattle Nomads of Oyo North, Nigeria

Aderemi Suleiman Ajala and Kayode Akinsete

Among the cattle nomads of Oyo north, healthcare system is challenged by a lot of environmental factors such as soil aridity, making access to water and regular green vegetation difficult; strenuous cattle grazing that induces some health risks; and residence in the jungle (distant bush) that makes healthcare facilities in Yoruba towns inaccessible to the nomads. Living mostly with their animals, making infections from animal diseases possible, and exposure to predators like snakes, scorpions, and so on create potential health risks associated with long distance cattle flocking. Combating these challenges require recognition and cognition of the environment, identification of potential resources within the environment and employment of those potential resources in the invention of healthcare strategies. While these negotiation processes abound in all human societies, in migrant populations like the Fulani cattle nomads of Oyo north in southwestern Nigeria, the process of negotiation becomes interesting and more challenging, reflecting exposure to health risks, exploration and exploitation of the environment, acculturation with and adaptation to the "new" environment and invention of "new" healthcare strategies.

Although there are other variations of cattle nomads in southwestern Nigeria such as Yoruba cattle nomads and mixed blood (Yoruba-Fulani) cattle nomads, mostly, the Fulani cattle nomads populate the semiarid region of Oyo north, a space covering about 305 square kilometer with sparse and low green vegetation (Onyima, 2019). Emergence of predominantly cattle rearing by Fulani in Oyo north is traced to 1836 (Ajala, 2013) when the Fulani migrated to a section of Old Oyo empire with the intention of spreading Jihad caused by Uthman Dan Fodio in 1804 in northern Nigeria. Being traditionally pastoralists who had migrated from Futa D'jallon Island in west coast of Senegambia in Africa, the Fulani moved with their cattle from northern Nigeria predominantly arid territory to where a better pasture could be secured for their cattle. In Oyo north, the pastoralists numbered about 18,000 people living in about 173 pastoral bands dispersedly located (Ajala, 2017) in bucolic environment with wet grassland having an average rainfall and humidity in Oyo north, southwestern Nigeria (Onyima, 2019).

Havilland (1975) once defined culture as reprocessing of natural environment to accommodate human existence and survival, suggesting that cultural actions are formed through negotiation with the environment. Such cultural actions as related to healthcare behaviors involve cognition of the environment, perception of the environment and invention of healthcare strategies. Negotiation also has to do with managing cultural challenges in the environment and recreation of new cultural patterns to deal with the challenges. Such processes can result in either abdication from the challenging environment or resilience against the challenges and living in the environment, and inventing new cultural patterns or modifying old patterns.

Humans, in time and space, have always engaged themselves in a continuous search for survival and, in the process, they have always strived to understand the nature of their environment. In effect, humans have always tried to develop cultural means of striking a balance with environment (Steward, 1955; Rappaport, 1968; Lee, 1969; Harris, 1968; Bernnet, 1976). Enshrined in the basic premise of ecological anthropology is the point that the environment is a socio-physical component of culture from which all biological organisms, including humans, produce a highly complex set of conditions and possibility of adaptation (Ellen, 1994). The complex condition and adaptation reflect so much on human capacity to favorably negotiate with the environment. Negotiation involves having the knowledge of the environment, cognition of resources in the environment, exploration of the use of the identified resources for human survival and creating effects on the environment. The processes of negotiation in turn alter the original positions of the two actors (human and environment) in such a way that new forms of cultural actions are invented. Every human being has to negotiate with the environment to secure survival. However, the capacity to negotiate differs across human settlements due to differences in environment, technological capacity and capability, knowledge of the environment and challenges posed against survival. In other words, as opined by ecological anthropology (Steward, 1955; Ellen, 1994), invention of new cultural patterns is a product of negotiation and adaptation to given environmental conditions.

The above discourse significantly plays out on the invention of healthcare strategies in Oyo north of southwestern Nigeria among the pastoral nomads where a combination of primary and newly created healthcare strategies is employed by the nomads to secure their health and treat diseases encountered in their settlement. Arising from the above includes an explanation of how the pastoral nomads in Oyo north negotiate in their environment. More importantly, critical to discourse on cultural negotiation and invention of new healthcare strategies is the identification of the pattern of cultural negotiation in nomads' healthcare system and the definition of the emerging patterns of health behaviors among the nomads of Oyo north. Similarly, it is imperative to identify the implications of the new health culture on sustainable human livelihood. Answering these questions prompted an ethnographic data collection among the cattle nomads in Oyo north, designed to examine how processes of negotiation can lead to invention of new healthcare strategies among the pastoral nomads of Oyo north in southwestern Nigeria. Thus, this chapter is based on fieldwork conducted between December 2018 and August 2019 among the pastoral nomads of Oyo north, southwestern Nigeria.

METHODOLOGY

Although both qualitative and quantitative methodologies were used, the aspect of the study being reported in this chapter dwells largely on the qualitative. Oyo north is one of the three senatorial districts into which the Oyo state in southwestern Nigeria is politically structured. Traditionally, the people of Oyo north are predominantly Oke-Ogun Yoruba brand, being one of the twenty-two subgroups of the Yoruba people of southwestern Nigeria. Oyo north occupies ten local government councils out of thirty-three such local political units in the Oyo state. The region is permissible to large settlement of nomadic bands, since the vegetation is mostly grass and shrubs with unwooded trees. The nomadic occupation of the region is dated to around 1836 following the spread of Fulani Jihad to most part of the Yoruba land in southwestern Nigeria (Ajala, 2013). The earliest nomads in the region were mainly the Bororo nomads, who were said to have migrated from Sokoto and Niger Republic with their cattle. The region now has other brands of cattle nomads such as mixed blood nomads (Yoruba-Fulani) and very limited number of Oke-Ogun natives who are gradually getting into cattle nomadism.

There are three types of band settlements: Permanent band settlement among the Oke-Ogun natives who practice cattle nomadism (they are limited in number and do not engage in transhumanism), semipermanent bands mostly among the mixed blood nomads who live in their bands for a period of time and upon exhaustion of grass and shrubs move to create a new band, and sedentary bands common among the Bororo nomads who do not settle at all in one place (they live in a band for a very short time and move to create new bands elsewhere). Among all the three bands, a common pattern of competition with environment exists. They all negotiate with their local environment to adapt to the environmental pressure and create new cultural patterns used to maintain their healthcare system.

Data collection relied on qualitative methods using participant observation, key informant interviews and focus group discussions (FGD). The study engaged 51 key informants selected through cluster sampling from 17 out of 173 bands located in Oyo north; 17 sessions of FGD and observation of 9 healthcare cases and disease tracking. Guided by the study's objectives, data collection procedures produced interview scripts in the form of field diaries which were carefully analyzed to form the research findings.

FINDINGS

Nomadic Socio-environment and Health Challenges

Cattle nomads in Oyo north are mostly the Fulani (Fulbe) who began to appear in the region starting from the 1836 when the people moved southward of Nigeria from northern Nigeria. Following the success of 1804 Jihad led by the Fulani, the Fulani who dominate pastoralism in Nigeria occupied most part of the northern Nigeria where they controlled the government (emirate) and pastoralism in the region. Their southward movement later occurred with the intention of spreading the Jihad further and taking over the southern region of the present-day Nigeria. Fulani Jihad had two purposes: to gain the political control and to propagate Islamic religion in their conquered territories. Penetrating the Yoruba land in southwestern Nigeria through the northern border of the Yoruba region in the ancient city of Ilorin, the Fulanis by the 1830s conquered Ilorin, which was then the Yoruba's northern border post. While the attempt was partially made possible since only the Yoruba ancient city of Ilorin fell under the control of the Fulani, the Fulani only succeeded in strengthening Islam and introduced cattle nomadism in southwestern Nigeria. In spite of the checkmating of the Fulani in Ilorin from total political control of the Yoruba society in southwestern Nigeria by the Yoruba warriors in 1836 (Ajala, 2013), movement of the Fulani to Yoruba hinterland did not seize. As at the 2020s, no part of the Yoruba society fails to have Fulani nomads. While official data do not yet exist about the accurate census of the Fulani nomads in southwestern Nigeria, it is estimated that about 20,000 Fulani nomads are located in Oyo north mostly engaging in cattle nomadism (Ajala, 2017) and living in bucolic environments of semiarid region, where they have established about 173 bands.

In Oyo north, apart from the pure Fulani that engage in cattle nomadism, there are also pockets of a mixed blood of Fulani and Yoruba and some original Yoruba engaging in cattle pastoralism. The mixed blood are the offspring of intermarriage between the Yoruba and Fulani, the agnatic relationship that began in Ilorin. Thus, they are commonly called the Ilorin Fulani. The Yoruba cattle pastoralists emerged recently when the Yoruba in Oyo north, mostly the Oke-Ogun subgroup of the Yoruba that dominates the Oyo north population, began showing interest in cattle nomadism. While the Fulani nomads are intensively involved in cattle nomadism featuring mono-economic practice in cattle rearing, long range transhumance and in temporary band settlements with larger flocks of cattle, the Ilorin Fulani operate semi-intensive system of cattle nomadism, with more permanent bands mostly located in the fringes of the semiarid region, and the Yoruba pastoralists often live very close to Yoruba towns and cities in Oyo north. Both the Ilorin-Fulani and Yoruba pastoralists practice mixed economy featuring farming and cattle rearing.

Oyo north is a plain land with suitable topography for cattle rearing. The region features average humidity and medium rainfall with abundant growth of grasses and shrubs suitable for good animal health. The forest is unwooded which allows for cattle rearing and tracking. The region is also fertile for farming. For centuries before the advent of cattle rearing in the region, the Yoruba inhabitants of Oyo north had been engaging in extensive farming in most parts of the region where crops like maize, millet, yam, cassava, groundnut, cotton, cowpea among others, and semi-intensive rearing of ruminants like goats and sheep were predominantly engaged. The practice still continues to date. Thus, right from the beginning, the advent of cattle rearing raises presumption of conflicts between the cattle herders and the farmers, which in itself constitutes a major health risk, since cattle nomadism in the region involves open grazing of animals that are likely to feed on farm crops.

Migration from north to the south defines nomads as strangers in Oyo north, and thus often excludes them from access to land in Oyo north. Among the Yoruba of Oke-Ogun in Oyo north, traditionally, land is incorporeal and right of possession rests on the kings and family heads who temporarily alienate the land on request to only those that will not take permanent possession. Traditional land tenure forbids outright sales of land; only gratuity in the form of farm proceeds, local wines, annual land rent and taxes are collected. Even with the promulgation of land use act in Nigeria in 1976, where land in Nigeria is presumed to be in the possession of the local and state governments in Nigeria, kings and family heads in Yoruba land still hold tight onto their land rights. In contrast, the Fulani holds the view that land is a natural resource created by God and made free to anybody who wants to use it. In one of the interviews with a Fulani key informant, the Fulani strong attachment to this land tenure belief is established: *Oga, who owns the land? Is it not God? If God creates land who then do I pay to acquire land?*[1] Conflict on land between the Yoruba farmers and cattle nomads is a common trend in Oyo north; thus, causing socioeconomic hostility between the Yoruba farmers and cattle nomads in Oke-Ogun. Based on the expression of perception and actual hostility, cattle nomads are excluded from access to government development programs. Mostly, cattle nomads perceive the hostility and thus ignore utilization of development projects sited in Yoruba towns and cities. Similarly, due to the remoteness and self-alienation of many of the nomadic bands in Oyo north, cattle nomads are excluded from the reach of many development projects. Thus, according to Aliyu in a key informant interview "*Government has neglected us. We do not also use the development projects in towns, because we are unfriendly with the Yorubas who live in towns.*"[2]

Oyo North Nomadic Environment and Associated Health Risks

Living in semiarid environment characterized by medium humidity, dispersed green grass and shrubs and unwooded trees and which has a relatively low access to water due to medium rainfall expose the cattle nomads in Oyo north to three main health risks, which generate health-related behaviors different from what the cattle nomads were used to in their original habitation in northern Nigeria. The risks are health risks associated with cattle flocking, health risks associated with their social conducts in the new environment and health risks related with biological and medical interactions and seasonal climatic changes. Snake bites, falling in traps mostly set in hunting for animals by neighboring hunters and farmers, fatigue due to long distance trekking during cattle flocking, hunger suffered due to longtime flocking of cattle without access to enough food and uncommon ailments which the cattle nomads referred to as "spirit attacks" due to their low knowledge of sources of such ailments constitute health risks associated with cattle flocking.

Social conducts in the new environment instigate hostility from neighboring farmers who accuse the cattle nomads of farmland destruction due to cattle grazing and financial losses due to poor sales in cattle businesses, livestock mortality, human injuries, and occasional loss of life due to attacks from their neighboring farmers, robbery, and insecurity issues. Accusations of kidnapping and possession of small and light weapons (guns) also attract police arrest, detention, conviction, and huge fines which in turn cause health risks. Nomads claim that these social conditions trigger biomedical health problems such as hypertension (high blood pressure), restlessness, insomnia, headache and other associated illnesses, and in extreme cases even deaths especially when hunters mistook nomads for animals and shot them. Cattle nomads in Oyo north are exposed to arthritis, cold, malaria, chicken pox, yellow fever, typhoid, and diarrhea due to biological and medical interaction with the new environment, while seasonal climatic change causes severe cold (*pewol*), cough (*douru*, *chowuru*), and catarrh (*mura*, *dambi*) during the wet and cold season, and child convulsion (*sukaabel/chukapil*, *palte*), measles (*duudu*, *pultei*) and body heat and rashes (*pinni*, *serungo*) are commonly experienced during the dry season. As shown in table 8.1, among all these, the most common are tuberculosis, malaria, typhoid, and bilharzia.

Healthcare Systems in Oyo North Nomadic Settlement

Commonly practiced among the cattle nomads in Oyo north are four types of healthcare system featuring modern healthcare, faith-based healing, self-medication and quack doctors, and drug hawkers. Conceptualization of disease largely determines the choice of healthcare systems. Cattle nomads construct the germ theory of the causation of disease used in the explanation of certain diseases, according to majority of our key informants (73 percent) that are not beyond ordinary. Diseases are beyond ordinary when the cause cannot be explained and, in most cases, when the disease is stubborn to control. Unexplainable diseases are thus linked with preternatural forces such as witchcraft and enemies either within or outside the bands. While the belief in witchcraft existence within the band is common, yet among the volatile polygynous bands, accusations of bewitchment among the co-wives are often expressed. Thirteen percent of our women key informants expressed that their co-wives in the bands bewitch their children with small pox and cholera. Cattle nomads generally often create the impression that the "hostile" Yoruba farming neighbors can poison the nomadic bands with pestilence and disease. In this case, the occurrence of such diseases is beyond the ordinary and such diseases will defy treatment from modern healthcare system. In cases where the causation of disease is clearly defined within the realm of pathogenic causation such as infusion of germs and bacteria, overworking and stress, modern healthcare system, quack doctors, and drug hawkers are approached to access the use of modern drug in the healing.

Perceived severity of disease, accessibility, and availability of care and perceived belief in the outcomes of choice of care also play major roles in the choice of healthcare system among the cattle nomads of Oyo north. Severe symptomatic expression of disease exists when the actors are incapable of self-supporting and are grossly incapable of discharging everyday

Table 8.1 Common Diseases among the Nomads of Oyo North

S/N	*Diseases*	*Prevalence in %*
1	Tuberculosis	13.3
2	Malaria	9.7
3	Typhoid	5.2
4	Bilharzia	3.2
5	Others (measles, rashes, convulsion, catarrh, cough, etc.)	7.2

Source: Fieldwork conducted among the Nomads of Oyo North, 2019.

engagements such as flocking the cattle and milking the cows. Such occasions occur at the critical stage of illness and point of death when doubt for survival is expressed. In such instances, all efforts are made to approach modern healthcare system in towns and cities irrespective of the remoteness of the band locations from the towns and cities. The belief is that modern drugs are quicker in restoring damaged life. Table 8.2 explains the utilization patterns of different healthcare systems among the pastoral nomads of Oyo north.

Pathway to healing among the people is determined by the actual severity and beliefs associated with disease and health. While the actual severity in most of the diseases are often difficult to determine, healing processes in most diseases often begin with self-medication. Through lay referrals and experiences gathered from drug hawkers, individuals in the band have knowledge of drugs needed to use on the occasion of any disease. Immediately, the symptoms become apparent and such are communicated to lay referrals who could be family members, friends, and customers that come to the band to purchase dairy products, drugs are self-prescribed for use. Mostly, actors abandon clinical test and medical prescription. Often, this results in complications in cases like pregnancy and infant illness. When complications occur, recourse is made to clinics and hospitals in town. In cases of malaria, through cultural adaptation with Oyo north, cattle nomads are knowledgeable of local herbs used in treatment. Such local herbs include *Ewé Òrúwo*, *Dóngóyárò*, *Èèpo Mango (back of Mango)*, *Kóko Oba (Lemon grass)*, and *Ewé Osàn Weere (Lime leaves)*. The medication is of common knowledge as those plants are planted in the bands as decoration and ornamental plants. They are therefore preserved for easy access.

Quack doctors and unlicensed drug retailers are common in the bands. They patronize the bands from neighboring Yoruba communities offering healthcare services for the cattle nomads and selling drugs without medical prescription. Quack doctors and drug sellers prescribe drugs for the cattle nomads without medical test. Prescription is often based on narratives of illness behaviors from the cattle nomads. Figure 8.1 explains the pathway for care among the cattle nomads in Oyo north.

However, the pathways to healing among the cattle nomads are flexible. The belief associated with the efficacy of each of the systems, availability

Table 8.2 Healthcare Systems in Nomadic Settlements of Oyo North

S/N	*Utilization of Healthcare Systems*	*Prevalence in %*
1	Modern clinics and hospitals	13
2	Faith-based and traditional herbal healing	27
3	Self-medication	32
4	Quack doctors and drug hawkers	28

Source: Fieldwork conducted among the Nomads of Oyo North, 2019.

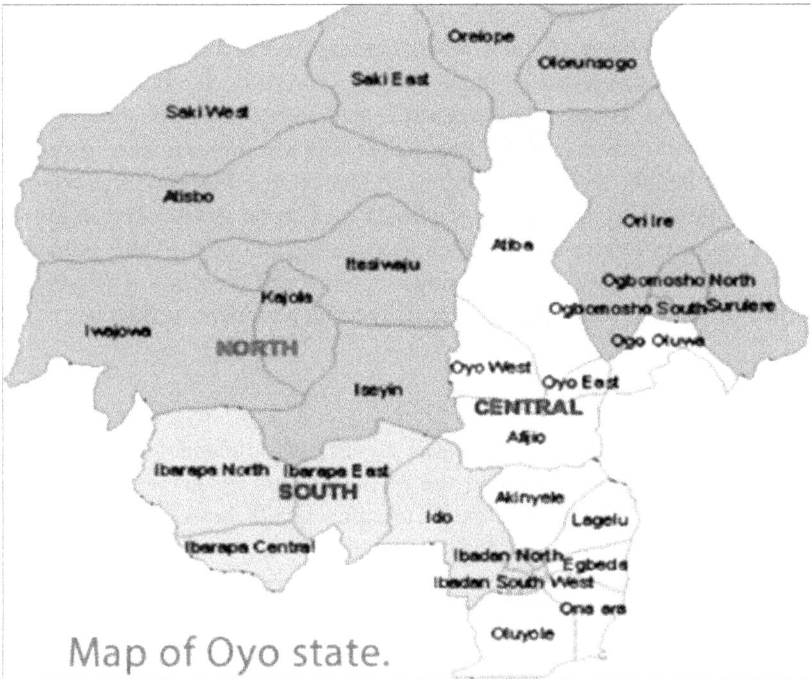

Figure 8.1 Map of Oyo. Authors' Conceptualization from Fieldwork Data among the Cattle Nomads of Oyo North, 2019.

and access to each determine the choices of the healing path among the cattle nomads. While mostly the Bororo cattle nomads who live in forests far away from Yoruba towns least patronize quack doctors and drug retailers due to ethnic suspicion and fear related to Yoruba/Fulani relationship in Oyo north, the Yoruba who mostly constitute the team of medical doctors and drug retailers patronizing the Fulani bands for service would rarely visit the far distant Fulani bands mostly occupied by Bororo Fulani due to distance and fear of attack by the Bororo Fulani. Thus, the Bororo cattle nomads take to self-medication using local herbs as the first path to healing, and when the first path fails or is inadequate to solve the problem, they shift or combine with faith healing and when the two options totally fail and patients resume critical condition of ill health, a recourse is then made to a clinic in town.

The Ilorin Fulani and Yoruba cattle nomads who live close to towns and who have regular relationships and contacts with Yoruba residents in town have low expression of fear and suspicion against the Yoruba who engage in quack healthcare services and drug retailing. Thus, the first path among these groups of cattle nomads is self-medication in local herbs. Then they shift to the use of quack doctors and drugs dispensed by unlicensed drug retailers. In both ways, generally among the cattle nomads in Oyo north, there is more attachment to the use of faith-based healing and self-medication in local herbs and drugs dispensed by unlicensed drug retailers. Interestingly too, the path shift is also witnessed between self-medication and utilization of clinic in town, mostly, among the affluent cattle nomads. Among these people, in physical ill health, the use of herbs commences the healing path, which is usually followed by utilization of clinics in Yoruba towns. The fluidity in healing pathway reflects the perception of healing among the cattle nomads in Oyo north. Due to poor access to modern clinics and hospitals in neighboring Yoruba towns, the cattle nomads rarely patronize modern health care.

Emerging Health Behaviors

Environmental forces and associated health risks related to cattle-rearing practices in Oyo north have led the cattle nomads in the region to invent some healthcare strategies as their emerging health behaviors. The use of herbs based on availability of local fauna and flora is an invented healthcare strategy, developed from cognition of local herbs grown in nomadic environments of Oyo north. Knowledge of the potency of the herbs is gathered and transmitted mostly through mouth-to-mouth transmission between the cattle nomads and some Yoruba who are seen as threats and mostly the original inhabitants of the environment. Having tried the herbs and the efficacy is confirmed, the herbs then become a household healthcare strategy, but with local modification and adaptation. For instance, *Ewé Òrúwo* is soaked in O*mi Ògì* (fermented water from millet or corn) instead of local gin and palm wine commonly used among the Yoruba. Since cattle nomads drink less wine due to religious inhibition, the use of O*mi Ògì*, lime juice, and *Omi wàrà* (fermented water from baked cheese) are preferred in extraction of medicinal contents in *Ewé Òrúwo.* There is also the use of cow urine in soaking some mixtures of herbs to prepare herbal remedy against child convulsion and chest cold.

Anther invented healthcare strategy among the people is the use of mobile phone to seek medical help from colleagues living in distant bands, inform members of the household while in health problems during cattle flocking and to seek healthcare services from their medical doctors in Yoruba towns. Also commonly engaged health-seeking behavior among the affluent nomads is occasional medical checkup in towns. Affluent nomads often register in private clinics in Yoruba towns like Shaki, Eruwa, Tede, Igangan, Iseyin, Kishi, and Lanlate where they engage in routine medical checks. More women are also engaged in ante-natal care mostly in private clinics in towns, and the use of mosquito nets and anti-malaria drugs and analgesics are common health behaviors that have also emerged among the cattle nomads of Oyo north.

The utilization of immunization against diphtheria, whooping cough, marasmus, measles, and polio myelitis for children between ages 0 and 5 years become prevalent in nomadic bands of Oyo north. Nursing mothers were captured in Primary Health Care (PHC) schemes through which they are given appointment dates to access immunization for their children. Bands are also covered in routine house-to-house immunization. While it was difficult to have wider coverage and participation at first, with wider health education and promotions through media campaigns and health incentives, over the years, there has been improvement in immunization coverage among the cattle nomads in Oyo north. The data sourced from the Office of the Director of Oyo State Primary Health Care Board, in table 8.3, shows the trends of five years (2014–2019) immunization coverage among the cattle nomads of Oyo north.

Building permanent settlements near towns among cattle nomads in Oyo north seems to be an emerging health behavior, which was caused by potential health risk and the need to have access to basic amenities that can enhance quality health among the people. With access to potable water, electricity, and better community sanitation, residence in settlements closer to towns tends to improve the health of the cattle nomads. They also enrich their nutrition with locally made factory foods such as beverages, indomie noodles, wheat (semovita), rice, and bread.

With semipermanent bands springing up in Oyo north, the cattle nomads are also engaging in subsistence farming with the cultivation of yams, millet, cassava, vegetables, and pepper, among others. Apart from yielding more household incomes as complements to sales from dairy products, farm produce, especially food crops, supplements their food intake, which in turn improves health care of the people.

The above discussed emerging healthcare strategies among the cattle nomads of Oyo north suggest some implications to the people's healthcare system. Although while official morbidity and mortality data are still absent, it seems, from casual observations and information collected through interviews, that while morbidity is high, there is apparently low mortality rates, especially among children and pregnant women. Mallam Yisa of Gaa Yisa stated that "we fall sick but die less. Our children do not die of convulsion and cholera again. Our women also do rarely die of pregnancy problems since we have started patronizing clinics in towns."[3] The emerging health culture also suggests improved access to modern health care especially in the use of preventive care as observed in immunization, medical checkups in clinics, use of anti-malaria devices, and utilization of ante-natal care. While the use of quack doctors and unlicensed drug retailers are on the increase among the low-income cattle nomads, the use of faith-based healing and local herbs are predominantly engaged when the causation of disease and illness is linked with preternatural causes.

Table 8.3 Immunization Coverage among Cattle Nomads in Oyo North, 2015–2019

Years	Percentage Coverage (%)
2015	27
2016	32
2017	46
2018	51
2019	63

Source: Fieldwork conducted among the Nomads of Oyo North, 2019.

DISCUSSIONS AND CONCLUSION

Culture is a response to environmental challenges which establishes links between humans and the environment involving negotiation. And negotiation is defined as choice of cultural action based on the struggle to survive. In threatening conditions, negotiation involves difficult exchange of values between two cultural actors. In the case of inventing "new" healthcare strategies as presented above, the two actors involved are the environment and cattle nomads of Oyo north in southwestern Nigeria. The cattle nomads live in semiarid environment, which presents threatening conditions against the well-being of the nomads. While the nomads engage the environment for their subsistence, the nomads have to negotiate with the environment by building resilience to threat and evolving new patterns of cultural actions, among which healthcare strategies are involved. The process of negotiation and resilience has far-reaching implications on healthcare systems of the pastoral nomads of Oyo north.

The above-presented findings suggest three interplay of variables. The first variable is the relations between the exploitative and productive (explorative) technology. The second is the emerging patterns of behavior involving appropriation through specific technology in a migrant environment of Oyo north, and the third is the extent to which behavior patterns are involved in healthcare systems and how such patterns influence other aspects of culture. Thus, among the pastoral nomads of Oyo north, variables such as population density, cattle nomadism, technology, settlement pattern, and social organization relate together to form social conditions acting on environmental physical components such as fauna, flora, water access, and other biological organisms to pose threat to health security. Attempt to survive brings about cultural negotiation and makes invention of "new" healthcare strategies possible.

From the foregoing, the relationship between humans, their environment and invention of new cultural patterns can easily be understood from daily reality of getting a living. Among the pastoral nomads of Oyo north, the invention of new healthcare strategies is a product of cultural negotiation between humans and the environment. Since health risks associated with the semiarid environment of Oyo north are a threat to pastoralists' survival, the pastoralists regularly negotiate with the environment to invent "new" healthcare strategies.

NOTES

1. All the respondents whose names are mentioned here have waived their anonymity. Key informant interview with Alfa Abdul in a band settlement known as *ago Abdul* near Tede. Interview held on 17 July 2019.
2. Interview with Aliyu on 17 July 2019 at Ago Abdul in Tede area.
3. Interview from Malam Yisa held on 19 July at Gaa Yisa near Tede.

REFERENCES

Ajala, Aderemi Suleiman. 2013. *Yoruba Nationalism: Culture, Politics and Violence in Southwestern Nigeria*. Cologne: Ruddiger Koeppel Verlag.

Ajala, T.Q. 2017. Parental and School Factors as Determinants of Enrolment, Attendance and Completion of Primary Education among the Fulani Nomads in Oyo State, Nigeria, 2010–2015. An Unpublished Doctoral Dissertation in Early Childhood and Educational Foundation, University of Ibadan, Nigeria.

Bennett, J.W. 1976. *The Ecological Transition: Cultural Anthropology and Human Adaptation*. New York: Pergamon Press.

Ellen, R. 2008. "Forest Knowledge, Forest Transformation: Political Contingency, Historical Ecology, and the Renegotiation of Nature in Central Seram". In Dove, M. R. and Carpenter, C. (eds.), *Environmental Anthropology: A Historical Reader*. Oxford: Blackwell Publishing.

Harris, M. 1968. *The Rise of Anthropological Theory: A History of Theories of Culture*. London: Routledge & Keegan Paul.

Havilland, J. 1975. *Nature and Culture: Studies in Cultural Anthropology*. New York: Applecroft.

Lee, R.B. 1969. "Kung Bushman Subsistence: An Input and Output Analysis". In Damas, D (ed.), *Contribution to Anthropology Ecological Essays*. Ottawa, National Museums of Canada Bulletin, 86: 3–94.

Onyima, B.N. 2019. "Inter-sectoral Identities and Access to Health-Oriented Ethnography among the Pastoralists in South-western Nigeria". *African Ethnography*, Vl.1(1): 13-42.

Rappaport, Rou A. 1969. "Some suggestions concerning Concepts and Method in Ecological Anthropology". In Damas, D (ed.) *Contribution to Anthropology Ecological Essays*. Ottawa, National Museums of Canada Bulletin, 230.

Steward, J. 1955. *The Theory of Culture Change*. University of Illinois Press: Urbana.

Chapter 9

Safe Food Systems for Better Health Outcomes

Emerging Food Safety Issues, Challenges, and Solutions in Sub-Saharan Africa

Marther W. Ngigi and Dominic Mureithi

The problem of health in sub-Saharan Africa cannot be addressed by the health sector alone, but through an integrative approach encompassing safe food systems as the majority of human diseases are foodborne or have an origin in animal agriculture (Cecchi and Slingenbergh, 2013). Safe food systems provide opportunities to improve nutrition, better health, improve income and drive economic growth, but food safety-related challenges may undermine these benefits. Furthermore, safe food systems, in essence, contribute to UN Sustainable Development Goals (SDGs). Food safety is vital in realizing SDGs goal three on good health and well-being by reducing the burden of foodborne diseases at national and global levels (Grace, 2017). Unsafe food and foodborne diseases are likely to affect human health, food systems, and have development implications on the economy at large. World Health Organization (WHO) estimates that, annually, more than 600 million people fall ill, 420,000 die, and 33 million become disabled from consuming contaminated and unsafe food (WHO, 2015).

The traditional food system is transitioning to a modern food system that is keen on food quality and safety. A safe food system is crucial because of the interlinkages between human and animal health and how these links affect the environment and sustainable food production (FAO and WHO, 2019). A safe food system considers aspects of food safety, healthy nutrition, and food security that have far-reaching implications for human health (High Level Panel of Experts, 2017; Walls et al., 2019). A food system reflects all elements of the environment, people, and the supply chain and activities along the chain and outcomes of these activities (High Level Panel of Experts,

2017). Integrating food security, food safety, and health presents a technical challenge that requires the collaboration of different actors and institutions, political will, and allocation of resources (Walls et al., 2019). However, Africa's food systems face notable challenges in production, distribution, and markets that lead to inadequate safe and nutritious food and is unable to meet the needs and expectations of rural and urban consumers.

Globally, the burden of foodborne diseases is largely borne in Africa, particularly in sub-Saharan Africa (SSA) (WHO, 2015). The African region has the highest per capita foodborne illnesses, with an annual estimate of 91 million people suffering from acute illnesses and 137,000 deaths from foodborne hazards (WHO, 2015). Hence, the challenge of food safety undermines the regions' agro-based development strategies including the Comprehensive Africa Agriculture Development Program (CAADP) and the 2014 Malabo Declaration that depend on increasing regional and global markets by assuring food safety is observed. The demand for safe and nutritious food in Africa is rising due to emerging middle class, urbanization, and population growth. Therefore, guaranteeing food safety is an important factor of sustainable and inclusive food systems (Global Food Safety Partnership, 2019).

This chapter prioritizes food safety in agri-food systems to provide positive health outcomes. Food safety risks in fresh vegetables, cereals, and animal source foods that have high demand and consumption as income and nutritional knowledge increase in Africa are reviewed and a case study of emerging risks of antibiotic residues in the milk supply chain in Kenya is presented. Some solutions to food safety concerns and their successful applications are also highlighted.

EMERGING FOOD SAFETY RISKS IN FOOD SYSTEMS IN SUB-SAHARAN AFRICA

Food Safety in Traditional Markets

The food system in sub-Saharan Africa (SSA) relies mostly on smallholder agriculture that produces mainly for traditional markets. Traditional markets include open-air markets, street vendors and kiosks that lack formal food systems, food hygiene, infrastructure, and good sanitary facilities (Global Food Safety Partnership, 2019). These informal markets face food safety challenges despite their vital contribution to food and nutrition security to low-income earners. Informal markets sell food at low prices and they are the most important source of milk, eggs, meat, and vegetables in SSA (Roesel and Grace, 2014). Evidence from East Africa shows that coliform and *Salmonella* are higher in fresh vegetables in the informal markets than they are at the farm level due to poor handling, hygiene, and sanitary facilities in the market (Kutto et al., 2011). Furthermore, the informal milk market presents higher microbiological hazards but could be less risky as milk boiling before consumption is widely practiced by consumers (Roesel and Grace, 2014). There is increasing formal markets such as supermarkets and specialty stores in SSA in response to urbanization and growing middle class, but these markets are not necessarily safe (Kutto et al., 2011; Roesel and Grace, 2014).

Mycotoxin Contamination

Another challenge facing food systems in SSA is mycotoxin contamination along cereal grain, groundnuts, milk, meat, and the animal feed supply chains. Aflatoxin contamination is a serious problem in SSA since dietary diversity is low, while most of the households rely on staples like maize. Aflatoxin is a metabolite produced by fungus *Aspergillus flavus* and *Aspergillus parasiticus*. Aflatoxins start at the farm due to poor pre- and post-harvest management, and enter the food chain through processing to consumers. Recent evidence shows that 64 percent of sampled milk in Nairobi have aflatoxin of 84 ng/kg, exceeding EU recommended limit of 50ng/kg, although over 80 percent of farmers are aware of risks of aflatoxin (Kagera et al., 2019). A study in Ethiopia shows that milk and feed samples had Aflatoxin B_1 (AFB_1) beyond the recommended levels that resulted in the rejection of milk at market points by consumers (Gizachew et al., 2019).

Consumption of milk and food contaminated with aflatoxins leads to negative health and nutritional status. Recent evidence in SSA shows that Aflatoxin M_1 (AFM_1) exposure in children aged between 6 and 12 years contributes to immune suppression, growth impairment and interferes with vaccine efficiency that increases the risk of children to infectious diseases (Sirma et al., 2019; Wangia et al., 2019). Maternal aflatoxin exposure during pregnancy result is associated with low birth weight, smaller head circumference, and stillbirth as shown by studies in Uganda and Kenya (Hoffmann et al., 2018; Lauer et al., 2019).

Long-term exposure to aflatoxins leads to liver cancer and worsens Hepatitis B infection. AFM_1 in milk contributes to a small proportion of Hepatocellular carcinoma (HCC) cases in Kenya (Sirma et al., 2019). In the dairy sector, contamination of feed with aflatoxin leads to direct and indirect economic losses such as decreased trade due to rejection of contaminated animal products, death of animals in acute mycotoxicosis, reduced growth and reproduction, and decreased immunity leading to more cases of animal diseases (Kemboi et al., 2020).

Residue of Agricultural Chemicals

Agricultural intensification and commercialization through the use of agricultural pesticides increase food availability and affordability and improve nutrition. Agrochemicals use has enabled Africa to make huge strides in reducing food insecurity and in improving livelihoods and income. Use of agricultural pesticides in Africa is, however, of concern because of weak regulation, compliance, and enforcement and inadequate knowledge of pesticide hazards among farmers and handlers that leads to pesticide poisoning (Loha et al., 2018). There is a growing market for insecticides and a notable increase of misuse of harmful pesticides in Africa. Harmful insecticides such as neonicotinoids that faced a ban in 2018 by the European Union (EU) have found their markets in most countries in Africa (ASSAf, 2021). There is evidence of neonicotinoid residues in honey, contamination in soils and in water and sediment in agricultural areas that threaten human health and ecosystems (Loha et al., 2018). Evidence in Kenya and Ethiopia shows that honey samples contain pesticides, among them neonicotinoids (ASSAf, 2021).

Exposure to pesticides is linked to health risks in humans including dermatological, gastrointestinal, neurological, carcinogenic, respiratory, reproductive, and endocrine problems. In Ghana, residual levels of organochlorine pesticides in marketed fruits and vegetables exceed the maximum residue limits (MRLs) that could result in systemic toxicity in children and health hazards in consumers (Donkor et al., 2016). Evidence in Zimbabwe shows that workers in commercial farms experience occupational hazards through poisoning by organophosphate due to excessive exposure to harmful agrochemicals since they are not provided with protective equipment (Magauzi et al., 2011). Furthermore, levels of pesticide residues such as organochlorines are found in soils and water bodies thus interfering with ecosystems.

Wastewater Use

Food safety is also linked to the quality of water used along the food chain from production to consumption. Wastewater is ever more being used in agriculture due to increasing freshwater competition and scarcity linked to industrialization and climate change. Use of wastewater for irrigation has been linked to increased cases of foodborne diseases and deaths among children in developing countries (FAO and WHO, 2019).

Wastewater used in peri-urban and urban farming contains pathogens, toxic organisms, heavy metals, inorganic particles, pesticides, and organic compounds that cause health risks to consumers and farmers. Leafy vegetables grown using wastewater contain a high level of *Salmonella* and fecal coliforms (Kutto et al., 2011) and high toxic levels of boron, copper, manganese, lead, and zinc (FAO and WHO, 2019). Wastewater exposes agricultural workers, children, farmers, and consumers to health risks. Agricultural workers and family members suffer occupational risks of skin diseases and helminthic infections (Adegoke et al., 2018). Foodborne outbreaks are reported from vegetables and fruits irrigated by wastewater due to contamination of fecal coliforms and *Salmonella* in developing countries (FAO and WHO, 2019).

Antibiotic Residues in Animal-Source Foods

Antibiotics use in animal production have contributed to improved animal health and increased productivity hence more availability of nutritious, high-quality and low-cost animal products. The dairy and meat value chain has the potential to provide animal protein, calories, and essential minerals for health outcomes in infants, children, and expectant mothers and to increase birth weight (Hjertholm et al., 2017). Regardless of these benefits, there are concerns of growing antibiotic resistance, food safety risks, and weak regulatory measures in the use of antibiotics in food-producing animals in SSA. The overuse and misuse of antibiotics in livestock production, transportation, and marketing contribute to antimicrobial resistance globally (FAO 2016).

Continued exposure of consumers to antibiotics in food and animal products may result in allergic reactions, hypersensitivity, and antibiotic resistance (FAO, 2016). Antibiotic residues in milk also reduce the economic value and quality of milk by interfering with bacterial cultures used in the processing of yogurt and cheese. Milk contaminated with antibiotic residues reduces farmers' income due to frequent rejections at selling points. Evidence in Ghana, Ethiopia, and Nigeria shows that antibiotic residue levels in meat, milk, and eggs are beyond recommended limits (Addo et al., 2011; Basulira, Olet, and Alele, 2019; Olatoye, Daniel, and Ishola, 2016). The main driver of antibiotic residues in milk is mastitis therapy which is associated with failure to keep the udder clean, especially in the wet season and poor floor conditions which encourage the accumulation of mastitis-causing bacteria (Mureithi and Njuguna, 2016).

Antibiotic residues in food produce are worsened by low awareness level of health risks of residues, selfish business behavior to prolong shelf life, and failure to observe antibiotic withdrawal period after therapy. The case study in this chapter shows that failure to keep treatment records of animals and high cost of production are the main drivers of the risk of antibiotic residues in milk.

CASE STUDY: RISK OF ANTIBIOTIC RESIDUES IN DAIRY SUPPLY CHAIN IN KENYA

The dairy industry is important to African rural setting in terms of income, employment, poverty reduction, and improved health outcomes. Milk improves children's growth, cognitive performance as well as physical activity, while milk intake by expectant women is associated with increased birth weight. The dairy supply chain is an important source of livelihood to women and youth in both rural and peri-urban settings in developing countries. However, the dairy supply chain poses health and food safety risks due to misuse and overuse of antibiotics by farmers and traders as discussed in the previous section.

This section uses the case study of Kenya dairy farmers in peri-urban areas to examine production practices that pose public health challenges and increase antibiotic residues in the milk supply chain. The study examines the production practices that increase the risk of antibiotic residues and the level of farmers' awareness about antibiotic residues in milk. Respondents were selected through a mixed-method sampling approach employing purposive and snowballing sampling. A semi-structured questionnaire was used to collect the data from 387 dairy farmers in the five wards of Githunguri Sub-County of Kiambu County in August 2018. Questionnaires captured information on farming enterprise characteristics, awareness of antibiotics residues, livestock management practices, delivery of animal health services, animal breeding practices, the occurrence of diseases and mortality, record keeping, and milk quality practices.

Farmers' Awareness about the Risk of Antibiotic Residues in Milk

The case study shows that 42 percent of dairy farmers are aware of the health and economic risks of antibiotic residues in milk. Awareness of risks of antibiotic residues is associated with dairy production behavior and the keeping of health records of animals. Awareness of risks of antibiotics is influenced by years of schooling, perceptions of food safety, and frequency of milk testing at collection points.

Lack of knowledge and awareness in milk value chain creates a perfect breeding condition for milk contamination with antibiotic residues and other impurities. Lunner-Kolstrup and Ssali (2016) similarly show that low awareness level of the use of antibiotics can jeopardize human health and food safety in Uganda. Low awareness of risks associated with antibiotic residues makes farmers secretly sell milk rejected at the collection point by companies to brokers or give it to pets and calves. Hence, raising awareness of the risk of antibiotic residues among actors in the dairy supply chain is an essential step toward reducing antibiotic residues and other contaminants in milk.

Drivers of Antibiotic Residues in Milk

The study pinpoints three drivers of antibiotic residues in the dairy supply chain—farm level (i) failure to withhold milk from all quarters during mastitis therapy; (ii) failure to observe withdrawal period for the recommended time; and (iii) failure to keep treatment records. These sources of antibiotics are elaborated in the subsections below.

Failure to Withdraw Milk from All Quarters

Antibiotic residues in milk are associated with mastitis treatment in lactating cows when withdrawal period is not properly observed. This study shows that 76.5 percent of the farmers reported that they only withhold milk from the quarter treated with intramammary infusion during the management of mastitis (see table 9.1). This poses risks of antibiotic residues since antibiotics infused into one quarter can spread to the other untreated quarters through the bloodstream. Hence, the milk needs to be discarded for all quarters of a treated animal. Farmers claimed that milk from their convalescent cow will eventually be bulked with milk from other producers thus diluting the level of antibiotic residues and hence there is no need to discard the milk.

Failure to Withhold Milk for the Recommended Time

While milk containing antibiotic residues is not safe for human consumption, consumers and farmers might be exposed to risks because of failure to discard the milk after treatment. Table 9.2 shows that a low proportion of farmers observe recommended withdrawal period, where only 38.5 percent withdraw milk after injection and 16.8 percent after intramammary infusion. About 15.5 percent of dairy farmers do not withhold milk for the full period claiming that the withdrawal period is too long. Besides, 34 percent of dairy farmers sell milk to cooperatives, middlemen, and neighbors during and immediately after treatment of a dairy animal with antibiotics. However, about 32 percent of dairy farmers discard the milk during and after treatment, while 19 percent give milk to calves, pigs, or dogs. Interestingly, 14 percent of farmers consume milk at household level from treated animals that pose a health risk of antibiotic residues to them and their families.

Table 9.1 Withdrawal of Milk during Mastitis Treatment

Withdrawal of milk during mastitis treatment (N = 387)		
Variables	*Frequency*	*%*
Withdraw milk from treated teat during treatment of mastitis?		
Withdraw milk from only treated teat	296	76.5
Withdraw milk from all teats	91	23.5

Source: Generated from Authors' own survey data of dairy farmers in Githunguri sub-County of Kiambu County, August 2018.

Table 9.2 Withdrawal of Milk during Treatment

Withdraw of milk during treatment (N = 387)		
Variables	*Frequency*	*%*
When do you practice withdrawal period?		
After injection	149	38.5
After intramammary infusion	65	16.8
Both	175	44.7
Not withdrawing milk for the recommended time	60	15.5
What do you do with milk during or after treatment?		
Take milk to cooperative or sell to neighbors or middlemen	133	34.4
Give milk to calves, pigs, or dogs	75	19.4
Discard milk	125	32.3
Consume milk at home	54	13.9

Source: Generated from Authors' own survey data of dairy farmers in Githunguri sub-County of Kiambu County, August 2018.

Farmers indicated that they fail to observe the withdrawal period because of the high cost of production, and the great need to break-even. They also reported that it is a waste of resources and that they are not given advice by the animal health provider and the duration recommended by a veterinarian is too long which leads to loss of income.

A recent study in northern Tanzania shows that 93 percent of agro-pastoralists do not observe a withdrawal period of milk and meat after animals are treated with antibiotics (Caudell et al., 2017). Previous studies show that failure to observe withdraw period by farmers is the main contributor to antibiotic residues in animal food products (Beyene, 2016; Mureithi and Njuguna, 2016). The decision by dairy farmers to observe withdrawal period is influenced by the level of education and knowledge of the risk of antibiotics by farmers and the frequency of screening of milk at collection points by dairy cooperatives and companies.

Failure to Keep Treatment Records

Keeping treatment records and regular updating of records after each treatment is important in capturing the use of antibiotics hence lower the risk of residues that could ensure food safety. About 61.5 percent of dairy farmers do not keep farm and treatment records at all. Notably, 65 percent of dairy farmers with a record book indicated that veterinarians often fail to update the records after treatment or farm visit, which presents an opportunity for improvement.

Farmers reported that poor records lead to milkers bulking milk from animals treated with antibiotics. Beyene (2016) found that failure to keep a proper treatment records was among the major drivers of antibiotic residue accumulation in food-producing animals. The treatment record should contain treatment date, animal identification, diagnosis, treatment therapy used, duration of therapy, withdrawal time for milk and the individual who administered the drug (National Milk Producers Federation, 2019). Therefore, dairy farmers should be encouraged to maintain good treatment records, while animal health providers should update the treatment details to reduce antibiotic residues, ensure effective herd health plan, reduce liability, reduce cost, and to improve the effectiveness of the animal health provider.

INTEGRATED APPROACHES TO MANAGE FOOD SAFETY ACROSS FOOD SYSTEMS IN SSA

As earlier highlighted about the emerging challenges of food safety and the health burden it presents, this section summarizes the approaches to manage food safety in food systems in SSA and the achievements or challenges likely to be encountered.

Food Safety Standards and Regulations

Government enacts laws and regulations responsible for surveillance and control of food systems. Both public and private inspection and testing services ensure actors across the value chains comply with food quality regulations and manage the risks of foodborne diseases. However, surveillance and control of food systems in SSA are inefficient due to weak regulatory framework, dysfunctional laboratory systems and weak marketing infrastructure that lacks basic sanitation facilities (Morse et al., 2018; Roesel and Grace, 2014).

Considering food safety as an integral part of international trade in agri-food products, regional and international standards offer solutions to several food issues. Codex Alimentarius provides standards, guidelines, and code of practices to assure safety and quality of food products adopted at international food trade (FAO and WHO, 2019). The case study of food safety standards pinpoints that implementation of standards requires coordination and collaboration among actors, partners, and researchers. For example, Africa Aflatoxin Information Management System enables sharing of mitigation interventions of aflatoxins across agriculture, health, and trade sectors across the continent. Food safety acts as a barrier for export markets by smallholder farmers who face high transaction costs by adhering to private food-safety standards such as GlobalGAP standards.

Technological Innovations, Training, and Extension Services

There is a need to put measures to ensure food safety at the production level to reduce foodborne threats to the health of farmers, buyers, and consumers. Technologies that promote Good Production Practices (GAP) can reduce contamination of food from wastewater, aflatoxins, chemicals, and antibiotics. However, domestic GAP in SSA is low with limited information on uptake and impacts. The growing demand for vegetables due to urbanization leads to wastewater use in irrigation. Farmers should explore low-cost strategies such as water application techniques that reduce risks of wastewater-irrigated vegetables and other produce. To reduce the adverse effects of pesticides, herbicides, and other chemicals in crop production, effective regulatory measures need to be enforced to ban harmful chemicals. Besides, farmers should be supported to adopt integrated pest management (IPM) to reduce the use of agrochemicals.

Training farmers through extension services and farmer field school (FFS) encourages the diffusion of IPM that is effective in reducing the use of chemicals in crop production. Clausen et al. (2017) have shown that IPM training in Uganda through FFS reduced pesticide applications and farmers used more safety measures that reduced pesticide exposure and, hence, ensured better health outcomes. Evidence in Kenya shows that farmers trained on GlobalGAP and monitored for compliance use less harmful chemicals, which in turn leads to fewer health problems (Asfaw, Mithöfer, and Waibel, 2009).

Farmers should be encouraged to adopt safe production practices, technologies, and innovations to improve food safety and quality. Integrated pre- and post-harvest technologies including biological control, chemical, and improved storage materials provide solutions to reduce aflatoxins contamination in SSA. The use of low-cost hermetic containers and bags suppress fungi-causing aflatoxins and farmers reduce the use of harmful pesticides in the storage of cereals (Udomkun et al., 2017). Recent research shows that adding mycotoxin binders in animal feeds suppresses adsorption or encourages the excretion of mycotoxins-reducing aflatoxins in milk and meat. There is, however, no regulations or standards guiding their use in several countries in SSA like Kenya (Mutua et al., 2019).

To reduce the risk of antibiotic residues in milk and meat, implementing best management practices is essential. One of the potential ways is adopting One Health approach that promotes human, animal, and environmental health to prevent diseases occurrence and minimize the use of antibiotics in livestock supply chains (Garcia et al., 2019). This could include herd biosecurity, early diagnosis, and accurate immediate action to sick animals and separation of treated cows from the milking herd. This case study illustrates that keeping good treatment records will help record antibiotic use, drug withdrawal period, and separate treated animal from the milking herd. Adequate records should document treatment history of animal and drug used to prevent drug residue in food, which in turn will protect the consumer by ensuring the food on the fork is safe.

Improve Food Safety in Wet Markets

Strategies to improve food safety in the trade and markets are crucial. As food produce moves from production to market, there is a need for food safety measures and adherence to regulations. Most of the foodborne diseases in SSA are experienced by the majority who depend on informal wet markets, that is less regulated (Boto and Mafolo, 2018). Wet markets will continue to matter and supply about 50–70 percent of market demand by 2050 which needs interventions in food safety. Training of traders, raising awareness, and use of simple technologies like disinfectants, and water points could reduce the health risks of foodborne illnesses. Sensitization of food handlers and consumers in informal food markets is important since informal markets supply a larger proportion of food consumed in major cities in SSA. New evidence shows that training and certification program in informal milk markets in Kenya led to improved microbiological quality and hygiene practices (Boto and Mafolo, 2018).

The National Dairy Development Policy advocates education campaigns on the consumption of well-handled milk, training on milk testing, and stakeholder sensitization on the safe use of antibiotics and veterinary drugs. Training of traders in abattoirs in Nigeria improved microbiological quality of meat in the short term, but required enabling environment and stakeholder collaboration to improve food safety in wet markets in the long run (Grace et al., 2019). Modernization of infrastructure and provision of basic sanitation facilities in informal markets can improve food safety in these markets. This should ensure the supply of clean water, improved personal hygiene, and removal of waste from markets and points of sale.

Consumers Demand Food Safety and Healthy Diets

The pull approaches on reverse thinking about food systems should consider the consumer demand especially on food quality and healthy diets. Hence, the private sector needs to respond to the evolving demand for safer food, as well as, address other challenges such as malnutrition in food systems (Boto and Mafolo, 2018). To reduce foodborne diseases, consumers must be aware of risks and be willing to pay more for safer handling practices during purchasing, and food preparation and they must observe hygiene. Consumer awareness of food safety is an important driver of decisions made by consumers and producer.

Since most of food safety issues arise from asymmetric information between producers and consumers, certification of products and Hazard Analysis and Critical Control Point (HACCP) system is essential. Case studies in SSA pinpoint that consumers are willing to pay more for quality and safety attributes of fresh produce, maize, meat and milk, HACCP certifications and assurance labels of antibiotic-residue-free meat and fish products (Ngigi et al., 2011; Ragasa et al., 2019). Besides, consumers are willing to pay more for Aflasafe food products—a case of maize and groundnuts in Nigeria (Ayedun et al., 2017). However, there is no guarantee of safety through certification and labeling. Hence, consumers use brand names as a proxy for quality and safety (Global Food Safety Partnership, 2019). Further, consumers assess food safety based on trust that adequate risk management measures are considered upstream in production, processing, storage, and trade. Creating awareness of foodborne illnesses, increasing consumer demands and market pressures will thrust for safe food systems in SSA.

CONCLUSIONS AND POLICY IMPLICATIONS

Safe food systems provide opportunities to improve nutrition, health, and income and drive economic growth, while food safety risks could undermine the benefits of food systems in SSA. Food safety risks emerge across the food systems from the farm level to the fork, which requires diverse measures to address them. These include mycotoxins contamination, microbiological hazards, agricultural chemicals residues in fresh produce and antibiotic residues in animal-sourced foods.

The case study on antibiotic residues pinpoints the main drivers of antibiotics residue in the milk supply chain in Kenya. These include low awareness levels of health risks of antibiotic residues by farmers, and failure to withhold milk from all quarters during mastitis therapy, observe a withdrawal period, and to keep treatment records. These findings have far-reaching policy implications. There is a need to create awareness for farmers, extension officers and animal health service providers on health risks of antibiotic residues and to provide possible measures to reduce antibiotic residues in milk and other animal-source products. Awareness-raising can be done through farmers' field days, workshops, seminars, and sensitization through information communication technologies (ICTs) such as radio, television, and mobile phones that could reach wider actors in the dairy supply chain. Farmers' dairy cooperatives that most farmers are associated with is a good starting point for developing policies and guidelines to encourage dairy farmers to keep treatment records and to update them regularly for all dairy animals to promote milk safety and quality.

At the farm level, efforts by policy makers should aim to create awareness and to improve knowledge on risks of aflatoxins, wastewater use, antibiotic and pesticide residues. Furthermore, the efforts of the government should aim to promote affordable technologies and innovations that improve food safety such as IPM, hermetic containers and bags, and mycotoxin binders among others. The adoption of technologies can be promoted through training and awareness campaign to sensitize farmers through farmer field schools, farmer groups, and extension services.

Food safety is not only a public health concern, but it also affects access to domestic and export markets. In SSA, informal markets dominate and present opportunities for smallholder farmers to sell nutritious food items. Measures to improve food safety at the market level include investments in infrastructure such as road, warehousing, sanitation facilities, and information systems on market prices and demand. Training of traders and certification programs in informal markets will improve the microbiological quality of food and hygiene practices and support positive health outcomes and better livelihoods, especially for food-insecure households in SSA.

Measures at the consumer level need to enhance consumer awareness on food safety, handling of food and to ensure access to nutritious diets. This can be achieved through public campaigns, community-based nutrition education, and the use of information communication and technologies (ICTs) such as television, radio, and mobile phones.

Lastly, to improve food safety across food systems, there is a need to strengthen national regulatory frameworks to enhance laws and regulations in order to encourage adherence to food-safety standards by all actors in the food chain. The efforts of the government should seek to improve the actors' capacity to embrace food safety standards. Collaborations of actors need to be encouraged and to consider roles of smallholder farmers, input providers, researchers, traders, transporters, public health and nutrition practitioners. Since food safety from the farm to the fork is complex, collaborative and multidisciplinary interventions can ensure food safety across food systems and improve health outcomes for all.

REFERENCES

Addo, K. K., G. I. Mensah, K. G. Aning, N. Nartey, G. K. Nipah, C. Bonsu, M. L. Akyeh, and H. L. Smits. 2011. "Microbiological Quality and Antibiotic Residues in Informally Marketed Raw Cow Milk within the Coastal Savannah Zone of Ghana." *Tropical Medicine & International Health* 16 (2): 227–32.

Adegoke, Anthony A., Isaac D. Amoah, Thor A. Stenström, Matthew E. Verbyla, and James R. Mihelcic. 2018. "Epidemiological Evidence and Health Risks Associated With Agricultural Reuse of Partially Treated and Untreated Wastewater: A Review." *Frontiers in Public Health* 6: 337.

Asfaw, S., D. Mithöfer, and H. Waibel. 2009. "Investment in Compliance with GlobalGAP Standards: Does It Pay off for Small-Scale Producers in Kenya?" *Journal of International Agriculture* 48 (4): 337–62.

Academy of Science of South Africa (ASSAf), (2021). "Neonicotinoid Insecticides: Use and Effects in African Agriculture. A Review and Recommendations to Policymakers." doi: http://dx.doi.org/10.17159/assaf.2021/0069.

Ayedun, Bamikole, Godwin Okpachu, Victor Manyong, Joseph Atehnkeng, Adebayo Akinola, G. A. Abu, Ranajit Bandyopadhyay, and Tahirou Abdoulaye. 2017. "An Assessment of Willingness To Pay by Maize and Groundnut Farmers for Aflatoxin Biocontrol Product in Northern Nigeria." *Journal of Food Protection* 80 (9): 1451–60.

Basulira, Yake, Susan A. Olet, and Paul Erasmus Alele. 2019. "Inappropriate Usage of Selected Antimicrobials: Comparative Residue Proportions in Rural and Urban Beef in Uganda." *PLoS One* 14 (1): e0209006. https://doi.org/10.1371/journal.pone.0209006.

Beyene, Takele. 2016. "Veterinary Drug Residues in Food-Animal Products: Its Risk Factors and Potential Effects on Public Health." *Journal of Veterinary Science & Technology* 7 (1): 1–7.

Boto, Isolina, and Lebo Mafolo. 2018. "Food Safety: A Critical Part of the Food System in Africa." Briefing 52. Brussels: Technical Centre for Agricultural and Rural Cooperation.

Caudell, Mark A., Marsha B. Quinlan, Murugan Subbiah, Douglas R. Call, Casey J. Roulette, Jennifer W. Roulette, Adam Roth, Louise Matthews, and Robert J. Quinlan. 2017. "Antimicrobial Use and Veterinary Care among Agro-Pastoralists in Northern Tanzania." *PloS One* 12 (1).

Cecchi, G., and J. Slingenbergh. 2013. *World Livestock 2013: Changing Disease Landscapes*. Rome: Food and Agriculture Organization of the United Nations.

Clausen, Anna Sabine, Erik Jørs, Aggrey Atuhaire, and Jane Frølund Thomsen. 2017. "Effect of Integrated Pest Management Training on Ugandan Small-Scale Farmers." *Environmental Health Insights* 11: 1–10. https://doi.org/10.1177/1178630217703391.

Donkor, Augustine, Paul Osei-Fosu, Brajesh Dubey, Robert Kingsford-Adaboh, Cephas Ziwu, and Isaac Asante. 2016. "Pesticide Residues in Fruits and Vegetables in Ghana: A Review." *Environmental Science and Pollution Research* 23: 18966–87.

FAO. 2016. *Drivers, Dynamics and Epidemiology of Antimicrobial Resistance in Animal Production*. Rome, Italy: Food and Agriculture Organization of the United Nations.

FAO, and WHO. 2019. *Pesticides Residues in Food 2018: Joint FAO/WHO Meeting on Pesticide Residues: Report of the Joint Meeting of the FAO Panel of Experts on Pesticide Residues in Food and the Environment and the WHO Core Assessment Group on Pesticide Residues Berlin, Germany, 18-27 September 2018.*

Garcia, Sara N., Bennie I. Osburn, and James S. Cullor. 2019. "A One Health Perspective on Dairy Production and Dairy Food Safety." *One Health* 7: 100086. https://doi.org/10.1016/j.onehlt.2019.100086.

Gizachew, D., B. Szonyi, J. Hanson, and D. Grace. 2019. "Aflatoxin Contamination of Milk and Dairy Feeds in the Greater Addis Ababa Milk Shed, Ethiopia." *Food Control* 59: 773–79.

Global Food Safety Partnership. 2019. "Food Safety in Africa: Past Endeavors and Future Directions." Washington, DC: World Bank.

Grace, Delia. 2017. "Food Safety and the Sustainable Development Goals," Nairobi, Kenya. ILRI. https://cgspace.cgiar.org/bitstream/handle/10568/100694/SDGs%20and%20food%20safety.pdf?sequence=4&isAllowed=y.

Grace, Delia, Morenike Dipeolu, and Silvia Alonso. 2019. "Improving Food Safety in the Informal Sector: Nine Years Later." *Infection Ecology & Epidemiology* 9 (1). https://doi.org/10.1080/20008686.2019.1579613.

High Level Panel of Experts. 2017. "Nutrition and Food Systems. A Report by the High Level Panel of Experts on the Committee on World Food Security, Rome." HLPE Steering committee 12.

Hjertholm, Katrine G., Per Ole Iversen, Gerd Holmboe-Ottesen, Ibrahimu Mdala, Alister Munthali, Kenneth Maleta, Zumin Shi, Elaine Ferguson, and Penjani Kamudoni. 2017. "Maternal Dietary Intake during Pregnancy and Its Association to Birth Size in Rural Malawi: A Cross-Sectional Study." *Maternal and Child Nutrition* 14 (1): e12433.

Hoffmann, Vivian, Kelly Jones, and Jef L Leroy. 2018. "The Impact of Reducing Dietary Aflatoxin Exposure on Child Linear Growth: A Cluster Randomised Controlled Trial in Kenya." *BMJ Global Health* 3 (6): e000983.

Kagera, Irene, Peter Kahenya, Florence Mutua, Gladys Anyango, Florence Kyallo, Delia Grace, and Johanna Lindahl. 2019. "Status of Aflatoxin Contamination in Cow Milk Produced in Smallholder Dairy Farms in Urban and Peri-Urban Areas of Nairobi County: A Case Study of Kasarani Sub County, Kenya." *Infection Ecology & Epidemiology* 9 (1): 1547095.

Kemboi, David Chebutia, Gunther Antonissen, Phillis E. Ochieng, Siska Croubels, Sheila Okoth, Erastus K. Kangethe, Johannes Faas, Johanna F. Lindahl, and James K. Gathumbi. 2020. "A Review of the Impact of Mycotoxins on Dairy Cattle Health: Challenges for Food Safety and Dairy Production in Sub-Saharan Africa." *Toxins* 12 (4): 222. https://doi.org/10.3390/toxins12040222.

Kutto, E. K., M. W. Ngigi, N. Karanja, E. Kange'the, L. C. Bebora, C. J. Lagerkvist, P. G. Mbuthia, L. W. Njagi, and J. J. Okello. 2011. "Bacterial Contamination of Kale (Brassica Oleracea Acephala) along the Supply Chain in Nairobi and Its Environment." *East African Medical Journal* 88 (2): 46–53.

Lauer, Jacqueline M., Christopher P. Duggan, Lynne M. Ausman, Jeffrey K. Griffiths, Patrick Webb, Jia-Sheng Wang, Kathy S. Xue, Edgar Agaba, Nathan Nshakira, and Shibani Ghosh. 2019. "Maternal Aflatoxin Exposure during Pregnancy and Adverse Birth Outcomes in Uganda." *Maternal & Child Nutrition* 15 (2): e12701.

Loha, Kumelachew Mulu, Marja Lamoree, Jana M. Weiss, and Jacob de Boer. 2018. "Import, Disposal, and Health Impacts of Pesticides in the East Africa Rift(EAR)

Zone: A Review on Management and Policy Analysis." *Crop Protection* 112: 322–31. https://doi.org/10.1016/j.cropro.2018.06.014.

Lunner-Kolstrup, Christina, and Tonny Kiggundu Ssali. 2016. "Awareness and Need for Knowledge of Health and Safety among Dairy Farmers Interviewed in Uganda." *Frontiers in Public Health* 4: 137.

Magauzi, Regis, Bigboy Mabaera, Simbarashe Rusakaniko, Anderson Chimusoro, Nqobile Ndlovu, Mufuta Tshimanga, Gerald Shambira, Addmore Chadambuka, and Notion Gombe. 2011. "Health Effects of Agrochemicals among Farm Workers in Commercial Farms of Kwekwe District, Zimbabwe." *The Pan African Medical Journal* 9(1).

Morse, Tracy D., Humphreys Masuku, Sarah Rippon, and Hudson Kubwalo. 2018. "Achieving an Integrated Approach to Food Safety and Hygiene—Meeting the Sustainable Development Goals in Sub-Saharan Africa." *Sustainability* 10 (7): 2394.

Mureithi, D. K., and M. N. Njuguna. 2016. "Prevalence of Subclinical Mastitis and Associated Risk Factors in Dairy Farms in Urban and Peri-Urban Areas of Thika Sub County, Kenya." *Livestock Research for Rural Development* 28: 13.

Mutua, Florence, Johanna Lindahl, and Delia Grace. 2019. "Availability and Use of Mycotoxin Binders in Selected Urban and Peri-Urban Areas of Kenya." *Food Security* 11 (2): 359–69.

National Milk Producers Federation. 2019. *Milk & Dairy Beef Drug Residue Prevention. Reference Manual 2019*. Dairy Management Inc. Rosemont, Illinois, USA.

Ngigi, M. W., J. J. Okello, C. J. Lagerkvist, N. Karanja, and J. Mburu. 2011. "Urban Consumers' Willingness to Pay for Quality of Leafy Vegetables along the Value Chain: The Case of Nairobi Kale Consumers, Kenya." *International Journal of Business and Social Sciences* 2 (7): 208–16.

Olatoye, Isaac Olufemi, Oluwayemisi Folashade Daniel, and Sunday Ayobami Ishola. 2016. "Screening of Antibiotics and Chemical Analysis of Penicillin Residue in Fresh Milk and Traditional Dairy Products in Oyo State, Nigeria." *Veterinary World* 9 (9): 948–54.

Ragasa, Catherine, Kwaw S Andam, Sena Amewu, and Seth B Asante. 2019. "Consumer Demand and Willingness to Pay for Safe Food in Accra, Ghana. Implications for Public and Private Sector's Roles in Food Safety Management." *IFPRI* 01795: 43.

Roesel, K., and D. Grace. 2014. *Food Safety and Informal Markets: Animal Products in Sub-Saharan Africa | International Livestock Research Institute*. London, UK: Routledge.

Sirma, A. J., K Makita, D. Grace, D. Senerwa, and Johanna Lindahl. 2019. "Aflatoxin Exposure from Milk in Rural Kenya and the Contribution to the Risk of Liver Cancer." *Toxins(Basel)* 11 (8): 469.

Udomkun, Patchimaporn, Alexander Nimo Wiredu, Marcus Nagle, Joachim Müller, Bernard Vanlauwe, and Ranajit Bandyopadhyay. 2017. "Innovative Technologies to Manage Aflatoxins in Foods and Feeds and the Profitability of Application—A Review." *Food Control* 76 (June): 127–38.

Walls, H., P. Baker, E. Chirwa, and B. Hawkins. 2019. "Food Security, Food Safety & Healthy Nutrition: Are They Compatible?" *Global Food Security* 21: 69–71.

Wangia, R. N., D. P. Githanga, J. Wang, and O. A. Anzala. 2019. "Aflatoxin Exposure in Children Age 6–12 Years: A Study Protocol of a Randomized Comparative Cross-Sectional Study in Kenya, East Africa." *Pilot Feasibility Studies* 5 (141). https://doi.org/10.1186/s40814-019-0510-x

WHO, ed. 2015. *WHO Estimates of the Global Burden of Foodborne Diseases.* Geneva, Switzerland: World Health Organization.

Chapter 10

Indoor Air Pollution and Child Health in Africa

Gloria Afful-Mensah, Edward Nketiah-Amponsah, and Robert Kaba Alhassan

Household fuel use in developing countries is a major source of indoor air pollution. Many rural and low-income urban households rely substantially on solid fuels (e.g., wood, agricultural residues, and dung) for the supply of household energy needs. Reliance on such fuels coupled with the use of inefficient cooking stoves generates emission of toxic substances that can impair the cleaning ability of the lungs and hence pose threats to human health, particularly among children (Rana et al., 2019; Ranabhat et al., 2015; Lim et al., 2012; Baumgartner et al., 2011). The World Health Organization (WHO) reports nearly 7 million deaths worldwide yearly due to exposure to outdoor and household air population of which about 1 million occur in Africa (WHO, 2020).

The WHO also estimates that indoor air pollution from the use of dirty fuels account for nearly 4.3 million premature deaths annually around the world and further argues that the associated health risks are comparable to the effects of tobacco smoking (WHO, 2016). In fact, household air pollution (mainly from the use of solid fuels) was ranked the third leading risk factor for global disease burden among children below age 5 in 2010 (Lim et al., 2012). When the level of air pollution is reduced, the prevalence of heart-related diseases, lung cancer, stroke, and respiratory-related diseases will be reduced as well. Although there have been some improvements in access to clean fuels in developing countries, millions of households still rely on inefficient and dirty fuels for cooking, posing severe health hazards for women and children due to their high participation rates in cooking and household activities.

Using data from the Ghana Demographic and Health Survey for thirteen African countries, this study provides further evidence on the relationship between exposure to smoke from biomass fuels and acute lower respiratory infection among children aged below 5 years by categorizing cooking fuels based on their levels of pollution as documented in the literature.[1] Given that the emission of pollutants from cooking fuels varies along the energy ladder, this study carries out a series of empirical analyses. First, the effect of households' use of biomass fuels (wood, agricultural residue, and animal dung) relative to other "cleaner" cooking fuels on acute respiratory infection (ARI) is investigated by testing the hypothesis that biomass (dirty) fuels for cooking have negative effect on the health of children compared to the use of cleaner fuels. Although the ultimate aim of the sustainable energy transition is to move households to clean cooking fuels, given that almost all countries in the regions are developing economies with relatively lower household income levels, the transition to clean cooking fuels is expected to be gradual and possibly move along with improvement in income and living standards.

Compared to biomass fuels, charcoal/kerosene/coal/lignite are cleaner since the smoke is usually released outside because they are burned on stoves that are typically started in open areas and brought indoors once the fuels are burning cleanly (Mishra and Retherford, 1997). Contrariwise, wood/agricultural residue/animal dung are burned on indoor stoves which are typically immobile. In addition, stoves for biomass fuels need to be refueled during the cooking process thereby leading to continual exposure to smoke. Conversely, smoke from charcoal/kerosene/coal/lignite is usually one-off during the early minutes of ignition (Mishra and Retherford, 1997). Certainly, empirical evidence regarding whether or not the use of such fuels has any health benefit compared to biomass fuels is scant. While policy makers are concerned about how to move households to the ultimate step on the energy ladder, it is equally important to explore some medium-term solution(s) in terms of investigating any benefit associated with other less efficient but less polluting fuels. Hence, this chapter tests the hypothesis that the use of biomass fuels for cooking has more negative health effects than the use of charcoal/kerosene/coal/lignite. The identification of causal impact is highly constrained with observational data (see, e.g., Garcia-Huidobro and Oakes, 2017; Gertler et al., 2011; Nicholas, 2007; and Cameron and Trivedi, 2005). However, in an attempt to move closer to the causal impact that would otherwise emanate from experimental techniques, the instrumental variable (IV) approach is adopted by instrumenting for households cooking fuel decisions with population density and soil fertility. Admittedly, estimates from the IV strategy may still not be as deemed strictly causal. Nonetheless they offer a good insight into the association between cooking fuel and child health outcomes.

Findings from the paper reveal that children from households that rely on biomass fuels for cooking are more likely to suffer from ARI. This is even greater after accounting for country fixed effects. Even among less efficient cooking energy sources, the use of raw biomass as cooking fuels has more negative health effects than the use of charcoal/kerosene/coal. The study contributes to two strands of the literature. First, it contributes to the literature on household energy use and its associated implications on households' welfare (Ezzati and Kammen, 2002; Mishra, 2003; Duflo et al., 2008; Pope et al., 2010; Gordon et al., 2014; Agrawal and Yamamoto, 2015; Imelda, 2018). By exploiting the quasi-random variation in the implementation of a nationwide LPG program, Imelda (2018) finds that the transition to LPG led to a significant reduction in infant mortality (about 4 infants per 1,000 live births) in Indonesia. In an experimental study, Barron and Torero (2017) provide evidence on the effect of household electrification on indoor air pollution and ARI among children and found the ARI rates among children in electrified households were 8–14 percentage points lower than controlled households. The evidence from available studies suggests that exposure to particulate matter and smoke from incomplete combustion of cooking fuels poses severe health risk to people, particularly infants.

Second, the paper contributes to the strand of the literature on the effects of ambient environmental quality on child health (Chay and Greenstone, 2003; Neidell, 2004; Currie and Neidell, 2005; Jayachandran, 2009; Chen et al., 2013; Bruederle and Hodler, 2017). Jayachandran (2009), for instance, examines the impact of air pollution associated with wildfires in Indonesia on infant mortality. Findings from the paper suggest that exposure to air pollution results in high infant mortality. Even though the present study does not explicitly focus on the mortality consequences of exposure to air pollution, it provides a mechanism through which exposure to pollutants can result in mortality: that is, by looking at the direct impact on child health.

EMPIRICAL FRAMEWORK

The first hypothesis is tested by categorizing household cooking fuels into biomass and cleaner fuels. "Cleaner" fuel here is broadly defined to include kerosene/charcoal/coal in addition to LPG, electricity, solar, and biogas. The set up for the second hypothesis compares biomass fuels to other less efficient but relatively "less polluting" fuels (charcoal/kerosene/coal) by restricting the empirical analysis to users of these types of fuels. The aim is to provide empirical evidence of health benefits (if any) associated with the latter as compared to raw biomass fuels. An empirical challenge in estimating these relationships using observational data is that the choice of cooking fuel is plausibly endogenous. For instance, households or individuals' preferences for cleaner fuel may be unobserved, making it difficult to control for all such determinants in a regression analysis. Again, people may differ in their extent of risk aversion and attitude toward activities that may affect their health such as the decision to use unclean fuels (which are typically cheap).[2] Therefore, neglecting the potential endogeneity of the cooking fuel variable might lead to invalid inference.

In this regard, the study adopted an Instrumental Variable (IV) approach using proxies for forest productivity and competition for forest products as instruments for households' reliance on biomass fuels for cooking. Specifically, population density and soil fertility are used as instruments. Population density is a key determinant of the demand for goods and services including land.[3] Given the finite supply of land, a high population density increases the demand for land for housing and other economic activities, thereby hastening degradation of forest resources or the conversion of agricultural lands into nonfarm activities and, hence, a reduction in agricultural residues. Reduced availability of forest products such as wood fuel or agricultural residue therefore implies a lower probability of households' relying on biomass as main cooking fuel, all else equal. While densely populated areas may aggravate the spread of infectious diseases, the definition of ARI (cough and short rapid breadth) makes it less likely to be spread this way. Also, soil quality is an important determinant of the productivity of forest(s) in providing wood used as firewood and/or agricultural activities. Therefore, areas with soil nutrients that support forest growth are more likely to have productive forest, increased supply of wood products and, hence, a high probability that households will rely on less fuel-efficient cooking energy sources. While trade in these cooking energy sources could imply that areas with less productive forest will still have high prevalence of less efficient cooking fuels conditional on location and time fixed effects, these will absorb locational differences in price and supply of cooking fuels. Hence, the instrument suffices to explain exogenous variations in household choice of cooking fuels.

To this end, the first stage IV equation is specified as:

$$1\left[BiomassFuel_{ihct}\right] = Z_{hct} + X_{ihct}\delta + \phi_{ct} + \varepsilon_{hct} \quad \text{(1)}$$

Where LHS is an indicator variable equal to 1 if an ith child in household *h* and in country *c* surveyed in year *t* relies on biomass cooking fuel such as wood, agricultural residue, or animal dung as the main cooking fuel; and 0 if otherwise. (Note that in testing the second hypothesis, users of LPG/electricity/solar are excluded from the analysis such that the indicator variable is equal to 0 if a household uses charcoal/kerosene/coal.)

Z_{hct} is a vector of IVs, X_{ihct} is a vector of characteristics of the ith child (i.e., age, gender, birth order); mother or caregiver (age, education, smoking status); and the household (size, gender of household head, place of residence [rural/urban], place for cooking, wealth).[4] The paper also controlled for country and survey year fixed effects, $ø_{ct}$. Country fixed effect is useful in absorbing cross-country heterogeneity in the determinants of ARI among children in the study countries. These may include quality of healthcare in the respective countries, and domestic policies on cooking fuels.[5] Survey year fixed effect also absorbs temporal variations in the ARI rates across the study countries, which could otherwise confound the results. ε_{hct} is the residual term.

Consequently, using the predicted probabilities from equation 1, the second stage IV model is estimated using the specification in equation 2.

$$1[ARI]_{ihct} = \alpha \times 1\sum BiomassFuel_{hct} + X_{ihct}\beta + \phi_{ct} + \mu_{ihct} \text{......................} (2)$$

where the LHS is an indicator variable equal to 1 if child *i* in household *h* and in country *c* surveyed in year *t* reports experiencing ARI in the two weeks prior to the survey. All other variables remain as previously defined; and μ_{ihct} is the residual term. The coefficient of interest is α, which measures the local average treatment effect of household use of biomass cooking fuel on the probability of a child experiencing ARI.

Even though the outcome variable(s) is (are) binary, this study opted for the standard linear (i.e., OLS) approach to estimating the IV model rather than nonlinear estimators such as logit/probit type IV-estimators.[6] The main advantage of logit/probit type estimators in estimating models with binary outcomes over the limited probability model (LPM) estimation using OLS is that the former ensures predicted probabilities fall within the interval 0 to 1. In spite of this, there are at least three advantages of OLS-type estimators over the nonlinear estimators. First, the logit/probit estimators are prone to the so-called incidental parameter problem when estimating equations with fixed effects (Greene, 2004; Bellemare et al., 2015). This "incidental parameter" is associated with a downward bias in the asymptotic standard errors, and hence may lead to type 1 errors (Greene, 2004; Bellemare et al., 2015). Second, the nonlinear models (logit and probit) are associated with interpretive difficulties and so rely on the computation of the marginal effects. Estimates from the standard IV, however, lend themselves to easy interpretation as the coefficients can be interpreted directly as marginal effects without the need for any further transformation. Meanwhile, as a robustness check, a biprobit model estimation with endogenous dummy using identical model specifications as used under the LPM, is also carried out. The empirical analysis uses robust heteroscedastic standard errors clustered at primary sampling unit (enumeration area) level.

DATA

Data from the standard Demographic and Health Surveys (DHSs) were used to carry out the empirical analysis. The DHSs are nationally representative household surveys that provide data on fertility, family planning, maternal and child health, gender, HIV/AIDS, malaria, and nutrition that are useful for monitoring and impact evaluation in the areas of population, health and nutrition (DHS, 2020). The main survey instrument is the use of questionnaires and the DHSs collected primary data by using four main standard model questionnaires: Household Questionnaire, Woman's Questionnaire, Man's Questionnaire and Biomarker Questionnaire.[7] Since this study focuses on ARI infections among children below 5 years, it relied on the data from the Woman's Questionnaire which contains information on the health of children aged 0 to 4 years. The DHS data are geocoded at the enumeration area level, thus allowing us to spatially match the data with other datasets.

Our sample is made up of data from Burundi, Comoros, Democratic Republic of Congo, Gabon, Ghana, Kenya, Lesotho, Mozambique, Namibia, Nigeria, Rwanda, Sierra Leone, and Zambia. The main measure of child health outcome is ARI. Following the conventional literature (see, e.g., Rana et al., 2019; Admasie et al., 2018; and Kilabuko and Nakki, 2007), definition adopted by the DHS and recommendations by the WHO on the definition of ARI, a child is classified as suffering from ARI if that child experienced cough accompanied with rapid short breath during the survey's two-week recall period.

Regarding the type of household cooking fuel, the focus is on households' responses to questions on the "main type of fuel used for cooking." Admittedly, households in developing countries often practice fuel stacking—a phenomenon where households rely on multiple cooking fuel sources.

However, the data only captures the main cooking fuel type. From the data, the main household cooking fuel types are electricity, liquefied petroleum gas (LPG), natural gas, biogas, kerosene, coal/lignite, charcoal, wood, straw/shrubs/grass, agricultural crop, animal dung, or solar. Given their fuel efficiency, combustion properties and existing studies, cooking fuel is classified as cleaner (electricity, LPG, natural gas, biogas, kerosene, coal/lignite, charcoal, solar) or biomass (wood, straw/shrubs/grass, agricultural crop and animal dung).[8] However, where biomass fuels are compared to other less efficient but less polluting fuels (as in the second hypothesis), the indicator variable for cooking fuel is equal to 0 if a household's cooking fuel is charcoal/kerosene/coal, referred to as "semi-clean." Whether or not a child experiences ARI may be influenced by other characteristics either at the household or individual level. In addition, there may be country-specific factors that may exacerbate ARI infection. At the individual (child) level, the study controlled for age (in completed years); gender and birth order number of the child. Given that this study looks at children under age 5, the "age" variable is made up of five categories (0, 1, 2, 3, and 4); and children below age 1 (i.e., "0" group) are used as the reference category. The gender of a child (male/female) is simply a dummy indicating the sex of a child and this is to account for any influence on the response variable as a result of gender differences. The birth order of a child is made up of four categories (1, 2, 3, and 4+ [i.e., 4 or above]); and the first category is used as the reference group.

Since children at this age cannot make meaningful decisions regarding their well-being, certain characteristics of the mother (or caregiver)[9] considered to be important for this analysis are controlled for in the empirical estimation. The first is the mother's formal education in completed years. Formal education is expected to make a person relatively more informed about good health practices. Therefore, all other things being equal, one more year of formal education of the mother or caregiver may lower probability that her child will be exposed to certain preventable health risks such as the combustion of biomass fuels. The age of the mother (in completed years) is also controlled for as a continuous variable in the analysis. The paper argues that, all things being equal, having more experience and better knowledge as regards caring for a child comes with age so that teenage or younger mothers may not be relatively well versed in their caregiving responsibilities as mothers. The particulates released from smoking cigarette may also have negative consequence on the child if exposed to it. Therefore, the empirical analysis includes a dummy indicating whether or not the mother (or caregiver) smokes cigarette and non-smoking mothers (or caregivers) are used as the reference group.

The study further controlled for some household-level characteristics: wealth, number of household members, gender of household head, and place for cooking. The DHS data do not record information on income or consumption either at the individual or household level. Rather, using principal component analysis, the data provides a measure of households' wealth status in five categories. Therefore, the regression model controlled for the living standard of households as five-categorical dummies (poorest, poorer, middle, richer, and richest) and the poorest category is used as the reference group. The inclusion of SES is to account for any possible interpretation that some households use biomass fuels for cooking because of their relatively lower standard of living. All things being equal, wealthier households are expected to use relatively more efficient fuels and so children from such households may be less likely to report ARI symptoms. The number of household members (household size) is included as a continuous variable to account for any possible effect on the response variable through, for example, congestion[10] or long cooking hours because of large quantities of food to be cooked[11] and, hence, longer period of exposure to the smoke. The inclusion of gender of household head is to account for its effect(s) on the outcome variable given that (s)he may be primarily responsible for decisions made in the household which include the health of all members. Female-headed households are used as the reference group.

Where applicable, the "place for cooking" is controlled for as four-categorical variables (indoors, different building, outdoor, and other) in order to account for proximity of kitchen to dwelling place and the degree/extent of ventilation in the cooking environment. Children in households with indoor kitchen are used as the reference category and it is expected that children in such households using biomass fuels will have a higher probability of experiencing ARI. Data on soil fertility indicators and population density are further included as instruments for households' choice of biomass cooking fuels. Specifically, the study used data on soil organic carbon content obtained from the African SoilGrids 250m GeoTiffs dataset (Hengl et al., 2015; Berazneva and Byker, 2017), and population density from the Socioeconomic Data and Applications Center (SEDAC).[12]

SUMMARY STATISTICS

The summary statistics[13] is carried out by first using the entire sample, and then by household's cooking fuel type (biomass or cleaner fuel) in order to highlight any important disparities among respondents which may not be obvious in the case of the entire sample. Generally, there are not many variations among the samples with respect to child's age, gender of child, and mother's current smoking status. The age distribution of children is almost even among the ranges considered, with slightly more children (21 percent) being less than a year old. The gender distribution of the children is almost even in both the full sample and the respective subsamples.

Meanwhile, there are some appreciable differences with respect to mother's education, households' standard of living (in terms of wealth), and place of residence. Thus, on average, among biomass fuel users, a woman has just about four years of formal education, indicating very low level of formal education. On the other hand, a woman in the sample of cleaner fuel has on average, eight years of formal education. The use of biomass fuel decreases with improvement in household's standard of living. For instance, one in every three persons in the poorest wealth quintile (33.71 percent) uses biomass fuels. The use of biomass fuel is also very common in the rural areas (83.27 percent), probably reflecting the standard of living in these areas given that this is a cheaper option. Another point worth noting is that female smoking appears to be uncommon given that less than 1 percent of mothers (or caregivers) smoke cigarette. This may not be very surprising since most typical African settings frown on such practices and in some cases, women who engage in the act are stigmatized. Since the data is sourced from thirteen countries, some descriptive for the outcome variable (acute respiratory infection [ARI]) and the key explanatory variable (type of cooking fuel) with respect to these countries are further provided (see table 10.1).[14]

In table 10.1, for each country, the 1st row figures provide percentage distribution of the variables within that country and the 2nd row figures compare the percentage distribution of the variables across the countries that make up the data.[15] For instance, in the case of Burundi, the 1st row presenting the distribution of cooking fuel and ARI symptoms shows that about 85.67 percent of households rely on biomass fuel for cooking and nearly one out of every

Table 10.1 Descriptive Statistics of the Main Variables by Country (in Percentages)

	Type of Cooking Fuel		*ARI Symptoms*		
Country	*"Cleaner"*	*Biomass*	*No*	*Yes*	*Survey Year*
Burundi	14.33	85.67	70.80	29.18	2010/11
	3.00	6.34	4.40	15.02	
Comoros	19.69	80.31	93.03	6.97	2012
	1.48	2.13	2.09	1.30	
DR Congo	22.70	77.30	87.44	12.56	2013/14
	10.50	12.62	11.77	14.01	
Gabon	67.20	32.80	84.59	15.41	2012
	9.73	1.68	3.53	5.32	
Ghana	41.42	58.58	93.51	6.49	2014
	6.48	3.23	4.41	2.54	
Kenya	26.25	73.75	83.46	16.54	2014
	14.89	14.76	14.37	23.58	
Lesotho	32.04	67.96	90.92	9.08	2014
	2.57	1.92	2.10	1.73	
Mozambique	20.12	79.88	95.09	4.91	2011
	5.73	8.02	7.94	3.40	
Namibia	34.30	65.70	86.33	13.67	2013
	4.59	3.10	3.27	4.28	
Nigeria	20.60	79.40	95.95	4.05	2013
	17.06	23.21	22.79	7.98	
Rwanda	16.93	83.07	88.35	11.65	2014/15
	3.65	6.32	5.79	6.32	
Sierra Leone	15.55	84.45	88.34	11.66	2013
	4.99	9.56	7.76	8.49	
Zambia	43.25	56.75	93.07	6.93	2013/14
	15.34	7.10	9.79	6.03	
Total	35.72	101.20	111.74	13.49	
	26.09	73.91	89.23	10.77	

The 1st (2nd) row presents the percentage distribution of the variable within (across) country.
Source: Authors' own construct based on the DHS data for the respective countries.

three children (29.18 percent) in Burundi had ARI in the two weeks preceding the survey. This obviously is a matter of public health concern. Again, comparing Burundi to the other countries, biomass fuel users from Burundi constituted 6.34 percent of the sample and recorded about 15 percent of all ARI cases (see 2nd row statistics for Burundi).

Although biomass fuel is the main source of cooking fuel in almost all the countries considered, the situation in Gabon is different and worth noting given the importance of SDG7. That is, households in Gabon predominantly (67.20 percent) use cleaner fuels in cooking. This is expected to have a positive effect on their environment. Meanwhile, a few countries (Ghana, Zambia, Lesotho, and Namibia) appear to be doing well regarding the use of relatively cleaner fuels, whereby close to half of the households sampled use cleaner cooking fuels. Comparing across countries, Kenya, Burundi, and Democratic Republic of Congo are the countries that recorded the most episodes (i.e., over 10 percent of children) of ARI (see table 10.1). Even more worrying is the fact that out of the total ARI experiences among the thirteen countries considered in this study, Kenya alone accounted for 23.58 percent of all cases with respect to the recall period. Comoros and Lesotho recorded the least rates of ARI (1.30 percent and 1.73 percent respectively) within the same recall period.

RESULTS AND DISCUSSION

The paper estimated variants of equations 1 and 2 using the 2SLS regression approach to test both hypotheses stated. While the focus here is on the results from the 2nd stage IV, it is important to highlight some findings from equation 1. As expected, the study finds a negative correlation between population density and households' adoption of biomass cooking fuels, and areas with fertile soils have a higher chance of households relying on biomass cooking fuels. The strength of the instruments is also high as indicated by the Kleibergen-Paap first stage F-statistics.

Now, to address the first hypothesis, table 10.2 presents regression results from three specifications that vary with the inclusion of individual and household level of variations, place of residence of respondent, and country fixed effects.

The results suggest that children in households that rely on biomass fuels for cooking are more likely to suffer from ARI compared to their counterparts in households using cleaner cooking fuels. This statistically significant association remains evident and even higher in the augmented models. That is, the effect of biomass cooking fuel on ARI is even higher in the unrestricted model (i.e., model 3) which accounts for country FE. Here, relative

Table 10.2 Cooking Fuel Use and ARI: Second Stage IV Regression

	Model 1	*Model 2*	*Model 3*
Type of cooking fuel			
biomass	0.0993***	0.1090***	0.2365***
	(0.0266)	(0.0281)	(0.0381)
Child's age (in years)			
1	0.0177***	0.0175***	0.0168***
	(0.0037)	(0.0037)	(0.0037)
2	−0.0074**	−0.0075**	−0.0094***
	(0.0036)	(0.0036)	(0.0036)
3	−0.0245***	−0.0246***	−0.0265***
	(0.0035)	(0.0035)	(0.0035)
4	−0.0344***	−0.0344***	−0.0354***
	(0.0035)	(0.0035)	(0.0036)
Mother's age	−0.0011***	−0.0011***	−0.0009***
	(0.0003)	(0.0003)	(0.0003)
Gender of child			
female	0.0001	0.0002	0.0006
	(0.0022)	(0.0022)	(0.0022)
Child's birth order (number)			
2	0.0013	0.0021	0.0012
	(0.0034)	(0.0034)	(0.0034)
3	0.0033	0.0048	0.0047
	(0.0039)	(0.0040)	(0.0040)
4+	0.0091*	0.0122**	0.0114**
	(0.0052)	(0.0053)	(0.0052)
Mother's education (in years)			
	0.0035***	0.0034***	0.0023***
	(0.0005)	(0.0005)	(0.0004)
Wealth status			
poorer	0.0075*	0.0088**	0.0137***
	(0.0041)	(0.0041)	(0.004)
middle	0.0166***	0.0187***	0.0273***
	(0.0057)	(0.0059)	(0.0057)
richer	0.0292***	0.0339***	0.0596***
	(0.0112)	(0.0118)	(0.0118)
richest	0.0495**	0.0591***	0.1118***
	(0.0202)	(0.0214)	(0.0223)
Current smoking status of mother			
smokes	0.0473***	0.0456***	0.0189
	(0.0151)	(0.0151)	(0.0151)
Household size	**NA**	−0.0010	−0.0033***
		(0.0007)	(0.0008)
HHH Male	**NA**	−0.0170***	−0.0047
		(0.0032)	(0.0033)
Place of residence			
urban	**NA**	**NA**	0.0665***
			(0.0123)

(*Continued*)

Table 10.2 Cooking Fuel Use and ARI: Second Stage IV Regression (*Continued*)

	Model 1	*Model 2*	*Model 3*
Survey year fixed effect	Yes	Yes	Yes
Country fixed effect	No	No	Yes
F-Statistic	146.77	137.53	76.024
Obs.	125,208	125,208	125,208

*** p<0.01; ** p<0.05; and * p<0.1. Robust standard errors in parentheses. Dependent variable is a dummy equal to 1 if the child exhibited symptoms of ARI; and 0 if otherwise.
Source: Authors' own estimations based on Demographic and Health Survey Data from Measure DHS.

to children in households relying on cleaner cooking energy sources, the probability of suffering from ARI is about 23.7 percentage points higher for children from homes relying on biomass fuels as the main cooking fuel. This result corroborates earlier findings in the literature (see, e.g., Rana et al., 2019; Ranabhat et al., 2015; Mishra, 2003; Mishra et al., 2005; and Kilabuko and Nakki, 2007).

The results from comparing biomass fuel to other less efficient but relatively less polluting fuels (charcoal/kerosene/coal) are presented in table 10.3. As earlier argued, though the transition to clean fuels (LPG, electricity, solar, etc.) is the ultimate, the prevailing low living standards in most countries especially in rural areas and the issue of culture and acceptability of cleaner fuels are real impediments. Therefore, as regards the second hypothesis, this study found that children in biomass fuel-reliant households are more likely to experience ARI compared to their counterparts in "semi-clean" fuel homes. Though the effect is not as high as that found earlier, one thing is obvious: the probability of experiencing ARI among children in biomass cooking fuel homes increases from about 7.2 percent in model 1 to about 18.92 percent in model 3. These are statistically significant at all conventional levels. This finding is in contrast with an earlier finding by Kilabuko and Nakki (2007) in Tanzania who found the effect of biomass fuel on ARI to be the same as the effect of charcoal and kerosene. Their work may be criticized based on their failure to account for the potential endogeneity of the cooking fuel variable in their empirical analysis. However, the results here should be interpreted carefully given that the magnitude of the effect is not very substantial.

Other covariates found to be statistically significant in explaining ARI among children are child's age, wealth status, and mother's smoking status and formal education. Regarding child's age, compared to children below the age of one year, those who are a year old are more likely to suffer from ARI. Meanwhile, their older counterparts (2–4 years old) are less likely to suffer from the infection. This finding is comparable to earlier findings (Mishra et al., 2005; Kilabuko and Nakki, 2007). The direction of the association

Table 10.3 Cooking Fuel Use and ARI: Second Stage IV Regression

	Model 1	*Model 2*	*Model 3*
Type of cooking fuel			
biomass	0.0717***	0.0776***	0.1892***
	(0.0260)	(0.0275)	(0.0418)
Child's age (in years)			
1	0.0140***	0.0140***	0.0128***
	(0.0038)	(0.0037)	(0.0038)
2	−0.0097**	−0.0097**	−0.0126***
	(0.0038)	(0.0038)	(0.0038)
3	−0.0233***	-0.0233***	−0.0261***
	(0.0036)	(0.0036)	−0.0036
4	−0.0349***	-0.0348***	−0.0382***
	(0.0038)	(0.0038)	(0.0039)
Mother's age (in years)	−0.0008***	0.0009***	−0.0005*
	(0.0003)	(0.0003)	(0.0003)
Gender of child			
female	0.0018	0.0019	0.0027
	(0.0023)	(0.0023)	(0.0023)
Child's birth order (number)			
2	0.0018	0.0023	−0.0001
	(0.0036)	(0.0036)	(0.0036)
3	0.0063	0.007	0.0049
	(0.0043)	(0.0043)	(0.0042)
4+	0.0053	0.0064	0.0020
	(0.0047)	(0.0049)	(0.0048)
Mother's education (in completed years)	0.0044***	0.0043***	0.0014
	(0.0005)	(0.0005)	(0.0011)
Wealth status			
poorer	0.0071*	0.0078*	0.0183***
	(0.0043)	(0.0043)	(0.0054)
middle	0.0097	0.0109*	0.0251***
	(0.0060)	(0.0062)	(0.0073)
richer	0.0082	0.0112	0.0324***
	(0.0106)	(0.0111)	(0.0112)
richest	0.0161	0.0217	0.0801***
	(0.0192)	(0.0203)	(0.0248)
Current smoking status of mother			
yes, smokes	0.0446**	0.0437**	0.0257
	(0.0192)	(0.0192)	(0.0190)
Place of residence			
urban	**NA**	**NA**	−0.0021***
			(0.0008)
Household size	**NA**	−0.0001	0.0361***
		(0.0007)	(0.0135)
HHH Male	**NA**	−0.0114***	−0.0019
		(0.0034)	(0.0035)

(Continued)

Table 10.3 Cooking Fuel Use and ARI: Second Stage IV Regression *(Continued)*

	Model 1	*Model 2*	*Model 3*
Place for cooking			
different building	−0.0164***	−0.0176***	-0.0391***
	(0.0061)	(0.0062)	(0.0079)
Outdoor	−0.0181***	−0.0187***	−0.0315***
	(0.0039)	(0.0039)	(0.0056)
Other	0.0109	0.0114	−0.0071
	(0.0359)	(0.0357)	(0.0399)
Survey year fixed effect	Yes	Yes	Yes
Country fixed effect	No	No	Yes
Variable interactions	No	No	Yes
F-Statistic	191.06	180.57	83.27
Obs.		92,070	

***p<0.01; **p<0.05; and *p<0.1. Robust standard errors in parentheses. Users of LPG/electricity/biogas/solar/solar are excluded from the analysis and the dependent variable is a dummy equal to 1 if a child exhibited symptoms of ARI; and 0 if otherwise.
Source: Authors' own estimations based on Demographic and Health Survey Data from Measure DHS.

regarding the age of the child and probability of suffering from ARI may be because children below age 1 are typically kept indoors and are brought out when they start to crawl and/or walk. Therefore, those below age 1 are unlikely to be exposed (or have little exposure) to combustion of biomass fuel. Once they are exposed, those within age 1 may be more susceptible to infections given that, all things being equal, immunity to diseases and infections develop with age up to a certain stage in life. Despite being practiced by only a few, maternal smoking habit is positively significant, suggesting that children whose mothers (or caregivers) smoke are about 5 percentage points more likely to suffer from ARI compared to non-smoking mothers or caregivers (see table 10.3). However, this association disappears when an adjustment is made for country fixed effects (see model 3 of tables 10.2 and 10.3).

It is puzzling to find that the probability of suffering from ARI is higher for children from relatively wealthier households and also increases with maternal education. However, given that the surveys rely on women's recall and responses to questions, the latter may be because the educated mothers may be relatively more knowledgeable and attentive to changes, signs or symptoms in their children. If this assertion holds, then ARI report will be higher among children whose mothers have more years of formal education. Since the analysis carried out in this study relied on data provided by responses to ARI-related questions, it cannot rule out the possibility of underreporting by respondents (e.g., from groups with lower wealth quintiles, lower level of education, etc.).

Again, the ARI-related information collected in the data does not include children who might have died from ARI during the recall period. If such deaths are concentrated among the lower wealth quintile households or women with lower level of education, then this may explain the results. Finally, another possible reason may be attributed to the fact that households typically practice fuel stacking. Therefore, children from varying backgrounds such as wealthier or even more educated households may also be exposed to pollutants from the combustion of biomass fuel. Unfortunately, the DHS dataset provides information on only the main type of cooking fuel; hence, our inability to control for this practice.

As a robustness check, the study replicates the analyses using a biprobit model to test both hypotheses. Though the results from the biprobit regressions are not presented here, the results are qualitatively and quantitatively similar to this study's findings.

CONCLUSION

The combustion of biomass fuel releases pollutants that can impair the cleaning ability of the lungs and make them susceptible to infections (Mishra and Retherford, 1997) such as ARI and this is particularly serious among children. Some studies have been carried out in this area with varying empirical strategies in the literature. Given that this remains a public health concern that needs increased attention because it is a preventable health problem, this study provides an empirical evidence about the effect of cooking fuel choice on ARI prevalence in Africa by addressing some empirical issues such as the potential endogeneity of cooking fuel type (the variable of interest), and the modeling strategy and further accounts for fixed effects.

Generally, the study finds evidence of some association between the use of biomass fuels for cooking and ARI prevalence among children under the age of 5 years. This association remains evident even after accounting for country fixed effects and additional household characteristics, including the cooking environment. Based on the study's findings, the call for a transition from biomass to cleaner fuels is justifiable. This transition is expected to help reduce indoor pollution and mitigate climate change.[16] The shift to cleaner fuels (which are mostly renewable) may ensure long-term sustainability in household energy consumption. Unfortunately, across countries in Africa, cleaner fuels are relatively more expensive compared to the biomass fuels. Meanwhile, among those who use less efficient cooking fuels, using charcoal/kerosene/coal is found to have some health benefit (though marginal) over raw biomass fuels. Therefore, while the study advocates clean fuels such as LPG and electricity, having households even move a step up on the energy ladder (e.g., from animal dung to charcoal) may be a step in the right direction toward the ultimate goal of clean fuel transition which may bring about some health benefits and also provide policy makers with the flexibility or opportunities to define clear policies or perhaps a piecemeal policy approach toward achieving the ultimate goal. Finally, to ensure the so-much talked about transition, there should be some form of incentives to make the usage of cleaner fuels competitive to the traditional fuels. This may be in the form of subsidy on cleaner fuels or the provision of improved stoves for cooking. There is also the need for increased sensitization programs to increase awareness about the health and environmental hazards associated with the combustion of biomass fuels.

NOTES

1. Or simply referred to as acute respiratory infection (ARI) in this chapter.
2. Besides, people have their own perceptions about cleaner fuels such as LPG and electric stoves given that accidents from such fuels are relatively more fatal. In addition, some people believe using biomass fuels to cook certain traditional dishes provide unique taste.
3. whether agricultural or any other purpose,
4. type or location of kitchen,
5. For instance, some countries may subsidize usage of cleaner cooking fuels such as LPG.
6. Ordinary least squares,
7. However, in adopting the standard model questionnaires, a country may add questions of particular interest to the respective country.
8. See for example: Mishra, 2003; Mishra et al., 2005; Kilabuko and Nakki, 2007.
9. where the mother is not available,
10. Congestion in households may facilitate the spread of say cough, which is one of the symptoms of ARI.
11. typically for households that practice the extended family system or where the man has more than one wife
12. See http://sedac.ciesin.columbia.edu/search/data?contains=population+density
13. For details about the summary statistics and other results, consult the authors.
14. The last column of table 10.1 shows the survey year for each country.
15. Note that where it is indicated "Total," the 1*st* row presents the number of observations for respective columns; and the 2*nd* row shows the respective column percentage.
16. especially because female smoking is uncommon among the countries considered in the data

REFERENCES

Admasie, Amha, Abera Kumie, and Alemayehu Worku. 2018. "Children under five from houses of unclean fuel sources and poorly ventilated houses have higher odds of suffering from acute respiratory infection in Wolaita-Sodo, Southern Ethiopia:

a case——control study." *Journal of Environmental and Public Health*, 2018, 9320603

Agrawal, Sutapa, and S. Yamamoto. 2015. "Effect of indoor air pollution from biomass and solid fuel combustion on symptoms of preeclampsia/eclampsia in Indian women." *Indoor Air*, 25(3), 341–352.

Barron, Manuel, and Maximo Torero. 2017. "Household electrification and indoor air pollution." *Journal of Environmental Economics and Management*, 86, 81–92.

Baumgartner, Jill, James Schauer, Majid Ezzati, Lin Lu, Chun Cheng, Jonathan A. Patz, and Leonelo E. Bautista. 2011. "Indoor air pollution and blood pressure in adult women living in rural China." *Environmental Health Perspectives*, 19(10), 1390—1395.

Bellemare, Marc, Lindsey Novak, and Tara L. Steinmetz. 2015. "All in the family: explaining the persistence of female genital cutting in West Africa." *Journal of Development Economics*, 116, 252–265.

Berazneva, Julia, and Tanya S. Byker. 2017. "Does forest loss increase human disease? Evidence from Nigeria." *American Economic Review*, 107(5), 516–521.

Bruederle, Anna, and Roland Hodler. 2017. "The effect of oil spills on infant mortality: Evidence from Nigeria." *Technical report, Navarra Center for International Development*, University of Navarra.

Cameron, Colin A., and Pravin K. Trivedi. 2005. *Microeconometrics—methods and applications*. Cambridge University Press: Cambridge, United Kingdom.

Chay, Kenneth, and Michael Greenstone. 2003. "The impact of air pollution on infant mortality: evidence from geographic variation in pollution shocks induced by a recession." *The Quarterly Journal of Economics*, 118(3), 1121–1167.

Chen, Yuyu, Avraham Ebenstein, Michael Greenstone, and Hongbin Li. 2013. "Evidence on the impact of sustained exposure to air pollution on life expectancy from China's Huai River Policy." *Proceedings of the National Academy of Sciences*, 110(32), 12936–12941.

Currie, Janet, and Matthew Neidell. 2005. "Air pollution and infant health: what can we learn from California's recent experience?" *The Quarterly Journal of Economics*, 120(3), 1003–1030.

Demographic and Health Surveys (2020). https://dhsprogram.com/What-We-Do/Survey-Types/DHS.cfm. Accessed, April 30, 2020.

Duflo, Esther, Michael Greenstone, and Rema Hanna. 2008. "Indoor air pollution, health and economic well-being." SAPI EN. S. *Surveys and Perspectives Integrating Environment and Society*, 1(1), 7–16.

Ezzati, Majid, and Daniel M. Kammen. 2002. "Evaluating the health benefits of transitions in household energy technologies in Kenya." *Energy Policy*, 30(10), 815–826.

Garcia-Huidobro, Diego, and Michael J. Oakes. 2017. "Squeezing observational data for better causal inference: methods and examples for prevention research." *International Journal of Psychology*, 52(2), 96—105.

Gertler, Paul, Sebastian Martinez, Patrick Premand, Laura B. Rawlings, and Christel M. J. Vermeersch. 2011. *Impact evaluation in practice*. The World Bank: Washington DC, USA.

Gordon, Stephen, Nigel G. Bruce, Jonathan Grigg, Patricia L. Hibberd, Om P. Kurmi, Kin-bong H. Lam, Kevin Mortimer, Kwaku P. Asante, Kalpana Balakrishnan, John Balmes, et al. 2014. "Respiratory risks from household air pollution in low- and middle-income countries." *The Lancet Respiratory Medicine*, 2(10), 823–860.

Greene, William. 2004. "The behaviour of the maximum likelihood estimator of limited dependent variable models in the presence of fixed effects." *The Econometrics Journal*, 7(1), 98–119.

Hengl, Tomislav, Gerald B. M. Heuvelink, Bas Kempen, Johan G. B. Leenaars, Markus Walsh, Keith D. Shepherd, Andrew Sila, Robert A. MacMillan, Jorge M. de Jesus, Lulseged Tamene, and Jerome E. Tandoh. 2015. "Mapping soil properties of Africa at 250 m resolution: random forests significantly improve current predictions." *PLoS One*, 10(6): e0125814. https://doi.org/10.1371/journal.pone.0125814

Imelda. 2018. "Indoor air pollution and infant mortality: A new approach." In AEA Papers and Proceedings, Vol. 108, 416–421. American Economic Association 2014.

Jayachandran, Seema. 2009. "Air quality and early-life mortality evidence from Indonesia's wildfires." *Journal of Human Resources*, 44(4), 916–954.

Kilabuko, H. James, and Satoshi Nakai. 2007. "Effect of cooking fuels on acute respiratory infections in children in Tanzania." *International Journal of Economics Resource Public Health*, 4(44), 283–288.

Lim, Stephen, Theo Vos, Abraham D Flaxman, Goodarz Danaei, Kenji Shibuya, Heather Adair-Rohani, Mohammad A. AlMazroa, Markus Amann, Ross H. Anderson, Kathryn G. Andrews, et al. 2012. "A comparative risk assessment of burden of disease and injury attributable to 67 risk factors and risk factor clusters in 21 regions, 1990–2010: A systematic analysis for the global burden of disease study 2010." *The Lancet*, 380(9859), 2224–2260.

Mishra, Vinod. 2003. "Indoor air pollution from biomass combustion and acute respiratory illness in preschool children in Zimbabwe." *International Journal of Epidemiology*, 32, 847–853.

Mishra, Vinod, Kirk R. Smith, and Robert D. Retherford. 2005. "Effects of cooking smoke and environmental tobacco smoke on acute respiratory infections in young Indian children." *Population and Environment*, 26(5), 375–396.

Neidell, Matthew. 2004. "Air pollution, health, and socio-economic status: the effect of outdoor air quality on childhood asthma." *Journal of Health Economics*, 23(6), 1209–1236.

Mishra, Vinod, and Robert D. Retherford. 1997. Cooking smoke increases the risk of acute respiratory infections in children. National Family Health Survey (NFHS) Bulletin, No. 8. Mumbai and East-West Center, Honolulu: International Institute for Population Sciences.

Nichols, Austin. 2007. "Causal inference with observational data." *The Stata Journal*, 7(5), 507–541.

Pope, Daniel, Vinod Mishra, Lisa Thompson, Amna R. Siddiqui, Eva A. Rehfuess, Martin Weber, and Nigel G. Bruce. 2010. "Risk of low birth weight and stillbirth associated with indoor air pollution from solid fuel use in developing countries." *Epidemiologic Reviews*, 32(1), 70–81.

Rana, Juwel, Jalal Uddin, Richard Peltier, and Youssef Oulhote. 2019. "Associations between Indoor Air Pollution and Acute Respiratory Infections among Under-Five Children in Afghanistan: Do SES and Sex Matter?" *International Journal of Environmental Research and Public Health*, 16, 2910.

Ranabhat, Chhabi Lal, Chun-Bae Kim, Chang-Soo Kim, Nilambar Jha, K.C. Deepak, and Fredric A. Connel. 2015. "Consequences of Indoor Air Pollution in Rural Area of Nepal: A Simplified Measurement Approach." *Front Public Health* 3, 5.

World Health Organization (WHO). 2014. https://www.who.int/mediacentre/news/releases/2014/air-pollution/en/, Accessed, May 20, 2020.

World Health Organization (WHO). 2016. *Burning opportunity: Clean household energy for health, sustainable development, and wellbeing of women and children.* WHO, Geneva, Switzerland.

Chapter 11

Pediatric Tuberculosis in Ghana

Understanding the Sociocultural Context to Increase Case Detection

Gloria Ivy Mensah

In Ghana, tuberculosis (TB) still presents a huge public health problem. The first ever nationally representative cross-sectional TB survey conducted in 2013 reported a prevalence of 264 cases per 100,000 population for all forms of TB and bacteriological prevalence of 356 per 100,000 population with smear-positive rate of 105 per 100,000 population (GHS, 2014, Bonsu *et al.*, 2020). This survey used only participants over 15 years old (Addo *et al.*, 2019). Hence, the prevalence of TB in children (under 15 years) is yet to be established. Globally, children constitute 10–11 percent of all TB cases. However, in Ghana, TB cases in children have always fallen short of this. From 2008 to 2017, figures from the National TB control program indicate that less than half of the expected number (10 percent of total number of new cases of TB) of childhood TB cases were detected.

In 2018, of the 13,978 incident cases of TB, representing 32 percent of expected cases detected in the country and notified by WHO (WHO, 2019), less than 6 percent were children. This indicates that many cases of TB in children remain undiagnosed within the clinical setting. To increase TB case detection in children, there is the need to focus more on targeted screening outside of the typical passive clinical setting. The results of the nationwide TB survey clearly show that the TB burden in Ghana is much higher (three-fold) in the population over 15 years than previously (92 per 1,000 population) reported (GHS, 2014). This means that the TB burden in children would also be higher because although transmission with children is possible, TB infection is mostly transmitted from infected adults to children (Munoz *et al.*, 2008) who share close contacts in households or schools. Children within the ages 0 to 4 years are the ones mostly at risk due to vulnerability of their

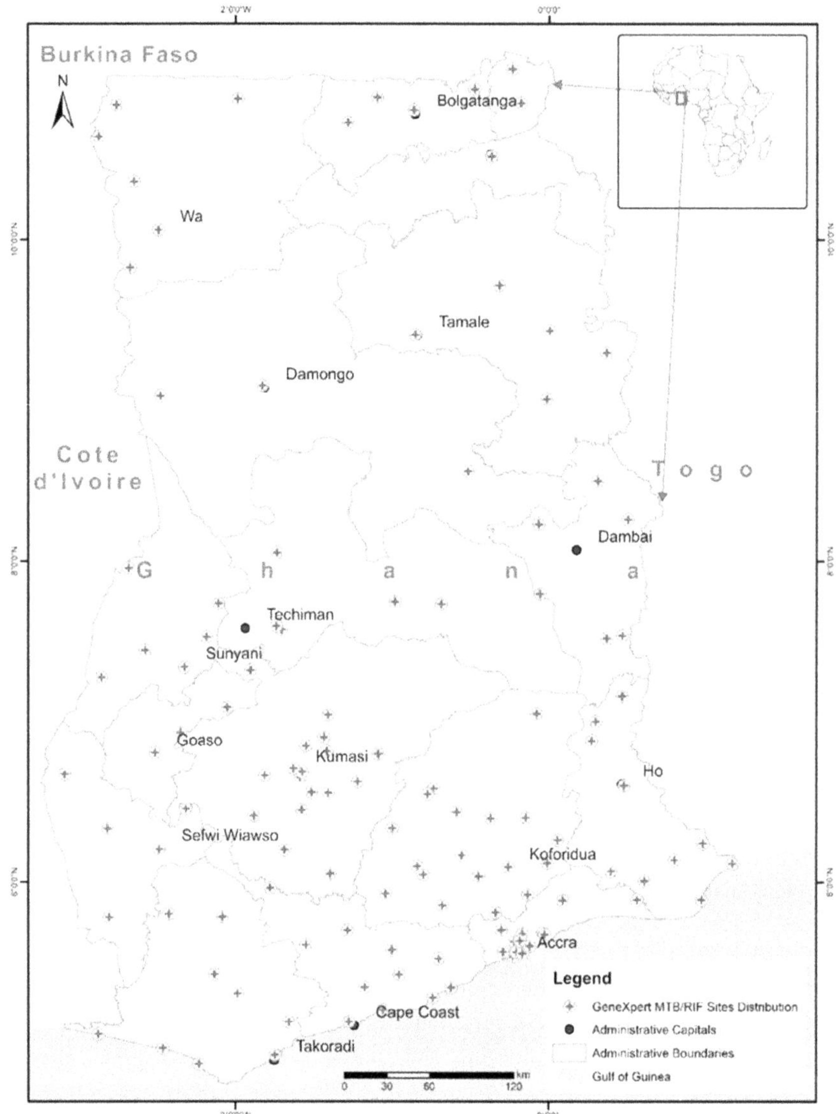

Figure 11.1 Map of GeneXpert Sites. Mensah et al. (Unpublished), generated based on information provided by the National Tuberculosis Control Program (NTP), 2019.

immune system (Attah *et al.*, 2018). Childhood TB is a marker of recent TB transmission in a community and a good indicator of how well the TB control program is doing (Seddon & Shingadia, 2014). In lieu of a TB prevalence survey, Ghana (2008) used a tuberculin skin test survey in children aged 6–10 years to determine the prevalence of TB infection (0.0 percent to 5.4 percent) as well as the annual risk of infection (ARTI) 0.0 percent to 0.6 percent in the country (Addo et al., 2010). The latest figures from the nationwide prevalence survey implies that the current systems for case detection are not optimum and there is the need for innovation to find undiagnosed and unreported cases (Bonsu *et al.*, 2020), many of whom may be children because of the difficulty in diagnosing TB in children.

TB is identified to be one of the main causes of death in children (Dodd *et al.*, 2014). In 2018, globally, more than half of the estimated one million cases of TB in children were not diagnosed (WHO, 2019); and in Ghana, only 43 percent (635) of the estimated 14,550 cases were diagnosed. Of the estimated 230, 000 children who died of TB in 2018, 80 percent were less than 5 years and 96 percent of deaths occurred before treatment started. It has also been established that when treatment is started early as a result of early diagnosis, treatment success rate is over 90 percent. A retrospective study of 3,704 TB cases in children under 15 years old in Accra (2010–2013) found that the proportion (90.7 percent) of children successfully treated for TB met the target of END TB Strategy treatment success indicator (Ohene *et al.*, 2019). On moral grounds it seems very unfair that a disease that has a cure should lead to the death of children just because the systems set in place are unable to identify all the infected. Interest in childhood TB (defined as TB in children less than 15 years old) has been ignited with the realization that if children with TB are not detected and treated, TB control cannot be achieved (Dodd *et al.*, 2014; Seddon & Shingadia, 2014). This is because children are highly vulnerable to chronic diseases and those with a latent TB infection may suffer disease reactivation when they become adults, thereby contributing to future epidemics (Newton *et al.*, 2008). What can we do differently in Ghana to enhance TB case detection in children based on our knowledge of the risk factors and the exigencies of the times?

The landscape of Ghana is changing and with its new status as a lower middle-income country, the social structure is changing with rapid urbanization, greater and free access to education, vaccination services, more churches due to the charismatic movement, more mosques, and an ever-increasing trading activity (buying and selling) at the market centers. It is important to capitalize on this new way of life to undertake active targeted screening of children for TB within and outside the clinical setting.

This chapter looks at how TB case detection in children in Ghana can be increased by taking advantage of the sociocultural characteristics of Ghana in 2020 and beyond.

TB, THE EVER-PRESENT DANGER

It has been over a century (1882) since Robert Koch made the discovery that *Mycobacterium tuberculosis* was the causative agent of tuberculosis, a disease that has been plaguing mankind dating back to thousands of years (Hershkovitz *et al.*, 2015). TB is one of the oldest diseases known to man, having had many monikers throughout history such as consumption, phthisis, and white plague. In the Akan language of Ghana, TB is referred to as *nsaman wo* (cough of the ghost) because of the notion that getting infected with TB is an implication of death sentence. However, today TB is a preventable and curable disease for which drugs are available for free (Raviglione and Sulis, 2016). Treatment is normally six to nine months, for a person infected with drug (Isoniazid and Rifampicin) susceptible TB; up to eighteen months for patients with rifampin-mono-resistant TB; and, following culture conversion, eighteen to twenty-four months for patients infected with a drug (isoniazid and rifampin) resistant TB (Bloomberg *et al.*, 2003).

The first drug for TB became available in the 1940s with the introduction of streptomycin. Due to the nature of the disease and its global spread, 24 March of each year is earmarked all over the world as World TB Day to draw attention to the need to deal with a disease that can affect us all.

It is, however, unsettling to acknowledge that in 2020, TB is still among the top ten causes of death due to a single infectious agent across all age groups and it is even ahead of HIV/AIDS (WHO, 2019). As expected, the rate of transmission differs across countries and even within regions in the same country, but epidemiological modeling suggests that one-third of the world's population is infected with the disease. This huge reservoir of individuals harboring a latent infection for which treatment is not recommended in many countries is one of the key reasons why elimination of TB remains a big global health problem. Latent TB is a major issue even though individuals with a latent TB infection are not infectious (they cannot spread the disease to others) because of the possibility of reactivation of the infection in old age or when one becomes immunocompromised. It is to avert this reactivation that in many countries now, people with HIV who are latently infected or uninfected with TB are given prophylactic TB treatment in the form of isoniazid. This Isoniazid preventive therapy (IPT) is also recommended for children who are contacts of adults infected with TB.

Out of the 10 million people infected with TB in 2018, 5.7 million, 3.2 million, and 1.1 million were men, women, and children, respectively; while the second largest number of TB cases was recorded in the African region with 24 percent after the Southeast Asian region with 44 percent (WHO, 2019).

GLOBAL TARGETS FOR TB CASE DETECTION; DREAMS DEFERRED OR UNMET

Many initiatives have been rolled out over the years with the aim of reducing the burden of TB through increased case detection and treatment success.

Notable among these are the millennium development goals (MDGs) and the Stop TB Initiative established in the year 2000. The bold ambition was to drastically decrease the global TB burden by 2015. What became known within the TB circles as target 6c of the MDG 6 was to "halt and reverse" TB incidence (WHO, 2015). A further boost was given to this goal through a partnership between WHO and the United Nations (UN) to target a reduction of TB prevalence by 50 percent. Through the DOTS (Directly Observed Treatment, Short course), many national TB control programs struggled to achieve the 70 percent case detection and 80 percent treatment success rates. The five pillars of the DOTS program were very clear and remain relevant: governments have to be committed to a sustained TB control program; case detected has to be improved through sputum smear microscopy; TB culture and drug susceptibility testing, provision of first line TB drug regimen for six to nine months, regular provision of anti-TB drugs and reliable recording and reporting system has to be in place (WHO, 2014b; Hargreaves *et al.*, 2011; Kanabus, 2019). In implementing DOTS, it became obvious that there was the need for interventions to support the vulnerable groups at risk of TB infection (Lo¨nnroth *et al.*, 2009).

With the help of the global fund for TB, HIV/AIDS and malaria, many countries were able to put in place an *enabler's package* as well as a system of treatment support. By 2015, it was clear that while many developing countries had met the target of 85 percent treatment success (Laghari *et al.*, 2019; Osman *et al.*, 2017; Tilahun & Gebre-Selassie, 2016), the 70 percent case detection was largely unattained and remains a great source of concern that needs to be addressed through active case finding (Kuznetsov *et al.*, 2014).

To keep the momentum, the sustainable development goals (SDGs) were promulgated. The SDGs have a more universal health goal to end epidemics of not only AIDS, tuberculosis, malaria but also neglected tropical diseases (NTDs), and waterborne and other communicable diseases. With the SDGs came the End TB Strategy which is geared toward ending the global TB epidemic. The most immediate targets set for 2020 to 2025 are to achieve a 35 percent and 20 percent reduction in TB deaths and incidence. Also, the target for 2030 is a 90 percent and 80 percent reduction in TB deaths and incidence while the target for 2035 is a 95 percent and 90 percent reduction in TB deaths and incidence respectively (WHO, 2016).

However, WHO itself acknowledges that realizing these goals will not be easy without identifying and addressing the health-related risk factors as well as social and economic aspects of TB (WHO, 2016). In fifteen years (2035), the next major target will be due, and we cannot achieve it without dealing with the TB cases in children for whom the available diagnostic options to detect the infection remains a challenge.

TB CASE DETECTION IN GHANA

The national tuberculosis control program was established in 1994 with the primary objective to reduce the incidence and prevalence of TB in the country and the Directly Observed Therapy Short course (DOTS) strategy was introduced the same year (Addo *et al.*, 2010). Since then, standardized monitoring and reporting of cases and treatment outcomes have been ongoing from facility to subdistrict through district to region and to national for onward transmission to WHO. By 2005, DOTS coverage had reached 100 percent in Ghana (WHO, 2006). However, the National Tuberculosis Strategic Plan for 2009–2013 projected low TB case detection rates as an issue that greatly affected the TB control program thus setting a new goal to increase TB detection from 45 percent in 2010 to 72 percent by 2013 (MOH, 2009). At present, cases are detected when patients walk into health facilities—both public and private—to seek treatment. If pulmonary TB is expected, the patient is asked to produce a sputum sample for the TB test; but if extra pulmonary TB (TB outside the lung) is suspected, tissue or fluid from the affected site is taken by a clinician for the test.

TB culture using LJ media remains the gold standard test for TB, and in Ghana, the year reference laboratories within the ten major regions of the country have the capacity to perform culture mainly using the MGIT system. However, for many years, smear microscopy was the main test for TB in many facilities. With the introduction of GeneXpert technology into TB diagnostics, Ghana is one of the countries that is gradually replacing smear microscopy with Xpert MTB/RIF as the primary diagnostic tool. Currently, there are over a 100 GeneXpert machines across the country (figure 11.2).

GeneXpert technology allows for detection of *Mycobacterium tuberculosis* DNA as well as resistance to rifampicin, which is one of the two most potent drugs for TB within 2.5 hours.

With this short turnaround time, prompt diagnosis is assured for presumptive TB cases which are presented to health centers and can also produce sputum for the test. This system works perfectly well for adults with TB but has challenges when it comes to diagnosis of children because TB disease presentation is markedly different in children.

TB Presentation in Children and the Diagnostic Difficulty

Just like in adults, exposure to TB does not always result in infection and even when it does, not every infection progresses to disease. However, 95 percent of pediatric TB that progresses to primary disease usually occur within twelve months. Therefore, TB disease occurring after twelve months is most likely post-primary regardless of age (Marais, 2011). TB disease in

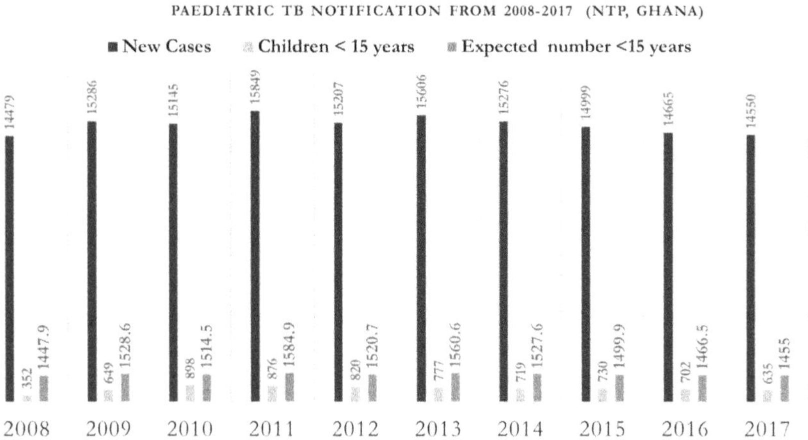

Figure 11.2 Pediatric TB Notification from 2008–2017. Graph generated using data provided by the National Tuberculosis Control Program (NTP), 2018.

adults has many distinctive signs and symptoms such as prolonged productive cough, night sweats, weight loss, anorexia, and fever. However, few children with TB present with these symptoms (Hoskyns, 2003) as childhood TB is associated with a variety of symptoms which makes diagnosis more difficult than in adults (Shingadia and Novelli, 2003). TB in children mimics many common pediatric diseases such as pneumonia, bacterial and viral infections, HIV, and malnutrition (Marais *et al.*, 2007).

The spectrum of presentation makes it difficult in many cases to use the standard microbiology methods such as sputum culture, smear microscopy, or the recently introduced GeneXpert and line probe assay (Kalu *et al.,* 2015) for diagnosis. This is because many children with TB cannot produce sputum required for these tests as the disease in children is paucibacillary or sometimes extrapulmonary. In some cases, gastric lavage or cerebrospinal fluid, or induced sputum may be taken for microbiological examination or Xpert MTB/RIF assay. Diagnosis of TB in children has, therefore, largely been based on a diagnostic algorithm which includes, X-rays, tuberculin skin tests (TST), and clinical parameters. Radiological methods play a critical role in assessing pulmonary TB in children. Chest radiographic features are often more definite even when clinical features are minimal. Common features suggestive of pulmonary TB include hilar and paratracheal lymphadenopathy, pulmonary infiltrations and consolidations, calcifications and tuberculomas (nodules) (Khatami *et al.*, 2008). Once diagnosed, treatment is initiated and lasts for six months. Targeted screening programs are very effective in helping to identify at-risk populations (Reznik & Ozuah, 2006). However, the existing strategies—where HIV positive children as well as child contacts of smear positive

TB cases are the main targets for testing through HIV clinics and contact tracing—are inadequate to pick all cases of TB. The Ghana Health Service Annual Report for 2016 reported a downward trend for the proportion of notified childhood TB cases (all forms) among the total number of cases reported. The proportion of childhood TB identified dropped gradually from 5.9 percent in 2010 to 4.8 percent in 2016. The report also indicates that interventions like improving capacity in pediatricians to make a diagnosis of TB as well as the introduction of PPD (purified protein derivative) are ongoing to increase TB detection rate among children (Ghana Health Service (GHS), 2017).

There is the need to cast the net wider since exposure to TB can occur outside the home environment. Scaling-up the existing contact-tracing strategy as well as looking for TB in other areas where children may congregate based on our present sociocultural context should include urban slums, immunization centers, schools, religious, and markets settings.

Improving Contact Tracing Using Digital Technology

Ninety-eight percent of all TB cases in children are acquired through the respiratory route (Kalu *et al.*, 2015) as a result of the inhalation of tubercle bacilli released in aerosolized droplets from an adult with active TB. As expected, the higher the bacillary load of the index case, the higher the risk of transmission making the proximity and continuous exposure to an infective adult with TB a real threat to children in the household setting (Singh *et al.*, 2004; Newton *et al.*, 2008). If not diagnosed early and treatment initiated, an adult with active TB can infect up to fifteen persons in a year (Zar *et al.*, 2012). Contact tracing is an easy way of identifying and testing child contacts to detect secondary cases of TB for treatment or to give prophylactic treatment to uninfected contacts under 5 years old. Children in contact with adult patients who have active TB are at the highest risk to getting infected. Therefore, there is the need for contact tracing for early detection (Altet *et al.*, 1996). Contact tracing mostly done in homes is tedious and inefficient due to the poor addressing systems in the country. However, this can now be made more efficient using digital technology.

With respect to digital technology, Ghana is way ahead of its neighbors in West Africa and is reported to be the best performing country in the region with the highest mobile phone penetration. By the end of 2019, mobile adoption stood at 55 percent, higher than the regional average which is at 44.8 percent (GSMA, 2020).

This means a huge number of people can be served through digital services and this, together with the introduction of the digital address system in Ghana, should make it easy to trace child contacts and have them tested for TB. In addition, contact tracing is usually done with paper forms, which may be limited by inefficiencies in data collection, storage, retrieval, and poor data quality. Data collection with a mobile app will be more cost effective. This mobile phone-based system of contact tracing is currently being used in Botswana (*Ha et al.*, 2016). There is also the need to focus more on the transmission than the close household contacts. If digital addresses of TB patients are taken and plotted, it can give an idea of the number of infections in an area (Hotspot) which can allow for active case search among children living within those areas.

Screening for TB during Postnatal (Immunization) Services

Childhood immunization is seen and recognized as an important component of health systems and an indicator of quality of care from vaccine-preventable infections (Olusanya, 2010). The Global Vaccine Action Plan of WHO demands that countries achieve 90 percent coverage for all antigens and at least 80 percent coverage in all antigens in 80 percent of districts by the year 2020 (WHO, 2012). As a result, there exists an active vaccination strategy with centers within many communities in Ghana—many of which are outside hospital settings. The Expanded program on immunization (EPI) covers children from birth up to age 5 years. These services offer an opportunity to do active case search for TB. NTP adapted symptoms questionnaires used in contact tracing can be used by the community health nurses who undertake the immunization services, and children found to have symptoms can be referred to the nearest health facility or laboratory for Xpert MTB/RIF test, TST, or chest Xray.

Following infection, several factors seem to affect the development of active TB disease. These include age, nutrition, vaccination, and immune health (Schluger, 2007). Malnutrition is a major risk factor for TB infection in children (WHO, 2014; Singh *et al.*, 2005; Munthali *et al.*, 2017) which can easily be identified at postnatal services as the weight of children is taken monthly on each visit and plotted in a growth chart in the *child health record book*. Malnutrition often results in children being underweight, anemic, and having diminished immunity against diseases (McNally *et al.*, 2009; Inamo *et al.*, 2011; Battersby e*t al.*, 2012; Bolursaz et al., 2016; Laghari *et al.*, 2019). If community health workers are given the proper training and tools, they should be able to pick out during each immunization day, children who have symptoms suggestive of TB for further testing. In hard-to-reach areas, samples can be sent to the hospitals for testing via drone technology and the same system can send drugs for treatment. The potential for drone use in clinical microbiology, infectious diseases, and epidemiology is vast and Ghana has already started this service through zipline®. Drones may help to increase access to healthcare for individuals that might otherwise not benefit from appropriate care due to remoteness and lack of infrastructure or funds (Poljak & Šterbenc, 2020). Identifying cases and offering treatment within the community will cut down transportation costs and inconveniences which have been identified as a barrier to some patients (Joseph *et al.*, 2008). However, it is important that if a child with TB is identified, investigations are initiated to ensure that the adult index case is also identified and treated. This will ensure that the child on treatment does not suffer from poor treatment response or relapse due to continuous exposure to the household index case. This is critical as it has been found that household contacts are the main risk for poor treatment outcomes in children (Alavi *et al.*, 2015).

The government through the district assemblies could implement policies to provide financial support to infected children and their immediate families as many countries are doing. For instance, cash transfers are used as incentive to ensure that patients adhere to TB treatment in Nigeria; Kenya is implementing a similar policy which includes medical insurance coverage and food support; Brazil is providing food baskets and nutrition support; while India, which has the highest number of TB cases in the world, is doing what is being done in Nigeria in addition to reimbursement of transport and food cost (Shete *et al.*, 2018).

These interventions are needed because TB is not just a disease, but a problem of social inequality and poverty (van Helden, 2003). There are myriad effects of poverty, all of which cannot be explored here. However, the main effects of poverty seen among TB patients are malnutrition and food, transportation challenges, and overcrowding (Joseph *et al.*, 2008; Pelissari & Diaz-Quijano, 2017). If all these interventions are targeted at children aged 0 to 5 who are the clients of the immunization programs, what happens to those between 5 years and 14 years who are also within the category of pediatric TB? This is the reason why there is the need to extend the active search to other sectors.

Active Case Search within the Educational System

The education policy of Ghana provides children with two years of free and compulsory kindergarten to ensure that young children are enrolled in school for early learning. This places Ghana ahead of the curve compared to other countries in sub-Saharan Africa. Preschool education has now been incorporated into the education system of Ghana. Many children begin their journey through the school system from as young as three months when mothers must resume work from maternity leave. These children usually spend long hours in the company of tutors and are at risk of infection (i.e., if any tutor has TB).

Many preschools admit children from 3 months to 5 years. Fifty percent of infants (1–5 years) with TB infections develop TB disease with considerably high morbidity and mortality risks as most of them develop disseminated TB and central nervous system TB (WHO, 2007). Taking a tuberculin skin test at the beginning of each academic year would be a strategic means of monitoring TB infection in preschools. Ghana has a system of Free Compulsory Universal Basic Education (FCUBE) for the ages of 6 to 15 years, and together with the school feeding program (for children from deprived communities to enjoy one free meal a day), the nation has seen an increase in school attendance. This makes screening for TB within the basic school system very critical for identifying children with TB. Again, this can be done at the beginning of each school year by a trained TB or district health official. With all these interventions there may still be some children who will not be in school. These children can still be found within the urban slum settlements and other social settings like the churches, mosques, and markets.

Active Case Detection within the Ghanaian Urban Slums, Social/Religious Structures

TB is aptly described as a social disease with medical aspect (Park et al., 2011). Therefore, any intervention that excludes the social, economic, and environmental aspects with accessible healthcare systems provided (Kjellstrom *et al.*, 2007) is bound to fail. It is for this reason that even the DOTs strategy, which focuses on "cutting infection transmission through early case detection, effective treatment and health systems strengthening," has recognized that social aspects of the disease cannot be ignored (Lo¨nnroth *et al.*, 2009). This need to understand the social determinants of health gave rise to the World Health Organization Commission on Social Determinants of Health framework. The framework is based on the belief that effective control of TB will best be achieved with social protection and urban planning interventions (Hargreaves *et al.*, 2011).

Generally, TB cases are identified in rural and semi-urban areas (Park, 2011). However, the new phenomenon of urban slums within some of the most urbanized areas in many developing countries requires that more targeted screening be done. Urban slums characterized by poverty, sanitation challenges, illiteracy, malnutrition, overcrowding and low socioeconomic factors are hot bed of TB transmission (Kalu *et al.*, 2015; Lo¨nnroth *et al.*, 2006; WHO, 2010). This is supported by the overwhelming evidence that a greater burden of TB cases are often found within clusters among disadvantaged groups of the society which often includes ethnic minorities (Hargreaves *et al.*, 2011). TB exposure in any setting is influenced by TB prevalence and age but in urban slums, social and cultural factors play a major role (Viney *et al.,* 2014). Such clusters are easily identifiable across Ghana and targeted screening within these communities for TB can detect children with TB.

Ghana is a secular country, but the nationals are very religious with more than 80 percent of the population being adherents of the Christian (71 percent) or Islamic (18 percent) religion (2010 population census). Those who practice the Christian faith worship on Saturdays and Sundays while practitioners of Islam worship on Fridays. Many of these religious congregations have special services for children. This also offers an opportunity for targeted screening of children with signs and symptoms of TB.

Open Markets are a social feature in most developing countries and many of the stalls are operated by women. This invariably means that many children can also be found in the market. Having health facilities attached to each market and setting a day for market women to bring their children for screening will also lead to the detection of more cases of TB. However, for all these strategies to lead to increased case detection, there will be the need to tackle stigmatization.

SENSITIZATION TO FIGHT STIGMA

Stigma, a phenomenon which happens when a characteristic of an individual is generally considered undesirable by society (Link & Phelan, 2001), is a very important social determinant of health (Heijnders & Van Der Meij, 2006). The victims of stigma often experience a sense of exclusion from the society, subconsciously adopting a set of attitudes and opinions of themselves as a result, with the major feeling of shame and guilt (Goffman, 1963). Treatment default which is of grave concern in TB is influenced by stigma (Jackson & Yuan, 1997; Sumartojo, 1993). Stigma has been cited as the reason behind people at risk of TB either refusing to seek treatment at DOTS clinics (Coreil *et al.*, 2010) or not allowing contact tracing in their homes because of fear that the presence of health workers would result in the family being stigmatized by the community (Gelaw *et al.*, 2001). Some families even cover up a TB-related death from their communities when that information will be critical for screening purposes. A study done in the western part of Ghana indicates that the main forces at play in TB stigma were fear of contracting the disease and loss of respect for the person with TB (Dodor *et al.*, 2008). While the former is easy to understand, the latter is mainly due to misconception that TB is acquired by people who have HIV (Ngamvithayapong et al., 2000), smoke or drink alcohol (Are *et al.*, 2004), or are poor, malnourished, and of low social standing (Westaway & Wolmarans, 1994; Baral *et al.*, 2007; Joseph *et al.*, 2008).

To deal with stigmatization, there is the need for greater sensitization using both the traditional media (print, TV, and radio) as well as social media (Facebook, Twitter, WhatsApp). Traditional authorities, religious leaders, and local celebrities can also be used to spread the message on the need to avoid stigmatizing people infected with TB. Due to the huge number of young people in schools, the formation of TB clubs in schools would be a great way to deal with stigma as it will lead to a generation of well-informed adults who would appreciate that TB is a disease condition that can affect anyone. There is evidence that TB clubs are effective in helping reduce negative attitudes in a community concerning TB infections, increasing the rates of treatment completion (Courtwright & Turner, 2010), and it could help make contact tracing easier.

CONCLUDING REMARKS

With the scaling-up of GeneXpert machines for rapid detection of TB and drug resistance in the country, Ghana is certainly on the brink of being able to detect TB cases that report to the health facilities with symptoms. What needs to be done in the case of finding the missing cases of TB in children is to take the giant leap of actively searching for cases outside the healthcare system by taking advantage of the emerging and existing sociocultural context of Ghana in 2020 and beyond. This is characterized by digital address systems, high mobile phone penetration, high preschool and basic school attendance, highly patronized community-based postnatal services, emerging urban slum settlements, bustling market centers and high church and mosque attendance. Within this context, children can be easily screened for TB, referred to the nearest health center for a TB test if necessary and treated at the community level with incentive packages to ensure adherence to treatment while putting in measures to prevent or minimize stigma.

REFERENCES

Addo K. K., Addo S. O., Bonsu C., Mensah E., Edusei S., Dedzo P., et al. 2019. Population-based tuberculosis disease prevalence survey in Ghana: The role and lessons learnt from the laboratory. *Journal of Tuberculosis Research*, 7(2): 95–108. Available from: http://www.scirp.org/journal/doi.aspx?DOI=10.4236/jtr.2019.72009

Addo K. K., van den Hof S., Mensah G. I., Hesse A., Bonsu C., Koram K. A., et al. 2010. A tuberculin skin test survey among Ghanaian school children. *BMC Public Health*, 10(1): 35. Available from: https://doi.org/10.1186/1471-2458-10-35

Alavi S. M., Salmanzadeh S., Bakhtiyariniya P., Albagi A., Hemmatnia F., Alavi L. 2015. Prevalence and treatment outcome of pulmonary and extrapulmonary pediatric tuberculosis in southwestern Iran. *Caspian Journal of Internal Medicine*, 6(4): 213–219. Available from: http://www.ncbi.nlm.nih.gov/pubmed/26644895

Altet MN, Alcaide J., Plans P., Taberner J. L., Saltó E., Folguera L., et al. 1996. Passive smoking and risk of pulmonary tuberculosis in children immediately following infection. A case-control study. *Tubercle and Lung Disease*, 77(6): 537–544. Available from: https://linkinghub.elsevier.com/retrieve/pii/S0962847996900520

American Thoracic Society/Centers for Disease Control and Prevention/Infectious Diseases Society of America. 2003. *American Journal of Respiratory and Critical Care Medicine*, 167(4): 603–662. Available from: http://www.atsjournals.org/doi/abs/10.1164/rccm.167.4.603

Attah C. J., Oguche S., Egah D., Ishaya T. N., Banwat M., Adgidzi A. G. 2018. Risk factors associated with paediatric tuberculosis in an endemic setting. *Alexandria Journal of Medicine*, 54(4): 403–409. Available from: https://doi.org/10.1016/j.ajme.2018.05.002

Baker M., Das D., Venugopal K., Howden-Chapman P. 2008. Tuberculosis associated with household crowding in a developed country. *Journal of Epidemiology and Community Health,* 62(8):715 LP—721. Available from: http://jech.bmj.com/content/62/8/715.abstract

Baral S. C., Karki D. K., Newell J. N. 2007. Causes of stigma and discrimination associated with tuberculosis in Nepal: a qualitative study. *BMC Public Health*, 7: 211. Available from: https://pubmed.ncbi.nlm.nih.gov/17705841

Battersby A. J., Kampmann B., Burl S. 2012. Vitamin D in Early Childhood and the Effect on Immunity to *Mycobacterium tuberculosis*. Rughetti A, editor. *Clinical Developmental Immunology,* 2012: 430972. Available from: https://doi.org/10.1155/2012/430972

Blankson H. 2012. *Economic burden of tuberculosis (TB) in Ghana, case of western region*. Kumasi.

Bolursaz M. R., Lotfian F., Aghahosseini F., Hassanzad M., Ghafaripoor H., Khalilzadeh S., et al. 2016. Characteristics of Tuberculosis among Children and Adolescents at a Referral TB's Hospital, 2006–2011. *Journal of Comprehensive Pediatrics*, 7: 3. Available from: http://comprped.com/en/articles/59822.html

Bonsu F. A., Hanson-Nortey N. N., Afutu F. K., Kulevome D. K., Dzata F., Ahiabu M-A, et al. 2014. The National Tuberculosis Health Sector Strategic Plan for Ghana 2015–2020. 2014. Available from: https://www.ccmghana.net/images/PRs/NTP/TB-health-sector-plan-2015-2020.compressed.pdf

Bonsu F. A., Hanson-Nortey N. N., Afutu F. K., Ahiabu M. A., Chimzizi R., Smith H., et al. 2009. The National Tuberculosis Health Sector Strategic Plan for Ghana [Internet]. Accra, Ghana; [cited 2020 Apr 29]. Available from: http://www.tbonline.info/media/uploads/documents/national_tb_health_sector_strategic_plan_2009-2013_2.pdf

Bonsu F.A., Addo K.K., Alebachew Z., Gyapong J., Badu-Peprah A., Gockah R., et al. 2020. National population-based tuberculosis prevalence survey in Ghana, 2013. *International Journal of Tuberculosis and Lung Disease*, 24(3): 321–328. Available from: https://www.ingentaconnect.com/content/10.5588/ijtld.19.0163

Coreil J., Mayard G., Simpson K.M., Lauzardo M., Zhu Y., Weiss M. 2010. Structural forces and the production of TB-related stigma among Haitians in two contexts.

Social Science and Medicine, 71(8): 1409–1417. Available from: http://www.ncbi.nlm.nih.gov/pubmed/20724052

Courtwright A., Turner A. N. 2010. Tuberculosis and Stigmatization: Pathways and Interventions. *Public Health Reports*, 125(4): 34–42. Available from: http://journals.sagepub.com/doi/10.1177/00333549101250S407

Dodor E. A., Neal K., Kelly S. 2008. An exploration of the causes of tuberculosis stigma in an urban district in Ghana. *International Journal of Tuberculosis and Lung Disease*, 12(9): 1048–1054. Available from: http://www.ncbi.nlm.nih.gov/pubmed/18713503

Gelaw M., Genebo T., Dejene A., Lemma E., Eyob G.. 2001. Attitude and social consequences of tuberculosis in Addis Ababa, Ethiopia. *East African Medical Journal*, 78(7): 382. Available from: http://www.ajol.info/index.php/eamj/article/view/9014

Ghana Health Service (GHS). Ghana Health Service 2013 Annual Report. 2014;

Ghana Health Service (GHS). Ghana Health Service 2016 Annual Report. 2017.

Goffman E. Stigma. 1963. *Notes on the Management of Spoiled Identity*. London: Penguin.

Global System Mobile Association (GSMA). 2020. Mobile for Development: The state of mobile in Ghana's tech ecosystem. https://www.gsma.com/mobilefordevelopment/blog/the-state-of-mobile-in-ghanas-tech-ecosystem/. Accessed on 16th April 2020.

Ha Y. P., Tesfalul M. A., Littman-Quinn R., Antwi C., Green R. S., Mapila T. O., et al. 2016. Evaluation of a Mobile Health Approach to Tuberculosis Contact Tracing in Botswana. *Journal of Health Communication*, 21(10): 1115–1121. Available from: https://www.tandfonline.com/doi/full/10.1080/10810730.2016.1222035

Hargreaves J. R., Boccia D., Evans C. A., Adato M., Petticrew M., Porter J. D. H. 2011. The social determinants of tuberculosis: from evidence to action. *American Journal of Public Health*, 101(4): 654–662. Available from: https://pubmed.ncbi.nlm.nih.gov/21330583

Heijnders M., Van Der Meij S. 2006. The fight against stigma: An overview of stigma-reduction strategies and interventions. *Psychology, Health and Medicine*, 11(3): 353–363. Available from: http://www.tandfonline.com/doi/abs/10.1080/13548500600595327

Hershkovitz I., Donoghue H. D., Minnikin D. E., May H., Lee O. Y. - C., Feldman M., et al. 2015. Tuberculosis origin: The Neolithic scenario. *Tuberculosis*, 95:S122–6. Available from: http://www.ncbi.nlm.nih.gov/pubmed/25726364

Hoskyns W. 2003. Paediatric tuberculosis. *Postgraduate Medical Journal*, 79(931): 272–278. Available from: http://europepmc.org/abstract/MED/12782773

Inamo Y., Hasegawa M., Saito K., Hayashi R., Ishikawa T., Yoshino Y., et al. 2011. Serum vitamin D concentrations and associated severity of acute lower respiratory tract infections in Japanese hospitalized children. *Pediatrrics International*, 53(2): 199–201. Available from: https://doi.org/10.1111/j.1442-200X.2010.03224.x

Jackson L., Yuan L. 1997. Family physicians managing tuberculosis. Qualitative study of overcoming barriers. *Canadian Family Physician*, 43: 649–655. Available from: https://pubmed.ncbi.nlm.nih.gov/9111981

Joseph H. A., Waldman K., Rawls C., Wilce M., Shrestha-Kuwahara R. 2008. TB Perspectives among a Sample of Mexicans in the United States: Results from an Ethnographic Study. *Journal of Immigration and Minority Health*, 10(2): 177–185. Available from: http://link.springer.com/10.1007/s10903-007-9067-5

Kalu E. I., Ojide C. K., Nwadike V. U., Korie F. C., Ibeneme C. A., Okafor G. C. 2015. Childhood tuberculosis in sub-Saharan Africa: A call to action. *Asian Pacific Journal of Tropical*, 5(10): 757–766. Available from: https://linkinghub.elsevier.com/retrieve/pii/S2222180815609288

Kanabus A. 2019. DOTS & DOTS-Plus, failed Global Plans. [cited 2020 Apr 18]. Available from: https://tbfacts.org/dots-tb/

Kjellstrom T., Mercado S., Sattherthwaite D., McGranahan G., Friel S., Havemann K. 2007. Our cities, our health, our future: Acting on social determinants for health equity in urban settings; Report to the WHO Commission on Social Determinants of Health from the Knowledge Network on Urban Settings . Kobe, Japan.

Kuznetsov V. N., Grjibovski A. M., Mariandyshev A. O., Johansson E., Bjune G. A. 2014. A comparison between passive and active case finding in TB control in the Arkhangelsk region. *International Journal of Circumpolar Health*, 73(1): 23515. Available from: https://www.tandfonline.com/doi/full/10.3402/ijch.v73.23515

Laghari M., Sulaiman S. A. S., Khan A. H., Memon N. 2019. A prospective study of socio-demographic, clinical characteristics and treatment outcomes of children with tuberculosis in Sindh, Pakistan. *BMC Infectious Disease*, 19(1): 82. Available from: https://doi.org/10.1186/s12879-019-3702-3

Link B. G., Phelan J. C. 2001 Conceptualizing Stigma. Annual Review of Sociology, 27(1): 363–385. Available from: https://doi.org/10.1146/annurev.soc.27.1.363

Lönnroth K., Jaramillo E., Williams B. G., Dye C., Raviglione M. 2009. Drivers of tuberculosis epidemics: The role of risk factors and social determinants. *Social Science and Medicine*, 68(12): 2240–2246. Available from: https://linkinghub.elsevier.com/retrieve/pii/S0277953609002111

Marais B. J. 2011. Childhood Tuberculosis: Epidemiology and Natural History of Disease. *Indian Journal of Pediatrian,* 78: 321–327.

Marais B. J., Graham S. M., Cotton M. F., Beyers N. 2007. Diagnostic and Management Challenges for Childhood Tuberculosis in the Era of HIV., 196(s1): S76–S85. Available from: https://academic.oup.com/jid/article-lookup/doi/10.1086/518659

McNally J. D., Leis K., Matheson L. A., Karuananyake C., Sankaran K., Rosenberg A.M. 2009. Vitamin D deficiency in young children with severe acute lower respiratory infection. *Pediatric Pulmonology,* 44(10): 981–988. Available from: https://doi.org/10.1002/ppul.21089

Munthali T., Chabala C., Chama E., Mugode R., Kapata N., Musonda P., et al. 2017. Tuberculosis caseload in children with severe acute malnutrition related with high hospital based mortality in Lusaka, Zambia. *BMC Research Notes*, 10(1): 206. Available from: https://pubmed.ncbi.nlm.nih.gov/28606173

Newton S. M., Brent A.J., Anderson S., Whittaker E., Kampmann B. 2008. Paediatric tuberculosis. *Lancet Infectious Diseases*, 8(8): 498–510. Available from: https://pubmed.ncbi.nlm.nih.gov/18652996

Ngamvithayapong J., Winkvist A., Diwan V. 2000. High AIDS awareness may cause tuberculosis patient delay: results from an HIV epidemic area, Thailand. *AIDS*, 14(10): 1413–1439. Available from: http://www.ncbi.nlm.nih.gov/pubmed/10930157

Ohene S. A., Fordah S., Dela Boni P. 2019. Childhood tuberculosis and treatment outcomes in Accra: a retrospective analysis, *BMC infectious Diseases,* 19: 749.

Olusanya B. O. 2010. Pattern and determinants of BCG immunisation delays in a sub-Saharan African community. *Health Research Policy and Systems*, 8: 1. Available from: https://pubmed.ncbi.nlm.nih.gov/20157426

Omondi G. 2020. The state of mobile in Ghana's tech ecosystem [Internet]. GSMA. 2020 [cited 2020 Apr 29]. Available from: https://www.gsma.com/mobilefordevelopment/blog/the-state-of-mobile-in-ghanas-tech-ecosystem/

Osman M., Lee K., Du Preez K, Dunbar R, Hesseling AC, Seddon JA. 2017. Excellent treatment outcomes in children treated for tuberculosis under routine operational conditions in Cape Town, South Africa. *Clinical Infectious Diseases*, 65(9):1444–1452. Available from: https://doi.org/10.1093/cid/cix602Park K. Park's textbook of preventive and social medicine. 22nd ed. New Delhi: Banarsidas Bhanot; 2013. 263 p.

Poljak M., Šterbenc A. 2020. Use of drones in clinical microbiology and infectious diseases: current status, challenges and barriers. *Clinical Microbiology and Infection*, 26(4): 425–430. Available from: https://linkinghub.elsevier.com/retrieve/pii/S1198743X19304999

Pelissari D. M., Diaz-Quijano FA. 2017. Household crowding as a potential mediator of socioeconomic determinants of tuberculosis incidence in Brazil. *PLoS One*, 12(4): e0176116–e0176116. Available from: https://pubmed.ncbi.nlm.nih.gov/28419146

Raviglione M., Sulis G. 2016. Tuberculosis 2015: burden, challenges and strategy for control and elimination. *Infectious Disease Reports*, 8(2): 6570. Available from: https://pubmed.ncbi.nlm.nih.gov/27403269

Reznik M., Ozuah P. O. 2006. Tuberculin skin testing in children. *Emerging Infectious Diseases,* 12(5): 725–726. Available from: http://wwwnc.cdc.gov/eid/article/12/5/05-0980_article.htm

Seddon J. A., Shingadia D. 2014. Epidemiology and disease burden of tuberculosis in children: A global perspective. *Infection and Drug Resistance*, 7: 153–165. Available from: https://pubmed.ncbi.nlm.nih.gov/24971023

Shete P. B., Reid M., Goosby E. 2020. Message to world leaders: we cannot end tuberculosis without addressing the social and economic burden of the disease. Lancet Glob Heal [Internet]. 2018 Dec 1 [cited 2020 Apr 20];6(12):e1272–3. Available from: https://www.thelancet.com/journals/langlo/article/PIIS2214-109X(18)30378-4/fulltext#.Xp1OnP-8L9o.mendeley

Singh M., Mynak M. L., Kumar L., Mathew J. L., Jindal S. K. 2005. Prevalence and risk factors for transmission of infection among children in household contact with adults having pulmonary tuberculosis. *Archives of Disease in Children*, 90(6):624 LP–628. Available from: http://adc.bmj.com/content/90/6/624.abstract

Shingadia D., Novelli V. 2003. Diagnosis and treatment of tuberculosis in children. *Lancet Infectious Diseases*, 3(10): 624–632. Available from: https://linkinghub.elsevier.com/retrieve/pii/S1473309903007710

Sumartojo E. 1993. When Tuberculosis Treatment Fails: A Social Behavioral Account of Patient Adherence. *American Review of Respiratory Disease*, 147(5): 1311–1320. Available from: https://doi.org/10.1164/ajrccm/147.5.1311

Tabong PT-N. 2017. Socio-cultural and health system factors affecting tuberculosis case detection and treatment in the Upper West Region of Ghana. University of Ghana Digital Collection [Internet]. [cited 2020 Apr 29]; Available from: http://ugspace.ug.edu.gh

Tilahun G., Gebre-Selassie S.. 2016. Treatment outcomes of childhood tuberculosis in Addis Ababa: a five-year retrospective analysis. *BMC Public Health*, 16(1): 612. Available from: https://doi.org/10.1186/s12889-016-3193-8

van Helden P. D. 2003. The economic divide and tuberculosis. Tuberculosis is not just a medical problem, but also a problem of social inequality and poverty. *EMBO Reports*, 4(Suppl 1): S24–S28. Available from: https://pubmed.ncbi.nlm.nih.gov/12789401

Viney K. A., Johnson P., Tagaro M., Fanai S., Linh N. N., Kelly P., et al. 2014. Tuberculosis patients' knowledge and beliefs about tuberculosis: a mixed methods study from the Pacific Island nation of Vanuatu. *BMC Public Health*, 14: 467. Available from: https://pubmed.ncbi.nlm.nih.gov/24885057

Westaway M.S., Wolmarans L. 1994. Cognitive and affective reactions of black urban South Africans towards tuberculosis. *Tubercle and Lung Disease*, 75(6): 447–453. Available from: http://www.ncbi.nlm.nih.gov/pubmed/7718834

WHO. The Global Plan to Stop TB 2011–2015. Geneva: WHO, 2010.

WHO. 2012. Electronic recording and reporting for tuberculosis care and control. Geneva: WHO.

WHO. 2014. Guidance for national tuberculosis programmes on the management of tuberculosis in children Second edition.[cited 2020 Apr 20]. Available from: www.who.int

WHO. 2014. Global Tuberculosis Report 2014. Geneva; [cited 2020 Apr 29]. Available from: https://apps.who.int/iris/bitstream/handle/10665/137094/9789241564809_eng.pdf?sequence=1&isAllowed=y

WHO. 2015. World Health Statistics 2015 [Internet]. WHO: Geneva, 2015 [cited 2020 Apr 29]. Available from: https://apps.who.int/iris/bitstream/handle/10665/170250/9789240694439_eng.pdf?sequence=1

WHO. 2015. Global Tuberculosis Report 2015 [Internet]. 20th ed. Geneva PP– Geneva: World Health Organization; Available from: https://apps.who.int/iris/handle/10665/191102

WHO. 2015. The END TB Strategy [Internet]. World Health Organization. 2015 [cited 2020 Apr 18]. Available from: http://www.who.int/tb

WHO. 2019. Global Tuberculosis Report 2019 [Internet]. [cited 2020 Apr 18]. Available from: http://apps.who.int/bookorders.

World Health Organization Country Office, Accra, Ghana. ohenes@who.int.; 2019. p. 749. Available from: http://europepmc.org/abstract/MED/31455234

Chapter 12

Maternal Nutrition and the Risk of Cardiovascular Diseases in Offspring

Translating Research into Practice in Sub-Saharan Africa

Richard Michael Blay

BACKGROUND AND DEFINITIONS

Cardiovascular diseases (CVDs) are the number one cause of death globally. Each year, about 17 million people, representing 31 percent of total deaths, die due to CVDs, according to the World Health Organization (WHO). The term "cardiovascular diseases" generally describes various conditions that affect the heart and blood vessels in humans. CVDs occur when fatty deposits build up in blood vessels resulting in a panoply of disorders such as coronary heart disease, cerebrovascular disease or stroke, and peripheral arterial disease. Over a long period of time, the build-up of fat in the arteries (known as atherosclerosis), narrows the lumen of the blood vessels and increases the risk of blood clot formation when the fat deposits begin to leak and release their contents into the bloodstream. The blood clots known as thrombus can then dislodge and block narrower vessels that supply blood to crucial organs like the heart or brain.

Coronary heart disease (CHD) occurs when blood flow to the heart is impaired due to the build-up of fat in the coronary arteries which are blood vessels that supply blood to the heart. Reduction of blood supply to the heart muscles results in ischemia leading to a heart attack, whose symptoms include chest pain, shortness of breath, discomfort in the arms and shoulders, and light-headedness or nausea. Cerebrovascular disease is another example of CVD resulting from lack of blood supply to the brain either due to blockage and ischemia or bleeding (hemorrhage) of the vessels. Stroke or cerebrovascular accident usually leads to deficits in the function of the brain resulting in impairments, including paralysis (Memetoglu et al., 2014).

Cardiovascular diseases have a complex pathophysiology. That is, they are not caused by a single known factor, but rather a combination of genetic and lifestyle risk factors which include age, family history, gender, diabetes, physical inactivity, unhealthy diet, high blood pressure, obesity, and smoking (O'Donnell and Elosua, 2008). The development of cardiovascular diseases takes place over a long period of time and can occur without warning signs. This makes prevention strategies, such as changes in lifestyle and diet, difficult to prescribe until it is too late.

Apart from the effects of lifestyle, family history and age on the occurrence of CVDs, reports have long existed that the environment and conditions that a developing fetus is exposed to in the womb may predispose a person to CVDs later in their adult life (Forsdahl, 1977; Barker and Osmond, 1986, 1988; Barker, 2004; Rodriguez-Rodriguez et al., 2018). This phenomenon of intrauterine life, suggested to play a key role in the development of CVDs by adults, is known as "fetal programming" or "developmental origins of health and disease" (DoHaD). This was first conceptualized by Dr. D. J. P Barker, an English physician and epidemiologist, who showed that low birth weight (LBW) due to poor nutrition by mothers during pregnancy was associated with hypertension and coronary heart disease in adult life of their offspring. Since then, several epidemiological and animal studies have provided evidence that support, help explain and extend the fetal programming hypothesis. However, translating the research into clinical practice by implementing interventions for the prevention and fight against CVDs remains challenging.

CVD as a sequel to atherosclerosis has an early onset as well as slow progression in the course of life but most cases are not detected or treated early enough. For this reason, CVD has been nicknamed "silent killer." This makes early detection and adoption of healthy lifestyle by expecting mothers important in order to ensure a healthy intra-uterine environment for developing babies. Prevention of CVDs has largely been focused on the adulthood period, by which time the foundations for developing the conditions may have already been firmly laid and is awaiting triggering conditions. Judging by the huge worldwide burden and cost of CVDs on economies, lives and livelihoods, there is a need to quantify the level of contributions of fetal environmental factors and adult lifestyle factors to the development and progression of CVDs in order to develop appropriate tandem and more effective preventive measures.

Burden of Cardiovascular Diseases in Sub-Saharan Africa

According to the WHO, in 2015, 82 percent of deaths were due to noncommunicable diseases (NCDs) and over three-quarters of deaths arising from

CVD occurred in low- and middle-income countries (LMIC). Historically, developed countries experience a higher percentage of cardiovascular diseases and the conventional perception was that CVDs were low in less developed regions of the world, including sub-Saharan Africa (SSA). However, in the last few decades, developing countries have witnessed a greater burden of NCDs, especially CVDs in a so-called epidemiologic shift from infectious diseases (Sun et al., 2015; Gillum, 2018). With the already existing burden of infectious diseases in SSA, the emerging increase of cardiovascular diseases presents a double challenge on the already inadequate and overstretched health systems and fragile economies.

Due to increase in urbanization, tobacco smoking, sedentary lifestyle, increased intake of the Western diet (high intake of saturated fats, sugar, and low fiber), alcohol consumption and psychosocial problems among populations in SSA, there is a surge in hypertension and heart attacks (Cappuccio and Miller, 2016). Although CVD mortality rates have reduced in high-income countries, low-income countries tend to experience higher mortality rates due to low capacity for early detection of disease, and poor accessibility to preventive, management, and treatment measures. The combined disease burden of infectious diseases and CVDs in SSA is a double jeopardy and calls for a more integrated and holistic approach to detection, prevention, and treatment (Cappuccio and Miller, 2016). Furthermore, the situation is expected to worsen as the prevalence of risk factors such as hypertension and obesity increase in LMICs, especially in SSA. With Africa having the highest prevalence of hypertension, the number one risk factor for CVDs in adults aged 25 and above, there is a huge impact on economic development due to loss of productive years of life and as such CVDs must be given high priority in SSA. In 2015, the estimated death rates due to ischemic heart disease for women/men aged 50–59 in Nigeria and South Africa per 100,000 were 81/127 and 134/294, respectively, as compared to 47/124 in Canada (Gillum, 2018). The same data also showed that death rates per 100,000 due to hemorrhagic stroke in women/men aged 50–69 in Nigeria and South Africa were 42/39 and 39/66 respectively as compared to 6/11 in Canada.

A serious cause for concern is that compared to the rest of the world, CVD deaths in SSA occur at a relatively younger age (Moran et al., 2013). This is worrisome as over 40 percent of Africa's population is young, and this signals a huge problem with far-reaching socioeconomic impact. A recent epidemiological study to determine the frequency and admission patterns of CVDs in Southwest region of Cameroon showed that about 16 percent of admissions in a referral hospital was due to CVDs. The highest affected age group was 50–59 years, with the length of hospital stay ranging from one to thirty-seven days (median stay of seven days) and in-hospital fatalities was about 16 percent (Nkoke et al., 2019). The high death rate due to CVDs in SSA may be due to a combination of factors including inadequate resources and healthcare system, lack of national prevention programs and lack of sustainable treatment therapies. All these lead to improper prevention, detection and control of CVDs in SSA populations.

According to the WHO's "Global action plan for the prevention and control of non-communicable diseases (NCDs) 2013–2020," two levels of strategies can be employed in combination to reduce CVDs. At the population level, countries can introduce comprehensive tobacco control policies, taxation to reduce intake of foods high in fat, sugar and salts, building walking and cycling paths to increase physical activity and providing healthy meals to children. A report published in 2017 indicates that Africa was totally off track in achieving the indicators set for reducing NCDs by the WHO and this calls for greater concern and awareness as we are already in 2020. Interestingly, despite the huge evidence supporting the contribution of fetal programming and developmental origins of health and disease, none of the indicators took into account preventive and control measures associated with optimal fetal environment and development. Given the precarious food security in SSA, where culturally women tend to have the least household provisions while doing the most household chores, efforts to optimize intrauterine environment by taking better care of pregnant women could make a huge impact on reducing occurrence of CVDs in future populations. The issue of displaced pregnant mothers fleeing armed conflicts in SSA could also be addressed to improve their well-being and that of their offspring with a view to addressing the DoHaD aspect of NCDs in the subregion.

One big challenge in SSA with the fight against increasing trends of CVDs is the lack of proper data to enhance the understanding of the disease and, therefore, making a case for the attention or focus of policy makers has been difficult (Mensah et al., 2015). The lack of national policies and measures has made deaths and disabilities due to CVDs to continually increase in countries like Ghana, Nigeria, Sudan, and Tanzania. Yet, it is still not regarded as a public health problem (Hamid, Groot, and Pavlova, 2019). In Ghana, however, in an attempt to reduce the burden of NCDs, the Ministry of Health introduced a shift from curative to preventive health services. A review and dedicated study may be needed to measure the extent of the benefit the program has yielded. What is undeniable is the strong indication that CVDs must be a top public health priority in SSA because of the impact it has on economies. This largely results from loss of life during peak productive years and the cost of healthcare and management.

Risk Factors of Cardiovascular Diseases in Sub-Saharan Africa and Their Socioeconomic Implications

Generally, the risks for CVDs are attributed to lifestyle factors such as smoking, unhealthy diet, physical inactivity, excessive alcohol consumption, and stress, which can lead to the development of high blood pressure and/or diabetes. High blood pressure and diabetes are the major underlying causes of coronary heart disease and stroke which account for about 60 percent of CVD deaths (Cappuccio and Miller, 2016). These lifestyle risk factors were known to be predominant in developed and high-income countries and this was clearly the case since the CVD burden had always been high in developed countries until about thirty years ago. There has been rapid urbanization of LMICs in Africa owing to socioeconomic forces within the past decades and this has led to a shift in lifestyle toward less physical activity, increased alcohol and tobacco consumption, and consumption of foods high in salt, sugar, and saturated fats (Amegah, 2018).

One often overlooked aspect of the Westernized acculturation in SSA has to do with changing occupations and increased intake of salt. Evidence exists that for many centuries, indigenes of SSA were farmers of perennial crops or nomadic livestock. These occupations requiring high manual labor and trekking daily, commenced from infancy and lasted throughout adult life. In those days, salt intake was very minimal because of unavailability of mined salt. Folk tales in the forest belt of Ghana indicate organized treks to the coast to batter head loads of salt with foodstuff, or purchasing from traders from the Saharan regions (Sanders, 2008). Consumption of salt was very strictly rationed among the forest-dwelling Akans in Ghana, for example. People obtained their salt requirements from meat supplemented with very little mined salt (Cartwright, 2019). In postcolonial SSA, the introduction of formal education, office jobs, and vehicles drastically has altered high mileage trekking and manual labor lifestyle to sedentary and less physically demanding labor. For high level executives, there is the added luxury of air-conditioned cars and offices which eliminate sweating as an excretory route for salt in the body. The combined effects of all these changes are hypertension, obesity, and related predisposition to CVDs.

The story gets even more complicated since it has been shown that the incidence, prevalence, and mortality due to CVDs are higher in black Africans compared to Caucasians, suggesting a genetic or environmental predisposition to cardiovascular risk factors (Opie and Mayosi, 2005; Mensah, 2018). The factors suggested by some authors for this difference are related to socioeconomic differences. The lack of access to high-quality healthcare and health-promoting services among poor communities in predominantly black communities may contribute to the high impact of CVDs among blacks. Another study examining the socioeconomic determinants of risk factors for CVDs in forty-seven LMICs found an inverse relationship between adult literacy and blood pressure. Moreover, female unemployment and literacy were positively associated with CVD risk factors (Sun et al., 2015). Poverty-related issues like inadequate housing, lack of potable water, poor sanitation, crowding, crime, air pollution, low education, job insecurity, unemployment, and transportation needs are potent predictors of poorer perceived health status and may contribute to increased risk for CVDs in SSA (BeLue et al., 2009). Putting all these together, SSA is at the point where two economic conditions merge to increase the incidence and burden of CVDs. In one direction, socioeconomic development is leading to increased access to unhealthy diet and lifestyle associated with CVDs and on the other hand, lack of good quality health services exacerbates the burden further. However, besides the lack of access to quality healthcare is a hitherto unrecognized risk factor for CVD due to poverty and low socioeconomic status: the fetal programming risk factor proposed by Dr. Barker (Barker et al., 1989; Barker, 2007; Barker and Osmond, 1988; Alsaied et al., 2017).

The fetal programming hypothesis (DoHaD) postulates that poor maternal nutrition during pregnancy could program a developing fetus for cardiovascular diseases later in adult life. Poor maternal nutrition during pregnancy is associated with low birth weight (LBW) in the newborn and birth weight is known to predict health status in infancy as well as later in life. One of the earlier studies to support the DoHaD conducted in the 1950s in Scotland shows that LBW is associated with a high incidence of coronary heart disease and stroke (Lawlor et al., 2005). Since it has also been shown by other studies that atherosclerosis begins very early in life and possibly even during fetal life (Napoli et al., 1999b, a), the implications of fetal programming for CVDs cannot be overlooked.

MATERNAL NUTRITION AND CHILD HEALTH; THE FETAL PROGRAMMING PHENOMENON, AND IMPLICATIONS FOR CVDs

The fetal programming hypothesis also known as "developmental origins of health and disease" suggests that the intra-uterine environment of a developing fetus and in early postnatal life can determine health and susceptibility to diseases later in life (Barker, 2007). This happens as a result of adaptive responses in the fetus, which leads to altered genetic expression. Malnutrition during pregnancy leads to fetal growth restriction, LBW and the development of hypertension, obesity, and diabetes later in life.

Predating the fetal programming hypothesis was the long-standing theory that coronary heart disease, stroke, and other cardiovascular diseases result from unhealthy lifestyle, Westernization, and genetics. However, this postulation alone does not explain fully the current rise in the disease and the reason why in an at-risk population some members are susceptible while others are not. Moreover, preventive measures based on the factors which underpin the antiquated thesis for predisposition to CVDs have not yielded significant results in many countries. In SSA, the rapid increase in CVDs and other NCDs may not be fully explained by the lifestyle risks due to urbanization (Mandy and Nyirenda, 2018). This disparity suggests that tobacco smoking, alcohol consumption, unhealthy diet, and physical inactivity among sub-Saharan Africans may not fully account for the surging rates of CVDs incidence and mortality currently being experienced in that part of the world.

Although in the last few decades, research scientists have given much attention to the study and understanding of mechanisms of DoHaD, much of the findings and knowledge have not influenced clinical management or preventive policies and programs for CVDs. Apart from the initial observations by Barker and Osmond (1988), other studies have shown that children born with low birth weight had a higher risk of type 2 diabetes, hypertension and coronary heart disease (Umer et al., 2019; Smith et al., 2016; Belbasis et al., 2016). Further contributions from other studies using data from regions exposed to famine have shown that adults who were exposed to a ten-week period of famine during gestation were three times more likely to develop hypertension than adults not exposed during fetal development (Calkins and Devaskar, 2011; Stein et al., 2006; Hoffman, Reynolds, and Hardy, 2017).

Maternal undernutrition during pregnancy may lead to fetal growth restriction and low birth weight (Kwon and Kim, 2017). It is known that in an attempt to adapt to the deficiency of necessary factors for the development of the fetus, some structural, physiological, and metabolic changes take place that may persist even after birth and enhance the development of CVDs in adult life. Putting all these together, the perinatal period is critical and its implications on cardiovascular diseases during adult life is evident. The efforts, therefore, to combat CVDs and their resulting mortality and morbidity will likely achieve significant results with the inclusion of measures that take into account the developmental origins of adult disease.

Looking at the socioeconomic situation in SSA, where most countries are in the low-middle-income bracket, undernutrition among pregnant women is most likely the number one cause of low birth weight. It is not surprising that in 2018, the prevalence of LBW in Burkina Faso, Ghana, Malawi, Senegal, and Uganda was 13.4 percent, 10.2 percent, 12.1 percent, 15.7 percent, and 10 percent, respectively, compared to about 7 percent in developed countries (He et al., 2018). In Ghana, the determinants of LBW include educational level, living alone during pregnancy, and anemia due to malnutrition in the first trimester (Adam et al., 2019). Maternal nutrition and health have profound influence on the health status of children both after birth and later in adult life and the evidence of association of maternal nutrition and cardiovascular diseases in children later in life is overwhelming. These indicators beg the questions: "to what extent does malnutrition during pregnancy in SSA women contribute to the rise in CVDs and to what extent is this incorporated in preventive measures at the national and sub-regional levels?"

MATERNAL NUTRITION AND CARDIOVASCULAR DISEASE RISK IN OFFSPRING

Maternal nutrition during pregnancy has long been known to affect fetal growth, birth weight, and infant morbidity and mortality (Hambidge and Krebs, 2018). With the huge evidence supporting birth weight's influence on childhood health status and, in addition, the risk of developing NCDs later in adult life, it has become evident that the effects of maternal nutrition during pregnancy extends beyond childhood. Although over nutrition and increased gestational weight may also have adverse effects on offspring in terms of cardiovascular risk, malnutrition is a more serious situation in many SSA countries due to under development and poverty (Onyango et al., 2019; Lartey, 2008).

Animal studies have been very useful in studying and understanding the effects of nutrition on fetuses during pregnancy and predisposition to risks for CVD development. Several studies were designed to restrict food intake or reduce specific nutrients during pregnancy and this resulted in offspring being hypertensive or obese later on (Mühlhäusler, Adam, and McMillen, 2008; Napoli et al., 2000; Rodríguez-Rodríguez et al., 2017). This data suggests that maternal nutrition is essential in fetal growth and development (Morrison and Regnault, 2016; Veena et al., 2016). The effects of maternal nutrition on the health status of offspring during adulthood have therefore led to the term "nutritional programming" (Hsu and Tain, 2019). Nutritional programming does not only predispose offspring to CVDs but has also been shown to increase allergic diseases, nonalcoholic fatty liver, kidney disease, metabolic syndrome, and cognitive impairment.

Nutritional programming is an opportunity for interventions and when well-designed can potentially reverse or reduce the risks of CVD development during adulthood. A huge challenge, however, is translation of animal studies into human studies and implementation in health programs and policies. Some of the manipulations and experimental designs (Blay et al., 2019) are practically challenging to repeat in humans and this has been a huge setback in translating the potentially useful research into clinical practice or human interventions.

Current Practices, Challenges, and Future of Translating Research into Practice

Although the evidence linking maternal nutrition and health with risk of CVD development in offspring later in life is well established, either by design or oversight or probably for lack of direction, both developed and developing nations have not implemented or included measures to account for this risk in their national health policies and programs (Hoffman, Reynolds, and Hardy, 2017). Preventive measures that may address DoHaD may help reduce the incidence of CVD risks, morbidity, and mortality thereby not only improving lives but also reduce the economic burden on nations brought about by the high cost of treatment and management and the burden on health facilities.

Many SSA countries like South Africa, Ghana, and Nigeria have suffered periods of famine and/or armed conflicts that internally displaced thousands of people in the past decades. It is suggested that children conceived during these times who may have been exposed to suboptimum conditions during *in utero* and developmental stages would be adults now with their higher predisposition to CVDs translating into increasing prevalence (Reddy and Mbewu, 2016). Public health programs must include an early screening of such "high risk" groups, because early detection is the key in managing CVDs. Interventions must also focus on improving nutrition and health in pregnant women in order to reduce the effect of DoHaD on the prevalence of CVDs in the future. For now, some social intervention programs currently being implemented may have some effects on the DoHaD. Examples of such programs include free secondary school education, health insurance for pregnant women, antenatal education on health and nutrition during pregnancy, and malaria prevention programs for pregnant women. More specific programs targeted at reducing undernutrition or malnutrition during pregnancy will be required to tackle fully the long-term effects of fetal programming for CVDs.

In spite of the huge body of research and literature on DoHaD and their implications for CVDs, most studies have focused on determining the associations of specific nutrients and substances and CVD risk and tried to elucidate the mechanism by which health and nutrition of mothers lead to genetic programming of CVD risks in later life of their offspring. This mechanistic information must lead unto studies exploring interventions that could be translated into clinical and nutritional interventions during pregnancy. Some animal studies have explored the supplementation of vitamin C, vitamin E, lipids, and antioxidants during pregnancy as a way to improve CVD risk or as a measure to combat factors that lead to LBW in children. Folic acid has showed positive results in reversing genetic changes in rats due to undernutrition during pregnancy (Lillycrop et al., 2005). Several other studies have demonstrated benefits of well-timed gestational or *in-utero* interventions in animals using proteins, vitamins, hormones, and growth factors. More studies are needed to explore interventions during pregnancy to reduce DoHaD and their translation into clinical practice and beneficial programs at national levels.

Several animal studies have shown that an intervention or practice during pregnancy to combat the fetal programming for CVDs may be able to achieve long-lasting benefits in the offspring. The use of antioxidants or drugs to lower the effects of maternal hypercholesterolemia (high cholesterol levels in pregnant mothers) has yielded significant results (Napoli et al., 2000; Blay et al., 2019). In this respect, natural cocoa powder, known to be rich in antioxidants and produced in several West African countries has shown some potential in reducing the effects of maternal nutrition on CVDs. With the huge amount of evidence showing how maternal factors, especially nutrition, can expose developing babies to adverse conditions that result in higher risk for CVDs, it should be a priority to establish the foundations of translating the research into clinical practice and national policies. However, this unfortunately has not been the case, not just in LMICs but also in developed countries. The focus of clinical practice is more to ensure the safety of mother and child, and safe delivery. The time has, however, come to think more of the future of these children and involve interventions, especially for high risk mothers. Sadly, as if by intention, developmental or fetal programming is not recognized or listed as a risk factor for CVDs by clinical practitioners and the traditional knowledge that lifestyle habits, age, and race are the risk factors for CVDs dominate. There are currently no guidelines for screening or treatment aimed at preventing deleterious programming of babies for diseases later in life. Even worse is the case for SSA countries due to the fact that clinicians are more occupied with dealing with infections and conditions that immediately may threaten the mother or child and, coupled with limited personnel, infrastructure and funds, there seems to be no space for considering the developmental origins of health and disease (Palinski, 2014).

A significant challenge to implementing treatments, screenings, or interventions against fetal programming is mainly the lack of evidence from long prospective human studies and clinical trials. Establishing the risk factors or conducting clinical trials in humans may require studies spanning most likely thirty to fifty years and this is expensive and logistically daunting. Another challenge is the establishment of verifiable and reliable physiological ranges for pregnancy to allow for screening. For example, it has been shown that high cholesterol levels during pregnancy may reduce birth weight and increase CVD risk, but there has been no studies to establish what the safe levels of cholesterol during pregnancy should be (Bartels and O'Donoghue, 2011). Moreover, there are no cholesterol-lowering drugs that can be assured to be safe for developing fetuses and any treatment or intervention must definitely be established to be safe to growing fetus. All these practical challenges, coupled with the cost of pharmaceutical intervention, point to the need for sub-Saharan African countries developing and adopting policies that achieve maximum results with minimum financial demands and hence public health programs and policies to have a broad benefit and at the same time to tackle the burden of CVDs. In this vein, our demonstration that prandial natural cocoa powder (NCP) mitigated predisposition of offspring of hypercholesterolemic rabbit mothers to aortic plaques (Blay et al., 2019) evokes inclusion of NCP in the diet of pregnant mothers as a public health policy. This is more so because NCP is a nutraceutical and has human anecdotal (Addai, 2010) and *in vitro* (Amponsah et al., 2012; Adika et al., 2016) as well as animal experimental (Aidoo et al., 2012) evidence of antimalarial activity, implying broad spectrum benefits of such a policy in cocoa-producing SSA.

Finally, clinical practice and the fight against increasing trends of CVDs will not succeed without strong scientific research. Sub-Saharan Africa needs to increase capacity and collaboration among countries when it comes to research and also to fight the phenomenon of brain drain. Governments must invest in research and see expenditure in this effort as investment in the health and well-being of their people and not cost, so that the fight against diseases and poverty in SSA will fully achieve intended or needed results. According to Palinski et al. (2014), the ingredients needed for a successful fight against CVDs include governmental will power, vigorous nongovernmental organizations, dedicated physicians, and fully trained nurses with technical support. Investing in human capacity and research is an important step for Africa in combating CVDs and developmental origins of health and disease (Volmink and Dare, 2005).

CONCLUSIONS

The current increase in CVDs cannot be fully explained by the conventional risk factors. Hence, the fight against CVDs may not be won without considering measures to address the conditions and the factors that lead to fetal programming for CVDs. The evidence supporting the developmental origins of health and disease and the effect of maternal nutrition on CVDs in offspring later in life is overwhelming and reproducible. This indicates the necessity of implementing clinical strategies and interventions during pregnancy in order to reduce the possibility of developing CVDs in adult life. In SSA where malnutrition is a significant challenge during pregnancy, it is inferential that the risk of fetal programming for CVDs or developmental origin of cardiovascular diseases may be accentuated. The main challenges have been the translation of animal studies into human interventions and the establishment of beneficial interventions during pregnancy as part of national policy and strategy. Beyond clinical and pharmaceutical therapies, nutritional interventions may hold significant promise. SSA governments and health services, as well as nongovernmental organizations, will need to muster the needed political and economic will to propel action. The medical fraternity, researchers, and public health officials and experts must also do more to collaborate within the region and come up with interventions that can be implemented to address the rising CVD prevalence.

In SSA, the strongest maternal risk may be malnutrition and this could be strongly tackled by public health policies for nutritional interventions as the search for pharmaceutical therapies during pregnancy is intensified. Compelling evidential reports support incorporation of natural cocoa powder as food supplement for pregnant mothers to mitigate predisposition of their babies to CVDs. It is worth mentioning that although no specific treatment or intervention to improve CVD risk later in life is being employed, the general effort by clinicians to ensure healthy mother and child may also have some CVD benefits for the child. But deliberate and targeted policies are required to slow the increasing prevalence of CVDs in SSA.

REFERENCES

Adam, Zakariah, Donne Kofi Ameme, Priscillia Nortey, Edwin Andrew Afari, and Ernest Kenu. 2019. "Determinants of low birth weight in neonates born in three hospitals in Brong Ahafo region, Ghana, 2016- an unmatched case-control study." *BMC Pregnancy and Childbirth* 19 (1):174. doi: 10.1186/s12884-019-2315-6.

Addai, F. K. 2010. "Natural cocoa as diet-mediated antimalarial prophylaxis." (1532-2777 (Electronic)).

Adika, Christopher, Fred Aboagye-Antwi, Regina Appiah-Opong, Nancy Duah, Ruth Ayanful, Sena Matrevi, Dorcas Osei-Safo, Ben Gyan, and Neils Quashie. 2016. "Assessment of the Effects of Natural Cocoa Extract on Erythrocyte Membrane and Asexual Erythrocytic Stage of Plasmodium falciparum." *Asian Journal of Ethnopharmacology and Medicinal Foods* 02:11–16.

Aidoo, Eric, Frederick K. Addai, John Ahenkorah, Bismarck Hottor, Kwasi A. Bugyei, and Ben A. Gyan. 2012. "Natural cocoa ingestion reduced liver damage in mice infected with Plasmodium berghei (NK65)." *Research and Reports in Tropical Medicine* 3:107–116. doi: 10.2147/RRTM.S33149.

Alsaied, Tarek, Khaled Omar, Jeanne F. James, Robert B. Hinton, Timothy M. Crombleholme, and Mounira Habli. 2017. "Fetal origins of adult cardiac disease: a novel approach to prevent fetal growth restriction induced cardiac dysfunction using insulin like growth factor." *Pediatric Research* 81 (6):919–925. doi: 10.1038/pr.2017.18.

Amegah, A. K. 2018. "Tackling the Growing Burden of Cardiovascular Diseases in Sub-Saharan Africa." *Circulation* 138 (22):2449–2451. doi: 10.1161/CIRCULATIONAHA.118.037367.

Amponsah, S. K., K. Bugyei, D. Osei-Safo, F. K. Addai, G. Asare, E. A. Tsegah, J. Baah, M. Ofori, and B. A. Gyan. 2012. "In vitro activity of extract and fractions of natural cocoa powder on Plasmodium falciparum." *Journal of Medicinal Food* 15 (5):1557–7600.

Barker, D. J. 2004. "The developmental origins of adult disease." *J Am Coll Nutr* 23 (6 Suppl):588S–595S. doi: 10.1080/07315724.2004.10719428.
Barker, D. J., and C. Osmond. 1986. "Infant mortality, childhood nutrition, and ischaemic heart disease in England and Wales." *Lancet* 1 (8489):1077–1081. doi: 10.1016/s0140-6736(86)91340-1.
Barker, D. J., and C. Osmond. 1988. "Low birth weight and hypertension." *BMJ* 297 (6641):134-5. doi: 10.1136/bmj.297.6641.134-b.
Barker, D. J., C. Osmond, J. Golding, D. Kuh, and M. E. Wadsworth. 1989. "Growth in utero, blood pressure in childhood and adult life, and mortality from cardiovascular disease." *BMJ* 298 (6673):564–567. doi: 10.1136/bmj.298.6673.564.
Barker, D. J. P. 2007. "The origins of the developmental origins theory." *Journal of Internal Medicine* 261 (5):412–417. doi: 10.1111/j.1365-2796.2007.01809.x.
Bartels, Änne, and Keelin O'Donoghue. 2011. "Cholesterol in pregnancy: a review of knowns and unknowns." *Obstetric Medicine* 4 (4):147–151. doi: 10.1258/om.2011.110003.
Belbasis, Lazaros, Makrina D. Savvidou, Chidimma Kanu, Evangelos Evangelou, and Ioanna Tzoulaki. 2016. "Birth weight in relation to health and disease in later life: an umbrella review of systematic reviews and meta-analyses." *BMC Medicine* 14 (1):147. doi: 10.1186/s12916-016-0692-5.
BeLue, Rhonda, Titilayo A. Okoror, Juliet Iwelunmor, Kelly D. Taylor, Arnold N. Degboe, Charles Agyemang, and Gbenga Ogedegbe. 2009. "An overview of cardiovascular risk factor burden in sub-Saharan African countries: a socio-cultural perspective." *Globalization and Health* 5 (1):10. doi: 10.1186/1744-8603-5-10.
Blay, R. M., S. K. Adjenti, K. K. Adutwum-Ofosu, B. A. Hottor, J. Ahenkorah, B. Arko-Boham, and F. K. Addai. 2019. "Natural cocoa inhibits maternal hypercholesterolaemia-induced atherogenesis in rabbit pups." *Cardiovascular Journal of Africa* 30:1–8. doi: 10.5830/CVJA-2019-019.
Calkins, Kara, and Sherin U. Devaskar. 2011. "Fetal origins of adult disease." *Current Problems in Pediatric and Adolescent Health Care* 41 (6):158–176. doi: 10.1016/j.cppeds.2011.01.001.
Cappuccio, F. P., and M. A. Miller. 2016. "Cardiovascular disease and hypertension in sub-Saharan Africa: burden, risk and interventions." *Internal and Emerging Medicine* 11 (3):299–305. doi: 10.1007/s11739-016-1423-9.
Cartwright, M. 2019. "The salt trade of ancient West Africa.", accessed 03/05/2020. https://www.ancient.eu/article/1342/the-salt-trade-of-ancient-west-africa/.
Forsdahl, A. 1977. "Are poor living conditions in childhood and adolescence an important risk factor for arteriosclerotic heart disease?" *British Journal of Preventive & Social Medicine* 31 (2):91–95. doi: 10.1136/jech.31.2.91.
Gillum, R. F. 2018. "The Burden of Cardiovascular Disease in Sub-Saharan Africa and the Black Diaspora." *Journal of Racial Ethn Health Disparities* 5 (6):1155–1158. doi: 10.1007/s40615-018-0474-1.
Hambidge, K. Michael, and Nancy F. Krebs. 2018. "Strategies for optimizing maternal nutrition to promote infant development." *Reproductive Health* 15 (1):87. doi: 10.1186/s12978-018-0534-3.

Hamid, S., W. Groot, and M. Pavlova. 2019. "Trends in cardiovascular diseases and associated risks in sub-Saharan Africa: a review of the evidence for Ghana, Nigeria, South Africa, Sudan and Tanzania." *Aging Male* 22 (3):169–176. doi: 10.1080/13685538.2019.1582621.

He, Zhifei, Ghose Bishwajit, Sanni Yaya, Zhaohui Cheng, Dongsheng Zou, and Yan Zhou. 2018. "Prevalence of low birth weight and its association with maternal body weight status in selected countries in Africa: a cross-sectional study." *BMJ Open* 8 (8):e020410. doi: 10.1136/bmjopen-2017-020410.

Hoffman, Daniel J., Rebecca M. Reynolds, and Daniel B. Hardy. 2017. "Developmental origins of health and disease: current knowledge and potential mechanisms." *Nutrition Reviews* 75 (12):951–970. doi: 10.1093/nutrit/nux053.

Hsu, C. N., and Y. L. Tain. 2019. "The Good, the Bad, and the Ugly of Pregnancy Nutrients and Developmental Programming of Adult Disease." *Nutrients* 11 (4). doi: 10.3390/nu11040894.

Kwon, Eun Jin, and Young Ju Kim. 2017. "What is fetal programming?: a lifetime health is under the control of in utero health." *Obstetrics & Gynecology Science* 60 (6):506–519. doi: 10.5468/ogs.2017.60.6.506.

Lartey, Anna. 2008. "Maternal and child nutrition in Sub-Saharan Africa: Challenges and interventions." *The Proceedings of the Nutrition Society* 67:105–108. doi: 10.1017/S0029665108006083.

Lawlor, D. A., G. Ronalds, H. Clark, G. Smith, and D. A. Leon. 2005. "Birth weight is inversely associated with incident coronary heart disease and stroke among individuals born in the 1950s: findings from the Aberdeen Children of the 1950s prospective cohort study." *Circulation* 112 (10):1524–4539.

Lillycrop, K. A., E. Phillips, A. Jackson, M. Hanson, and G. C. Burdge. 2005. "Dietary protein restriction of pregnant rats induces and folic acid supplementation prevents epigenetic modification of hepatic gene expression in the offspring." *The Journal of Nutrition* 135 (6):1382–1386.

Mandy, Mirembe, and Moffat Nyirenda. 2018. "Developmental Origins of Health and Disease: the relevance to developing nations." *International Health* 10 (2):66–70. doi: 10.1093/inthealth/ihy006.

Memetoglu, O. G., A. Taraktas, N. B. Badur, and F. U. Ozkan. 2014. "Impact of stroke etiology on clinical symptoms and functional status." *Northern Clinics of Istanbul* 1 (2):101–105. doi: 10.14744/nci.2014.40327.

Mensah, G. A. 2018. "Cardiovascular Diseases in African Americans: Fostering Community Partnerships to Stem the Tide." *American Journal of Kidney Diseases* 72 (5 Suppl 1):S37–S42. doi: 10.1053/j.ajkd.2018.06.026.

Mensah, G. A., G. A. Roth, U. K. Sampson, A. E. Moran, V. L. Feigin, M. H. Forouzanfar, M. Naghavi, C. J. Murray, G. B. D. Mortality, and Collaborators Causes of Death. 2015. "Mortality from cardiovascular diseases in sub-Saharan Africa, 1990–2013: a systematic analysis of data from the Global Burden of Disease Study 2013." *Cardiovascular Journal of Africa* 26 (2 Suppl 1):S6–10. doi: 10.5830/CVJA-2015-036.

Moran, A., M. Forouzanfar, U. Sampson, S. Chugh, V. Feigin, and G. Mensah. 2013. "The epidemiology of cardiovascular diseases in sub-Saharan Africa: the

Global Burden of Diseases, Injuries and Risk Factors 2010 Study." *Progress in Cardiovascular Diseases* 56 (3):234–239. doi: 10.1016/j.pcad.2013.09.019.

Morrison, Janna L., and Timothy R. H. Regnault. 2016. "Nutrition in Pregnancy: Optimising Maternal Diet and Fetal Adaptations to Altered Nutrient Supply." *Nutrients* 8 (6):342. doi: 10.3390/nu8060342.

Mühlhäusler, Beverly Sara, Clare L. Adam, and I. Caroline McMillen. 2008. "Maternal nutrition and the programming of obesity: The brain." *Organogenesis* 4 (3):144–152. doi: 10.4161/org.4.3.6503.

Napoli, C., C. K. Glass, J. L. Witztum, R. Deutsch, F. P. D'Armiento, and W. Palinski. 1999a. "Influence of maternal hypercholesterolaemia during pregnancy on progression of early atherosclerotic lesions in childhood: Fate of Early Lesions in Children (FELIC) study." (0140-6736 (Print)).

Napoli, C., C. K. Glass, J. L. Witztum, R. Deutsch, F. P. D'Armiento, and W. Palinski. 1999b. "Influence of maternal hypercholesterolaemia during pregnancy on progression of early atherosclerotic lesions in childhood: Fate of Early Lesions in Children (FELIC) study." *Lancet* 354 (9186):1234–1241. doi: 10.1016/S0140-6736(99)02131-5.

Napoli, C., J. L. Witztum, F. Calara, F. de Nigris, and W. Palinski. 2000. "Maternal hypercholesterolemia enhances atherogenesis in normocholesterolemic rabbits, which is inhibited by antioxidant or lipid-lowering intervention during pregnancy: an experimental model of atherogenic mechanisms in human fetuses." (1524–4571 (Electronic)).

Nkoke, C., A. M. Jingi, C. Makoge, D. Teuwafeu, C. Nkouonlack, and A. Dzudie. 2019. "Epidemiology of cardiovascular diseases related admissions in a referral hospital in the South West region of Cameroon: A cross-sectional study in sub-Saharan Africa." *PLoS One* 14 (12):e0226644. doi: 10.1371/journal.pone.0226644.

O'Donnell, C. J., and R. Elosua. 2008. "[Cardiovascular risk factors. Insights from Framingham Heart Study]." *Revista Española de Cardiología* 61 (3):299-310.

Onyango, A. W., J. Jean-Baptiste, B. Samburu, and T. L. M. Mahlangu. 2019. "Regional Overview on the Double Burden of Malnutrition and Examples of Program and Policy Responses: African Region." *Annals of Nutrition and Metabolism* 75 (2):127–130. doi: 10.1159/000503671.

Opie, L. H., and B. M. Mayosi. 2005. "Cardiovascular disease in sub-Saharan Africa." *Circulation* 112 (23):3536–40. doi: 10.1161/CIRCULATIONAHA.105.597765.

Palinski, Wulf. 2014. "Effect of Maternal Cardiovascular Conditions and Risk Factors on Offspring Cardiovascular Disease." *Circulation* 129 (20):2066–2077. doi: doi:10.1161/CIRCULATIONAHA.113.001805.

Reddy, S. P., and A. D. Mbewu. 2016. "The Implications of the Developmental Origins of Health and Disease on Public Health Policy and Health Promotion in South Africa." *Healthcare (Basel)* 4 (4). doi: 10.3390/healthcare4040083.

Rodriguez-Rodriguez, P., D. Ramiro-Cortijo, C. G. Reyes-Hernandez, A. L. Lopez de Pablo, M. C. Gonzalez, and S. M. Arribas. 2018. "Implication of Oxidative Stress in Fetal Programming of Cardiovascular Disease." *Frontier Physiology* 9:602. doi: 10.3389/fphys.2018.00602.

Rodríguez-Rodríguez, Pilar, Angel L. López de Pablo, Concha F. García-Prieto, Beatriz Somoza, Begoña Quintana-Villamandos, José J. Gómez de Diego, Perla Y. Gutierrez-Arzapalo, David Ramiro-Cortijo, M. Carmen González, and Silvia M. Arribas. 2017. "Long term effects of fetal undernutrition on rat heart. Role of hypertension and oxidative stress." *PLoS One* 12 (2):e0171544. doi: 10.1371/journal.pone.0171544.

Sanders, K. 2008. Sustainable Trade in Pre-Colonial Asante. Senior Honors Theses. 188. https://commons.emich.edu/honors/188.

Smith, C. J., K. K. Ryckman, V. M. Barnabei, B. V. Howard, C. R. Isasi, G. E. Sarto, S. E. Tom, L. V. Van Horn, R. B. Wallace, and J. G. Robinson. 2016. "The impact of birth weight on cardiovascular disease risk in the Women's Health Initiative." *Nutrition, Metabolism and Cardiovascular Diseases* 26 (3):239–245. doi: 10.1016/j.numecd.2015.10.015.

Stein, Aryeh, Patricia Zybert, Karin Bruin, and L. H. Lumey. 2006. "Exposure to famine during gestation, size at birth, and blood pressure at age 59 y: evidence from the Dutch Famine." *European Journal of Epidemiology* 21:759–765. doi: 10.1007/s10654-006-9065-2.

Sun, Li-Yuan, Eun-Whan Lee, Aqeela Zahra, and Jae-Hyun Park. 2015. "Risk Factors of Cardiovascular Disease and Their Related Socio-Economical, Environmental and Health Behavioral Factors: Focused on Low-Middle Income Countries- A Narrative Review Article." *Iranian Journal of Public Health* 44 (4):435–444.

Umer, Amna, Candice Hamilton, Lesley Cottrell, Peter Giacobbi, Kim Innes, George A. Kelley, William Neal, Collin John, and Christa Lilly. 2019. "Association between Birth Weight and Childhood Cardiovascular Disease Risk Factors in West Virginia." *Journal of Developmental Origins of Health and Disease* 11 (1):86–95. doi: 10.1017/S204017441900045X.

Veena, Sargoor R., Catharine R. Gale, Ghattu V. Krishnaveni, Sarah H. Kehoe, Krishnamachari Srinivasan, and Caroline H. D. Fall. 2016. "Association between Maternal Nutritional Status in Pregnancy and Offspring Cognitive Function during Childhood and Adolescence; A Systematic Review." *BMC Pregnancy and Childbirth* 16 (1):220. doi: 10.1186/s12884-016-1011-z.

Volmink, J., and L. Dare. 2005. "Addressing Inequalities in Research Capacity in Africa." *British Medical Journal*, 331 (7519):705–706. doi: 10.1136/bmj.331.7519.705.

Index

Page numbers in *italics* refer to Figures and Tables.

About the Editors and Contributors

EDITORS

Nketiah-Amponsah, Edward (PhD) is an associate professor at the Department of Economics, University of Ghana. He holds a bachelor of arts and master of philosophy degrees all in economics from the University of Ghana. He also holds a PhD with specialization in Development and Health Economics from the University of Bonn, Germany. He currently teaches Public Sector Economics and Health Economics at the graduate level. He has over seventy peer-reviewed publications to his credit, of which fifty-five appear in Scopus. He is an editor of the *Ghanaian Journal of Economics* and also serves on the editorial board of the BMC Public Health and Ghana Social Science Journal.

Odeku, Oluwatoyin A. (PhD) is a professor of pharmaceutics and pharmaceutical technology and the dean of the Faculty of Pharmacy, University of Ibadan, Nigeria. She holds a PhD degree in pharmaceutics from the University of Ibadan, Nigeria, and a certificate in Modern Higher Education Management and Leadership from the University of Applied Sciences, Osnabruek, Germany. She has been a recipient of many research fellowships and awards including UNESCO/Israel Co-Sponsored Post-Doctoral Fellowship, MacArthur Foundation Grant, CAS-TWAS Visiting Scholar Fellowship, DAAD visiting Fellowship, Alexander von Humboldt Foundation Fellowships among others. Her research interests include drug delivery, nanotechnology, indigenous excipients development and formulation of herbal medicinal products. She has over 100 articles in books, chapters in books, and journal articles to her credit. She is a fellow of the West African

Postgraduate College of Pharmacists, West African Research Association and the Nigerian Academy of Science.

CONTRIBUTORS

Afful-Mensah, Gloria (PhD) is currently a lecturer with the Department of Economics, University of Ghana; and a research associate with Agender for International Development (A-id). She holds a PhD in economics from the University of Milan. She also holds master of philosophy degree in economics and bachelor of arts degree in economics with geography and resource development, all from the University of Ghana. Gloria has a strong interest in empirical microeconomics, particularly issues concerning health outcomes and healthcare service utilization. She is also passionate about issues related to gender and economic development.

Ajala, Aderemi Suleiman (PhD) is a professor of medical anthropology, University of Ibadan, Nigeria. He teaches courses in anthropology and African studies in the Department of Archaeology and Anthropology, University of Ibadan. He is a recipient of British Academy Fellowship (UK), Rockefeller Fellowship (US), and Alexander von Humboldt Fellowship (Germany) and a research grantee of CODESRIA, Ford Foundation, Humboldt Foundation, and Economic and Social science Research Council (ESRC). His research interests include culture and health; nationalism and politics in Nigeria and sustainable development. He currently authors three researched textbooks and published extensively in journals and edited books.

Akinsete, Kayode (PhD) is a senior-ranked lecturer in medical and environmental anthropology, University of Ibadan, Nigeria, where he teaches courses in anthropology. His research interests are culture and health, logging culture and forest management in Nigeria. He has published in journals and contributed to chapters in edited books.

Akuffo-Henaku, Patricia Ohenewaa (MSc) is a researcher with interest in public health and social development. She holds a master of public health degree with a specialization in health policy, planning and management and a bachelor of arts degree in social work and sociology from the University of Ghana. She currently volunteers with a nonprofit organization, Hope Wheel Group, where she is the lead for the '*Develop Me*' community-wide project. Patricia's research interests are in health financing, elderly care and health policy development in sub-Saharan Africa.

Alhassan, Robert Kaba (PhD) is a senior research fellow at the Institute of Health Research, University of Health and Allied Sciences (UHAS), Ho, Ghana, and a registered general nurse. He obtained his PhD from the University of Amsterdam (medical faculty), Netherlands, with a specialty in medical technical quality care and health financing. He also has an MPhil in health services management and a bachelor's degree in nursing and psychology from the University of Ghana, Legon. Robert has over ten years cumulative clinical and nursing education experience with the Ghana Health Service and Ministry of Health. He was also the head of research at the health training institutions secretariat of the ministry health headquarters before joining UHAS as a lecturer and researcher. In UHAS has a served as a head of department and currently the acting dean of international programmes and also on several university committees.

Andoh-Adjei, Francis-Xavier (PhD), a public/allied health professional and educationist, is director of administration at the National Health Insurance Authority in Ghana. He has over thirty-five years of work experience in education and health sectors, holding positions at the policy and operational levels. He has provided consultancy services in health insurance design and implementation for the Republics of Zambia, Zimbabwe, and Liberia; and facilitated capacity-building workshops for health insurance personnel in Ethiopia, Ghana, Nepal, and Zimbabwe. Dr. Andoh-Adjei holds doctor of philosophy (PhD) degree in medical sciences, master of public health, master of science-health services planning & management, postgraduate diploma in research methods & skills, bachelor of arts (Hons) and teachers' diploma.

Asante, Felix Ankomah (PhD) is a professor in the Institute of Statistical, Social and Economic Research (ISSER) and currently the pro-vice chancellor in charge of Research, Innovation and Development, University of Ghana. He was the director of ISSER from August 2013 to July 2019. His research focuses on a broad range of themes in development economics relating to household food security; decentralization and provision of public goods and services; health issues; and climate change. He had both his bachelor of science (BSc) and master of philosophy (MPhil) in agriculture economics from the University of Ghana and the doctor of philosophy (PhD) in agriculture (agriculture economics) from the University of Bonn, Germany.

Blay, Richard M. (PhD) is a lecturer at the University of Ghana Medical School, Korle-Bu, Accra. He obtained his PhD at the Ludwig-Maximilians University, Munich. His research interest is the role of maternal nutrition during pregnancy in development of cardiovascular disease in offspring. He is also interested in the role of microRNAs in cardiovascular diseases. He is a Christian and mentors young people.

Codjoe, Emmanuel A. (PhD) holds a PhD in Economics from the School of Oriental and African Studies, University of London. He is a lecturer in economics at the Department of Economics, University of Ghana, where he teaches macroeconomics, development economics, and international economics at the undergraduate and graduate levels. His research interests are broadly within the area of development economics, especially the economies of sub-Saharan African countries. He has been part of many research projects and has several publications in peer-reviewed journals.

Dzudzor, Makafui I. (MSc and PhD Candidate) is currently a doctoral student at the Centre for Development Research (ZEF), University of Bonn, Germany. He holds MSc in agricultural bioengineering (professional focus) from the Université Catholique de Louvain in Belgium and MSc in business and economics (economics) from the Swedish University of agricultural sciences in Sweden. Makafui has engaged in a number of research activities in Ghana and other African countries. His current research activities are focused on food and nutrition security, food systems, and agricultural markets.

Fenny, Ama Pokuaa (PhD) is a research fellow with the Institute of Statistical, Social and Economics Research (ISSER) at the University of Ghana. She has researched and published in the area of developmental issues in health financing, health service delivery, and social protection. She is currently involved in research projects that identify strategic shifts to integrate government policies and service delivery systems in Africa. She has a PhD in health economics from the Department of Public Health, Aarhus University, Denmark, and an MSc in health, population & society from the London School of Economics & Political Science (UK).

Mensah, Gloria Ivy (PhD) is a research fellow of the Bacteriology Department, Noguchi Memorial Institute for Medical Research (NMIMR), University of Ghana. She has a PhD in Medical Research-International Health from the Ludwig Maximillian's University, Munich-Germany. Her research interests include host-pathogen interaction in tuberculosis (TB) and other bacterial zoonosis as well as novel diagnostics and biomarkers for TB. She is a part-time lecturer of veterinary microbiology at the School of Veterinary Medicine, University of Ghana. She is presently a postdoctoral fellow of Afrique One-ASPIRE, a One Health research consortium of institutions of higher learning in West and East Africa and Northern partners. Gloria has over fifteen years of research experience in TB that has led to several publications and conference presentations. Her current research focus is on immunodiagnostic tools for childhood TB.

Mureithi, Dominic (MSc and PhD Candidate) is a lecturer in the Department of Animal Sciences, Chuka University. Dominic has a MSc in pharmacology and toxicology and bachelor of veterinary medicine from University of Nairobi. He also holds a postgraduate certificate in molecular toxicology from Hokkaido University, Japan. Dominic does research in veterinary medicine with a focus on antimicrobial resistance, food safety, and one health. He has done research on assessing the presence of antibiotic resistance genes (ARG's) in commensal bacteria in wild baboons. He has also researched on milk safety and antibiotic resistance in milk and milk products. His current is on the use of enhanced antibiotic stewardship and development of guideline to improve prescribing in large animals in low resources settings.

Namuli, Proscovia (MSc) is a researcher as well as a monitoring and evaluation practitioner. She holds MSc in development evaluation and management from the University of Antwerpen–Belgium. She obtained a MA in Development Management from Ruhr University Bochum–Germany. Her bachelor's degree is in development studies. Her research interests are in gender, public health, poverty, and community development. Her major research focuses are reproductive health, domestic violence, and gender equality.

Ngigi, Marther W. (PhD) is a lecturer and a researcher in the Department of Agribusiness Management, Machakos University. She is currently working on improving nutritional outcomes of adults and children under 5 years using interventions in ICT. Before, she worked on domains of food safety, market development, gender dimensions of climate change, livestock diversification as a risk strategy, poverty, and food security in SSA. Marther has a PhD in agricultural and development economics from the University of Bonn, Germany, and MSc in agricultural and applied economics from the University of Nairobi, Kenya. Her research interests include food security and nutrition, gender economics, sustainable food systems, agricultural value chains, and poverty in developing realms.

Nwafor, Felix (MSc and PhD Candidate) is a researcher and PhD scholar at the Department of Pharmacognosy and Environmental Medicines, Faculty of Pharmaceutical Sciences, University of Nigeria, Nsukka. He obtained his BSc and MSc degrees from the University of Nigeria. He was trained in herbal medicine and field taxonomy at the International Centre for Ethnomedicine and Drug Development/Bioresources Development and Conservation Programme and is conversant with West African medicinal flora. His research interests revolve around plant taxonomy (chemotaxonomy), Bioprospecting of novel bioactive compounds, ethnomedicine, herbal formulations, indigenous knowledge, and pharmacognosy. He has over twenty publications (journal articles and book chapters) in these research areas.

Ola, Christie Bose (BPharm) is a registered pharmacist. She holds a bachelor of pharmacy degree from the University of Ibadan, Nigeria. She is a research assistant in the same faculty. Her research interest includes oncology and herbal pharmacotherapy.

Onyekere Pecucliar Feenna (MPharm) is a trained pharmacist, healthcare educator, lecturer, and researcher. He was a beneficiary of the DAAD In-country/In-region Scholarship during his masters program which he graduated with distinction in phytochemistry. He was a participant in the 2018 EARTHS Summer School at Hamburg University of Applied Sciences, Germany. Currently, He lectures in the Department of Pharmacognosy and Environmental Medicine at the Faculty of Pharmaceutical Sciences, University of Nigeria and is pursuing a doctoral degree in clinical pharmacognosy. With over fifteen publications in international journals and books, his research interest is on novel natural products for the treatment of diabetes and oxidative diseases.

Peculiar-Onyekere, Chioma (**MSc and PhD candidate**) is a trained microbiologist. She holds a master's degree in medical microbiology on distinction grade from the prestigious University of Nigeria. Currently, she is pursuing her doctorate degree in pharmaceutical microbiology and biotechnology. Her research interest is on antimicrobial resistance and tropical diseases. She has authored and coauthored journals and book chapter.

www.ingramcontent.com/pod-product-compliance
Ingram Content Group UK Ltd.
Pitfield, Milton Keynes, MK11 3LW, UK
UKHW020840290926
15470UKWH00004B/1457

9 781793 633699